**Kate Mosse** is the author of three works of non-fiction, three plays and six novels, including the No 1 multi-million international bestselling Languedoc Trilogy – *Labyrinth*, *Sepulchre* and *Citadel* – published to outstanding reviews and sold in more than 40 countries throughout the world in 38 languages. Her standalone novel, *The Winter Ghosts*, was also a No. 1 bestseller, confirming her position as one of our most captivating storytellers. Her collection of short stories, *The Mistletoe Bride & Other Ghostly Tales*, was published in Autumn 2013. In recognition of her services to literature, Kate was awarded an OBE in the Queen's Birthday Honours List in June 2013.

www.katemosse.co.uk

Praise for *Becoming a Mother*:

'It is refreshing to read a book which combines a great deal of interesting information with anatomy and physiology, some history and statistics from a wide range of continents. Most professionals could benefit from reading this book too because of the insights into parents' views and feelings'
*Midwifery Digest*

'An exploration of women's thoughts and feelings about what is happening to their minds and bodies during pregnancy, birth and their aftermath. I highly recommend it as an intelligent woman's pregnancy companion'
Amazon.co.uk reader review

## By Kate Mosse

*Becoming a Mother*

*The House: Behind the Scenes at the Royal Opera House,
Covent Garden*

*Chichester Festival Theatre at Fifty*

*Eskimo Kissing*

*Crucifix Lane*

*Labyrinth*

*Sepulchre*

*The Winter Ghosts*

*Citadel*

*The Mistletoe Bride & Other Ghostly Tales*

## Plays

*Syrinx*

*Endpapers*

*Dodgers*

# Becoming a Mother

## Kate Mosse

Third Edition revised and updated by
Martine Gallie

virago

VIRAGO

First published in Great Britain in 1993 by Virago Press
Revised edition published in 1997
Reprinted 2001, 2002
This updated paperback edition published in 2007 by Virago Press
Reprinted 2009, 2014 (twice)

A CIP catalogue record for this book
is available from the British Library.

ISBN 978-0-3490-0480-8

Typeset in Palatino by Palimpsest Book Production Limited,
Grangemouth, Stirlingshire
Printed and bound in Great Britain by
Clays Ltd, St Ives plc

Papers used by Virago are from well-managed forests
and other responsible sources.

MIX
Paper from
responsible sources
FSC® C104740

Virago Press
An imprint of
Little, Brown Book Group
100 Victoria Embankment
London EC4Y 0DY

An Hachette UK Company
www.hachette.co.uk

www.virago.co.uk

To Greg and Martha and Felix, with love

# Contents

# Acknowledgements

Although the opinions and choice of facts are mine, the contributions of a great many people have made this book what it is. For their honesty and generosity in sharing their experiences with me, I'd like to thank: Sharon Bull; Debbie; Debra; Lisa Dye; Fran Hanley; Jane; Jenny; Joanne; Lee Keating; Candida Lacey; Lynne; Caroline Matthews; Nicki Martin; Rachel; Tessa Ross; Sasha; Siân; Sue; Rose Summerhayes; Sarah Taylor; Pam Trigg.

I also want to thank my publisher Lennie Goodings, for her enthusiasm for the book in its various editions over the past fifteen years – and her assistant Vanessa Neuling for her hard work on this third new edition; my agent Mark Lucas and all at LAW; Sue Murray (RGN, RM, MA) who cast an expert eye over the first edition in 1993; my midwife Becky Reed – now a grandmother herself – who helped with facts and figures in 1997 for the second edition. Most especially, I want to thank Martine Gallie who has done a fantastic job of updating the science, medical procedures, social changes and generally knocked the third edition into shape, suitable for today's women going through – enjoying – pregnancy. It all seems a long time ago!

My love and thanks, as ever, to my parents, Richard and Barbara Mosse; to my sisters, Caroline Matthews – who'd been there and done that when I was pregnant, so was my oracle in all things – and Beth Huxley, who now has two lovely daughters of her own, Thea and Ellen; to my mother-in-law Rosie Turner, who continues to be the most energetic, supportive and fabulous granny. I was also lucky enough to have a handful of close friends with whom I gossiped and worried through every twinge of both my pregnancies, in particular Tessa Ross (who has added Louis, now nearly 10, to the Joe and Tilly mentioned in the book) and Lucinda Montefiore, mother to Rufus and Luke, and now in 2007, to two-year-old Sammy!

Finally, as always, my love and thanks to Greg. For everything.

# Preface to the Third Edition

When I sat down in 1997 to revise the original edition of *Becoming a Mother*, even though I was amazed at how much had changed medically in just four years, it was still a world I knew. My daughter Martha was nearly seven, my son Felix four. I allowed myself a week (or two) for revisions, a bit of updating of statistics, changes to maternity leave, extra bits about the new tests, but I had friends who were still going through pregnancies, and I inhabited spaces full of toddlers and babies. It was a familiar landscape.

Not so now. Martha is now seventeen, Felix fourteen. Instead, I inhabit the world of teenagers. It is an utterly different environment – a wonderful one – with distinct emotional and physical demands. In 2007, life is less about food and more about exams; it's less about that extra vest than Top Shop; it's less about being a nurse and more about running a taxi service. Most of all, it's about advice and conversation and negotiation rather than bedtime reading, bath times and breastfeeding. What I have learned in the past ten years is that this constant shifting of roles and responsibilities is one of the best kept parenting secrets of all – that, if you are lucky, how each year of your child's life becomes, de facto, the most interesting, the most rewarding, the most satisfying.

A decade is a lifetime in pregnancy and maternity care. Back in 1993, I didn't know any IVF children and now I know eight. I knew only three or four sets of twins, now I know many more than that. I didn't know any women who had either used the services of a surrogate or undertaken that role for someone else. As a parent-in-waiting in the early 1990s, there was plenty to read if you sought it out. In the mid 00s, it is hard to avoid advice, information, online services, GPs, midwives, editorials in newspapers and magazines. The medical advances have been huge, the availability of information – online, in person and in books – wonderful. I have also been lucky to have the help of a wonderful collaborator, Martine Gallie, who has brought the book into the twenty-first century.

Despite the enormous social and medical advances, it soon became clear that not so much has changed on the emotional and psychological landscape. The more I looked into it, the more I realised that my reason for writing the book in the early 1990s seemed as valid now as it was then, namely that when I was pregnant, I wanted an anecdotal, funny, honest record of what individual women – *real* women, not celebrities – felt about pregnancy, and maybe there were other women who felt the same. And, despite suffocating under a mountain of facts and figures and information, in 2007 – as back in 1993 and 1997 – most of us going through pregnancy and child-birth do not know what we will need or want until we get there! The human heart, with all its longing and expectations, remains much the same.

In 1993, pregnant friends said they wanted to know all the facts, but then wanted that little bit more. That moment of identification, that realisation that someone else out there felt as they did. *Becoming a Mother* has been in print pretty much ever since, and year after year the letters (and now emails!) from women and their partners have kept coming. Most of all, it's been an interesting – sometimes weird – experience to look back. To revisit the person I was before I was a mother. Being a parent is the most important, the most enjoyable, the most challenging, the most fabulous thing in the world. Nothing else comes close. For all of you just setting out on the adventure, good luck. And, most of all, enjoy it.

Kate Mosse
Spring 2007

# Introduction

> I told myself that I wanted to write a book on mother-
> hood because it was a crucial, still relatively unexplored,
> area for feminist theory. But I did not choose this subject;
> it had long ago chosen me.
>
> Adrienne Rich, *Of Woman Born*[1]

It wasn't that I really believed that if I stopped eating Brie,
had no caffeine or refined sugars or artificial additives, then
nothing could go wrong. I didn't in my heart of hearts think
that my partner Greg's sperm would be so very different if
he stopped drinking alcohol and eating twelve Jaffa Cakes a
day. It was more that, for me, pregnancy was at best a
haphazard business, at worst a dangerous one. I suppose I
felt that if we could at least try to stack the odds in our favour
then it would be harder for my body to ambush me.

I became pregnant for the first time in the stifling summer
of 1989. I was 28, and the baby was planned. My character
changed immediately, even though on the surface I appeared
to be the same woman. I couldn't shake off the sense of how
dangerous and unnatural it all was. Having always trusted

my body and my instincts, I woke every morning convinced something was wrong. The daily interminable wait for the baby's first movements was followed by the stubborn fear that I was going to give birth to a terribly disabled child. It was a miserable 36 weeks. Every stab and ache became symptomatic of the worst calamities my well-thumbed stack of pregnancy books could catalogue. Dread, guilt and embarrassment at being so entirely out of control were my constant companions, although few people realised. For the first time in my adult life I started a diary, partly because I hoped keeping a record might make it all less intimidating.

> 14 DECEMBER 1989: walking past the industrial estate this morning, I knew the baby was dead. The sky was that flat grey, no character. I couldn't understand why I was bothering to go to work. Standing on the train, 20 minutes later, little thumps made the protest at no one offering me a seat. The sense of relief nearly made my knees buckle. I feel stupid writing this now, because I'm overtaken by these waves of panic every day. But I felt so sure.

Women used to know about pregnancy from their friends, their mothers and their sisters. Although everyone had heard of so-and-so down the road whose baby had died, or the friend of an acquaintance whose agonising labour had gone on for three days, there was still the expectation that – though painful – childbirth would be relatively straightforward. Now some of us have never even held a newborn baby before giving birth to our own. Now many of us have nobody with whom to share the excitement, or to talk over those isolating fears and worries. Most of us do need knowledgeable friends who are genuinely interested in how our changing shape is undermining our self-confidence, who reassure that they too had nipples that felt as if they had been set about with a pair of pliers.

But once pregnant your emotions can swing wildly to and fro. Confident women may start to feel vulnerable just as less assertive women sense new personal strengths. Every woman changes. And most worry, if only from time to time. About what is happening to their characters and their bodies. Will you enjoy being a mother too much and never want to work again? Will you not enjoy it at all? Will that teenage obsession with weight loss sneak back up on you? How different will your partner's once-removed experience be from your intimate, internal one? Can your body actually do something so extraordinary as create another person inside of it? Why are all children's names so awful? A haphazard column of irrational thoughts marches endlessly through your mind.

For me, it was as if my body knew what to do but my mind had absolutely no idea. Hungry for facts, my undiscriminating appetite for pregnancy books grew week by week, although I binged in secret. I didn't want outsiders – friends, family, work colleagues – to know that I was spending so much time thinking about being pregnant. But once I'd digested all of the specialists' technical and practical information, I started to hanker after the tiny personal details, the stories behind the facts, the faces behind the figures. I still felt uninformed about what it meant to be pregnant. I had an almost naive belief that if only I could make sense of what I thought, then I would be confident about the changes I was physically experiencing. What I needed – and didn't find – was a literary map of this uncharted emotional territory to accompany me as I lay in the bath each night. I wanted a book that wouldn't glibly dismiss these new conflicting feelings as 'expected hormonal mood-changes . . .', or 'many women feel more emotional during pregnancy . . .' Even the most longed-for, planned conception isn't free of ambivalence, days when you really can't stand being pregnant any more. And for me there was the shock – resentment, even – when I realised our unborn baby had somehow become the most important single thing in my world.

Trawling the bookshops and libraries two years later when pregnant with Felix, my second child, I found an even broader range of handbooks, some good, some not, but still so little charting the emotional experience. This time I didn't feel such a novice so far as practical information was concerned, but I hankered for personal stories even more. And, because women tend to spend much less time thinking about their subsequent babies, there was a part of me that felt that Felix deserved new books, that I shouldn't simply skim through the now second-hand books I'd bought when pregnant with Martha. Every woman I talked to who had attended an ante-natal class – from those run by the local hospital to Active Birth groups – commented that one of the most valuable reasons for going had been to listen to other women talking about their pregnancies and births. Clearly I was not the only one who would welcome a more anecdotal book. I decided to write one.

During the summer of 1992 I interviewed a range of women, with thirty-six pregnancies between us (biograph-ical details are given on page 379). I did not attempt to assemble a representative cross-section of British society, but instead concentrated on including women who had experi-enced different sorts of pregnancies and births: heterosexual and lesbian women; those who first became mothers at the age of 19, those who waited until their forties; women who have one child, women who have two, three or four; those who have suffered miscarriage or abortion; those who conceived easily and those for whom it was extremely complicated; women who physically prepared themselves for conception to those who got unpleasant surprises some

12 weeks after a drunken night out; those opting for home, for hospital, even water; caesareans, forceps and white-coated technology; those who revelled in state-of-the-art drugs to those who had no pain relief whatsoever; trouble-free fairy-tale pregnancies and nine-month physical calamities with happy endings.

Because the book is about pregnancy not parenthood, my only decision was not to interview anyone whose baby had not survived. Just after I discovered I was pregnant with Martha, a close friend suffered a stillbirth. Statistically, I knew that I was more likely to be killed in a road accident than lose my baby in that way. I knew that thousands of women gave birth to healthy babies every week. But I still compared my pregnancy with hers every step of the way, as if somehow a coded warning of what was to come had been there in her physical symptoms all along. Many women read books for reassurance during their pregnancies, so in the end I felt it would be counterproductive to detail a seemingly normal pregnancy which had resulted in tragedy. For the same reason, I decided not to include anyone who had unexpectedly given birth to a severely disabled child.

I have swapped the usual structure of pregnancy books – divided trimester by trimester – for a more detailed twinge by twinge approach. What you feel at the beginning of week 4, after all, is very different from what you might go through in week 12. Medical, historical and physical facts are included – signposted by subheadings within the text – to provide the context in which the women interviewed lived their pregnancies.

Different things were of importance to different women. We all like to think that our decision to conceive is a uniquely personal one. But not only do families and friends play their subtle parts, society too exerts unseen, often unacknowledged pressures. From the number of children we are expected to have to the age at which we are expected to have them, we are unconsciously influenced. And judged.

Modern medicine, with its reluctance to accept that it cannot completely control or even understand nature, sometimes fosters an 'if only' approach to pregnancy. If only women prepared their bodies for conception, if only they ate the right things and none of the prohibited things, if only they kept away from all car fumes, aluminium pans and industrial chemicals, if only they took advantage of all prenatal testing available, if only . . . The message is that all babies could be perfect if only women took more care.

It is obviously no more than common sense for women to avoid any drugs that might be dangerous to an unborn baby, to eat a well-balanced diet that will help their bodies to function efficiently and provide the necessary energy to cope with the huge physical stresses of pregnancy. But many of us felt that this pre-natal – even pre-conceptual – burden of guilt was in many ways simply a prelude to the level of responsibility society expects its mothers to assume: a *woman* may make personal choices, but a *mother* should entirely subordinate her needs to those of her child.

There is no right and no wrong way to feel when pregnant. We all respond according to our expectations, our personal and professional situations and to the evidence of our own bodies. Partners of either sex can – and should – make a difference, though I have given them no space of their own here. Some women feel fantastic for the first six months, then depressed in the weeks leading up to the birth; others find the first 12 weeks mentally unbearable, then suddenly the cloud lifts and the 'bloom' appears. Any psychological shift, however small, is important to the woman experiencing it, and ambivalence and confusion are as natural components of pregnancy as are sore breasts and disappearing waistlines. The physical experience colours the emotional one and some physical symptoms do indicate problems whereas others do not. But all twinges assume equal significance if they are not given enough attention by time-pressed doctors, and can make pregnancy a frightening, undermining experience when it should be an enjoyable, exciting one.

I prevaricated about writing. Why a pregnancy book of all books, particularly since I didn't enjoy being pregnant? Maybe everything had already been said about the body, the mind and the politics. But even by 2007, pregnancy in print remains by and large the province of medical experts. To find out what ordinary women feel about being pregnant, who better to bear witness than women themselves? Childbirth educator and writer Sheila Kitzinger was encouraged by similar motivations:

> I was interested in childbirth long before I became pregnant myself because anything in books was written from a male point of view. I wanted to find out, I wanted to learn what women's lives were all about. I wanted to put it into words because women had no voice.[2]

I am not a specialist, just a woman who has twice been through the experience of pregnancy, who has found the process of giving birth exhilarating and who loves being a mother. If this book, in its turn, helps even one other pregnant woman put her thoughts into focus, then it will help fill that gap on the bookshelf.

# *If and When . . .*

## The Decision to Conceive

28 MAY 1989: A few weeks ago, when the issue of children came up – as it does quite a lot now – I quite confidently announced that we had decided that we didn't want to be parents, ever. My friend was equally sure that he *did* want to be a father one day. I've always shouted my mouth off about this, but suddenly only a couple of months later I'm not sure any more. It's not that I *do* want a baby, it's just that I'm not sure that I *don't*. Am I changing my mind, or is it simply a fear of missing out? What if I do now want a child and Greg doesn't? And how can I know if it's the right decision?

It is perhaps harder than ever before for today's women and men to decide when or if to become parents. For women in the industrialised world, who have access to contraception and safe methods of abortion, pregnancy has become a positive choice. Until the 1960s the majority of women expected – and were expected – to become mothers. Today there are fewer women for whom motherhood is synonymous with adulthood.

Caroline is a full-time mother and playgroup leader from Bognor in West Sussex. She conceived Emma when she was 18, three months after her marriage.

> Having children was always the only thing I wanted. I wanted two children when I got married, then when I'd had two I wanted four, and now I want six. Each time I got pregnant I hoped it might be twins. Twins are so special, and babies are lovely anyway so if one's asleep you've got another one to play with.

But increasing numbers of women are asking themselves whether, on balance, they really do want to have children at all. It's estimated that about 22 per cent of women born since 1990 will remain childless.[1] Maggie Rogers of the UK Council for Psychotherapy has estimated that the largest number of clients she has for therapy are women in their thirties who want to talk over the baby question. One such woman told me:

> I couldn't tell if it was my instincts telling me I wanted a baby or because I felt under pressure from my husband. Then there was his mother. She wanted grandchildren, but I had to have them for me not her. I thought someone with a fresh eye might help me get my ideas sorted out, even though I felt embarrassed and didn't tell anyone at the time, not even my husband.

The dramatic increase in the numbers seeking professional counselling is perhaps a symptom of the myriad of – often opposing – influences that affect women's decisions about whether or not to take the plunge.

## Outside Influences

What constitutes good mothering varies from country to country, from age to age, even from year to year. However personal our decisions may seem, it is within a social context that they are made. Increasingly since the 1990s, anxiety over the shape and size of 'the family' has filled the newspapers, bookshelves, the airwaves and television chat shows. Infidelities of MPs, irresponsible single parents jetting off to the Costa del Sol leaving their children home alone, antisocial adolescents, paedophiles on the Internet, all are held up as indications of society gone bad. The temptation is – as it has always been – to blame parents, mothers in particular, for working too hard; for scrounging off the State; for divorcing; for marrying too young; for not being there enough; for being too suffocating.

I suspect the media and peer group pressure on mothers is greater now than ever. Several of the women interviewed admitted to feeling uncomfortable that their decisions might be criticised by others. As one professional woman in her thirties put it:

> It wasn't that it made a difference to my decision, but it did make me worry about what people would think of me if I went back to work after having a baby. My husband assumed I'd stay at home when we started a family and it seemed that every time I opened the papers they backed him up. I just kept putting the decision off.

In a country where women are increasingly becoming the main family breadwinner, mothers are right to ask themselves why *they* are being exhorted to put their careers on hold while their children are young. One woman felt that her mother had been pressurised in this way back in the 1960s.

My mum wouldn't admit it, but she really wishes that she hadn't stopped working when she got pregnant. When I asked her why she didn't go back after we'd been born, she said that wasn't what people did then. She hated being at home with babies. But my dad and everyone would have said that she was a bad mother if she'd left us with someone else, and it's still the worst thing you can say to a woman, isn't it? But it made me determined to be me, and not to give everything up for my children.

One would have hoped that feminism would have buried once and for all the debate about whether mothers should or should not work. In many respects, it is largely a debate conducted *about* mothers rather than *by* them. The majority of new mothers do want to look after their babies when very young, but fewer women expect to become permanent full-time parents. Some make their choice for financial reasons, others because they are less willing to accept that women should have to choose between a career and a child when men do not.

In 1994, 51 per cent of married or cohabiting women with children under five were working. Ten years later, the figure had risen to 59 per cent. Now 67 per cent of women with dependent children (under 16) earn outside the home and in some 68 per cent of couples with dependent children both partners are working.[2] The death of the male 'job-for-life', part-time and flexi-working and job-sharing have radically altered the shape of employment for us all. In many parts of the country – Kent, East and West Sussex, Devon, Wiltshire, Oxfordshire, Gloucestershire and Somerset as well as many other regions – women employees now outnumber the men. A 1996 survey conducted by The Institute of Personnel and Development (IPD) discovered that even though 75 per cent of people stayed in their jobs for over a year, over half of them would leave before hitting the five-year mark.

What is extraordinary is that despite this there has been so small a psychological shift in the way working parents – especially working mothers – are portrayed. Guilt is still the overriding emotion of many parents who work, whatever their economic and practical needs.

## The Right Time to be Pregnant

Whatever the outside influences – practical, financial or emotional – the desire to be pregnant will override them. Few hearts are ruled by heads. But when will the time be right? According to Chinese myth, women take care not to conceive a child that would be born in the Year of the Firedragon since the auspices are so malevolent. The point when professional and financial auspices rule out pregnancy for the foreseeable future might also be the time when the longing for a child is strongest.

Tessa was 29, working as a script executive in Glasgow. She and her 32-year-old husband Mark wanted to have a large family. At the same time, they both had demanding full-time jobs which they enjoyed. At the end of the first year of their marriage they subconsciously acknowledged that professionally there was never going to be a 'right time'.

> It was a very easy thing to think about, but it was always going to be difficult to make the decision.

Awareness that there is no right time has led psychologists such as American Phyllis Ziman-Tobin to coin the phrase 'adaptive choice',[3] whereby a woman manages to combine unconscious impulses with a conscious assessment of her practical situation. Though her decision appears fraught with conflict, adaptive choice enables the woman to reach balanced decisions that take account both of her feelings and her common sense.

Some women can weigh the pros and cons and come to an 'adaptive' decision. Others never lose the sense that it would be irresponsible to try to conceive a child at this point in their working lives. This awareness, meshing subconsciously with the realisation that it will always seem irresponsible, leads many couples to take deliberate risks with contraception in order not to face it squarely. Paul Entwhistle, a biochemist researching infertility at Liverpool University, not only believes that many so-called accidents are unconsciously planned, but also that some women are unconsciously able to bring forward or delay ovulation in order to ensure conception.

Rachel, then 29 years old, works in the City. She admitted: 'I wasn't on the pill and we hadn't been using condoms. We hadn't owned up to the fact that we were aiming for me to get pregnant.'

## Losing Oneself

Timing is not just a question of common sense. More powerful in many ways is how a woman's sense of herself as a social and professional person may be at odds with the positive or negative image she has of motherhood. It is not simply the issue of freedom, although many women and men are reluctant to sacrifice their spontaneous, childless lifestyles. It is more a genuine concern that they might lose emotional contact with those closest to them, that their friends will be unable to identify with their changed lives. Almost every woman interviewed for this book had found that a relationship with a very important friend had been spoiled. One woman was even accused by her very oldest friend of 'selling out'.

> When I finally challenged her about not returning my calls – I was about five months pregnant at the time – she simply said that I'd changed and we didn't have anything in common any more. It was really upsetting at the time. Looking back, I think she was jealous and it made me angry that she assumed that I was suddenly a different person.

Up until the point that I acknowledged I might want to be pregnant, I had no interest in children at all. I resented adult areas, such as restaurants, being taken over with the sound of crying. I was frustrated by new parents' seeming inability to concentrate on a serious conversation. I was offended by being considered a childless woman – somehow incomplete – rather than a childfree one. So when suddenly I became able to visualise myself as a mother, one of my first emotions was guilt about my previous insensitivity and intolerance. Hard on its heels came the fear that parenthood would destroy the intimacy of my relationship with Greg, that we would never have time to ourselves again and that pregnancy and parenthood would ruin our sex life. I was sure that Greg shared these worries, but it was too elusive, too hypothetical to discuss. How can anyone imagine how they will feel, let alone how they will cope?

Some women feel that pregnancy will undermine profound aspects of their character. Sasha, a successful artist in her late thirties, had never seen herself as a mother, although she and her partner had discussed having a child in vague terms for about ten years. The situation was complicated by the fact that Lou had two children from a previous relationship. However, 'he was a very positive father and knew what it was like, and wanted me to have that experience.'

Even acknowledging that she might want to become a mother, Sasha always saw that day as belonging to an older, different sort of woman.

> My creativity comes from my inner child, all my outgoing positive energy comes from my child aspect and it was threatening for me to contemplate losing that. And if I became a woman I could get drawn into things that I associated with negativity, pessimism, depression and having to be a grown-up. My whole identity was at stake, and there was a big friction between producing a child as the fundamental creative act and going on being an artist, in other words going on being me.

Professionally there are similar issues to be addressed. Will one's work persona be destroyed by motherhood? Many successful women are aware that they are somehow perceived as not being quite like ordinary women. Like the women who appear on the hit BBC show *The Apprentice*, they are ambitious, tough, focused; more like one of the lads, in fact. They often feel guilty about being mentally manipulated into dividing the working world into three sexes – men, women and mothers – but at the same time they do feel different. In the past, some might even have used the badge of not wanting children as proof to the outside world of how seriously they took their careers. Eve, then 29, works as an editor and lives in Brighton: she feels she did this.

> I spent the whole of my second year at university making a great show of trying to get sterilised and I definitely didn't want children, ever, ever, ever. And then I felt that this was a wicked horrible thing to be trying to do.

## I Once Had an Abortion . . .

Eve's 39-year-old husband had always wanted children. Over their six years together they'd moved towards an amicable agreement that they would have a child at some stage in the future, although it was always a distant future for Eve. Then, because of a contraceptive failure, Eve became pregnant. She had no difficulty in deciding on an abortion at seven weeks. Physically and emotionally she took it all very much in her stride, went home after the operation, had a gin and tonic, organised a huge birthday party and started a new job the following week. But about seven months later, at about the time that the baby would have been born, she started to develop nausea and high temperatures on the first day of her period. She now attributes these physical symptoms to grief and guilt starting to rise to the surface. Subconsciously she started to prepare herself for conceiving and carrying a baby to term; consciously she reached no such decision and her ambivalence was as strong as ever.

> I knew logically there was no right time; but I felt very conscious of being so typical. Here I was, heterosexual, of child-bearing age, having a baby, causing disruption, giving everyone a lot of extra work. And I sort of felt it wasn't that trendy really.

Fran, then a 26-year-old teacher, felt that her six-week abortion was the only decision she could make in the circumstances. She and her partner Jim, a postman, had been living together for only three months. They didn't have a place of their own and she would not have qualified for any maternity benefit. However, 'it [the abortion] sort of kicked me off to having another baby, because I regretted it so much.'

Debra, who is now 35, had been with her partner Hugo – seven years her junior – for less than a year when she became pregnant by accident. Although she would have been happy to go ahead, Hugo was simply not ready to be a parent at such an early stage in his life.

> I'd rather have had him than a baby, actually. That was much more important, and I didn't want to mess it up. I could have just said right, that's it, been really brave and done the right thing – I thought I was doing the wrong thing – and I also worried that it would make it more difficult if I wanted to have a baby again, that I wouldn't deserve to be able to do it again.

Jane, a 31-year-old office administrator, chose to have a termination in a relationship she was unsure about, a relationship that did subsequently collapse. One of the ways she justified her action was by vowing to herself that she would never go through the experience again.

> Although I've always been a great supporter of abortion being freely available, it's not something that I'd ever wanted to go through. Yet I knew I was doing the right thing, even though it wasn't what I really wanted. I didn't think it was really fair to bring a child into the world that wasn't wanted by a parent, whose father didn't want it.

When she conceived for a second time – again by accident, but with a new partner – she was not only relieved that she was getting another chance but surprised to realise how strong her desire for a child had become.

Caroline stopped using contraception as soon as she got married at 18, partly because she was terrified that her

fertility had been affected by an abortion she'd felt forced
to have at the age of 15 when she was still at school. In
common with many women, Caroline's worry about being
unable to conceive again – either as a punishment for the
abortion or because of a medical error – was extremely
strong.

> I was worried something would have gone wrong, and
> I'd never be able to have them and that would have
> been my only chance of it. That's why I came off the
> pill so early, because I wanted to know that if I couldn't
> have any we could do something about it.

In fact infections are the most common problems with abortions. Approximately 1 in 10 women contract an infection
following an abortion, usually because there was already a
pre-existing infection present. Most of these can easily be
treated with antibiotics.

## Reaching the Point of No Return

When they had been together for three years Siân, a 28-year-
old television producer, and her husband discussed how
important children might or might not be to them.

> I can't say I'd always really wanted children. I was a
> youngest child, had never had much to do with chil-
> dren, had always found them a bit weird. We talked
> about whether it would matter if we didn't have them
> and had come to the conclusion that on the whole it
> wouldn't. That we could have quite happily led our
> lives doing other things despite the pressure from
> friends.

But Siân wanted to come off the pill and Peter hated condoms, so they decided to use the rhythm method. Siân feels that in some way this was a silent acknowledgement that it wouldn't be disastrous if she did conceive.

> It was hormones, I'm convinced, changed my mind. There were times when you'd feel passionately that you'd want a baby, for no apparent reason, because when your period came two weeks later you'd think, 'thank God for that'. It definitely wasn't me making the decision, it was my body. It was as if I'd been taken over by something.

Before we'd met neither Greg nor I had ever anticipated children being part of our adult lives. Together things were no longer so clear cut. It was only when a friend commented that I seemed to be reading round the subject rather a lot that I accepted that my picture of our future together had changed. In common with many people, we subconsciously turned to friends for help. Watching how those with children were coping, talking to friends who were pregnant – without betraying the fact that it was something we were considering – helped to set up the social context in which we could expect to become parents.

Once Greg and I had acknowledged this swirl of confused emotions, I developed an overwhelming need to go ahead immediately rather than live with the possibility of regret. Curiously neither of us believed that we would be able to conceive. I was only 28, Greg 29, but I was impatient. For some reason I already felt old. Perhaps I was infertile anyway? If so, I gloomily reasoned, the sooner we knew the sooner we could adjust to the idea. Lurking in the back of my mind was also a paranoid notion of how unfair it would be to have spent so much of my life fiddling around with unsatisfactory contraceptive devices of all shapes, colours and smells only to find that they'd never been necessary at all . . .

## The Biological Clock

Both women and men may not want to leave parenting too late for social reasons. Suddenly all your peers are expecting children and you realise that you want to be young enough to enjoy being a parent yourself. Men tend to be older than their partners and often feel pressure from their advancing years first. 'You are as old as you feel' is only true up to a point . . . But for women it is usually worry about one's body being unable to cope with pregnancy that tips the balance.

The average age of women conceiving for the first time in Britain has been steadily rising over the past ten years and now stands at about 28 years old. In 2007, women in their early thirties are more likely to be embarking on pregnancy than women in their twenties and the numbers of women in their early forties conceiving has doubled since 1981.[4] Almost 5 per cent of babies are now born to mothers over 35 years old.

This trend towards older motherhood has occurred despite alarmist and misleading statistics about the 'biological clock' or 'time-bomb' finding their way into medical and pregnancy books. Reproductive efficiency reaches a pinnacle in women between 17 and 19, but psychological and economic factors mean that for most women and their babies this is not the best time to become a mother. After the age of 35 the statistics of reproduction do begin to change and fertility starts a precipitous decline, but scientists have identified an interesting trend. Colloquially referred to as 'the last fling of the ovaries', there can be a sudden surge in fertility around the age of 39, briefly reversing the decline of previous years.

## Risks Over 35

Psychologists at Bristol's Institute of Child Health reviewed the medical literature in this field and carried out research of their own:

> Social and psychological factors were not taken into account and most research is out of date. We were also surprised at the sometimes very small samples that researchers used. The problem is that poor science of this type is then used to justify the label 'high risk'.[5]

The most publicised risk for mothers in their late thirties and early forties is the increased likelihood of having a child with Down's syndrome. A woman's eggs are as old as she is, so a woman of 38 conceiving does so with 38-year-old ova. The odds on the child having Down's spiral from 1 in 910 at the age of 30 up to 1 in 380 at 35 and 1 in 110 at 40.[6]

For older women there is also an increased likelihood of non-identical twins (where the ovary simultaneously releases two eggs which are both fertilised). The use of fertility drugs – Clomid (clomiphene) successfully induces ovulation in about 80 per cent of women treated; Pergonal (a brand name for the naturally occurring human menopausal hormone gonadotrophin) has a similar success rate – is also considered to contribute strongly to the high incidence of multiple pregnancies in women over 35. Estimates put the likelihood of a woman treated with Pergonal having twins or more as between 20 and 40 per cent.

Statistics also indicate that forceps and caesareans are more common for the over-35s, although this may be linked to the fact that older mothers are often considered 'high risk' even if their pregnancies are straightforward. The risk of miscarriage gradually increases as women get older and the risk of losing the baby during or after the birth appears to increase over the age of 35, too. It's important to remember, though, that the rate of stillbirth among pregnant women of all ages has dropped dramatically over the last 30 years.

## Advantages of Late Motherhood

> To be a good enough parent one must be able to feel secure in one's parenthood and in one's relation to one's child.[7]

Women leaving childbearing until later in life are more likely to fulfil Bruno Bettelheim's criteria above for being good parents. Emotional readiness is as important as physical preparedness. Many older women say that – so long as they don't get negative and frightened responses from their obstetricians – their confidence in their pregnancies is very high. Research psychologist Dr Josephine Green found that older mothers were generally better informed. When psychologists at the Bristol Institute of Child Health asked first-time mothers over 35 why they had had their babies when they did, far and away the most common response was because the time was right emotionally. In another sample only 5 per cent of mothers aged over 40 claimed to have delayed pregnancy for career reasons. Dr Zena Stein of the New York State Psychiatric Institute found in a seven-year study of over 50,000 women that the older the mother the higher the child's IQ.[8]

Pam had been with her husband for fourteen years before the marriage broke up. They had always talked about having children, but were enjoying their jobs and their lives too much and the time had never been right. She didn't worry about her biological clock – although friends clearly did – feeling that her fertility would last for ever . . . 'Then I got to the age of 41 and realised that if I didn't hurry up and do something about it, I could possibly miss out: and I didn't want to.'

## The Appliance of Science

There are various medical treatments now available to those suffering from sub-fertility or secondary infertility problems: IVF, where the ripe eggs are collected at the time of ovulation, assessed for quality, then mixed with the partner's sperm before being transferred back to the uterus; ICSI (intracytoplasmic sperm injection), where the sperm is injected directly into the egg before being placed in the woman's body; GIFT (gamete intra-fallopian transfer), where the eggs are mixed with fresh sperm outside the body before being reintroduced to the fallopian tube where the aim is for one or more of the eggs to be fertilised and implant in the uterus; and ZIFT (zygote intra-fallopian transfer) is a similar procedure to GIFT, except that the eggs and sperm are put back into the fallopian tubes at the zygote stage, after fertilisation. There is also donor insemination (DI) where donor semen from a sperm bank is placed in the vagina around the time of ovulation, and egg donation where another woman's egg is used for IVF, although the number of sperm and egg donors has dropped dramatically since the government lifted anonymity for donors in 2005.

The science of reproduction has become big business. In August 1992, a couple of months before I had Felix, a pregnant 61-year-old Italian woman, Lilliana Balocchi, was in the news. The debate asked: should age alone be a deciding factor or was maternal health as important an issue? British specialists lined up on opposite sides. Professor Robert Winston of the Fertility Unit at Hammersmith Hospital accused the private sector of taking unjustifiable risks. Professor Ian Craft of the London Fertility Centre insisted that non-smoking, non-drinking women with no history of high blood pressure or diabetes were at no greater risk than younger women.

Since then, the debate has moved on. Maternal age is no longer quite the headline-catcher it was. Instead, it is the ethics that preoccupy rather than the medicine, the sense of science out of control. For many, the worst science-fiction nightmares of uncontrolled genetic engineering have come true. Barely a day seems to pass without yet another sensationalised press report suggesting that Britain's hospitals and clinics are performing one implantation after another: surrogacy, payment for egg donation, grandmothers giving birth to children for their daughters, frozen embryos being destroyed en masse. It is, without doubt, one of the most pressing issues that we as a society have to deal with.

The fundamental disagreements between Professors Winston and Craft continue, perhaps echoing the world's rather schizophrenic attitudes to IVF. In one press interview, Winston expressed his disquiet at the lack of control and forethought in some of the decisions being made:

> We are dealing with a fragile technology which is easily
> brought into disrepute . . . the idea of treating children
> as commodities seems sleazy to me.[9]

Although more and more babies are being born thanks to medical technology, it's still an expensive business. Women aged between 23 and 39 can now have one cycle of IVF on the NHS, but many go on to fund further cycles privately. According to the Human Fertilisation and Embryology Authority, one cycle of IVF now costs up to £3,000, which doesn't include the cost of all the drugs needed to do the treatment.

Meanwhile, a cycle of IVF using a donated egg can cost in excess of £4,000. Eggs are implanted by Professor Craft for £5,400. Defending his corner, he admitted that he would much prefer people to donate out of altruism, but in the real world this doesn't happen often enough. If more eggs were made available, I could help so many more women to have the babies they long for.[10]

Obviously a full debate about the social, psychological and ethical issues surrounding IVF and related techniques is beyond the scope of this book. But, given that IVF treatment is now responsible for one in every eighty births, it is important to move to a situation where the uses of technology can, if necessary, be questioned without attacking individual children and their parents. After all, once pregnant, it is the baby or babies that matter, not the method of conception . . .

## An Only Child?

Many parents and couples with one child still find it hard to think of themselves as 'a family'. Families are things that appear in McDonald's advertisements or the *Radio Times*. Greg and I only really got used to the word after Felix, our second child, was born.

The transition from non-parent to parent is probably the most fundamental we will ever make, but many of the questions thrown up by 'if and when' persist beyond the first child. Once you have a child, issues of self-image are usually less preoccupying, but they are still there. So far you might have managed to prevent your career from suffering, but how will you cope with the remorseless demands of two children? As Hilary Land wrote in *Balancing Acts*:

When confronted (and I choose the word deliberately) with the possibility of having another child, I was frightened by the prospect. Exactly why, I do not fully understand. All I will say is two things: first, that I had realised how precarious my financial situation would have rapidly become had I wanted another child and had wanted to take as much maternity leave as I had taken (and felt I needed) the first time. Second, being a mother is about having a dependant. How then do mothers make room for other things they want to do, and how is a balance struck?[11]

British families are shrinking. In the industrialised world, the average birth rate dropped from 2.6 children per woman in the 1970s to 1.8 in the 1990s; in the developing world, the slide was from 5.9 children in the 1970s to 3.9 in the 1990s.[12] Leaving aside stepchildren and children brought into new relationships from previous ones, the most recent government figures suggest an average British family has 1.7 children. The average birth rate in France is 1.9, 1.4 in Germany and 2.0 in America.[13]

Many parents are concerned about their daughter or son being an only child. Fran had her first child, Matthew, when she was 26. Her daughter Rowan was born just over two years later. 'I was an only child, and I was absolutely positive that my child wouldn't be an only child.'

Debbie, a 26-year-old teacher living in rural Catholic Northern Ireland, also felt that not wanting her four-year-old son to be an only child was one of the decisive factors in becoming pregnant again. She and her 29-year-old husband Patrick had been together for six years. She had originally wanted four children, but Jack was a very sleepless, crying baby and Debbie suffered mild postnatal depression for 18 months after his birth; she revised her image of her family.

I felt that because we live in the country it was important that Jack had someone to play with really. I also

fancied being pregnant again, actually, and having time
off school.

Debra and Hugo both come from large, happy families and
enjoyed being part of a gang.

> I think it would be quite selfish to only have one, actu-
> ally. I do think it would be nice for them when they
> grow up to have brothers and sisters.

Other women, whilst not feeling happy with the idea of an
only child, still feel equivocal. Eve, whose daughter Annie is
now four, says

> I have sense of a feeling that I would like another child
> for Annie, but at the same time thinking I can't have
> another child for anyone else, whoever that person may
> be. It's got to be for me as well.

We spent a long time trying to decide whether to have another
baby. The prospect of Martha being an only child didn't bother
Greg, but I couldn't imagine life without my two sisters and
so I felt that Martha would treasure a sister or brother to play
with. I caught myself feeling sorry for children of five or six
sitting alone with their parents in restaurants, as if somehow
they would have been happier and healthier if they had a
sibling to kick under the table. I was also aware that because
we loved Martha so much we could run the risk of unwittingly putting too much pressure on her.

On the other hand I feared that the intimacy of our relationship with Martha would be spoiled if we had another
child. Miserably torturing myself, I felt that in some indefin-
able way she would think she hadn't been enough on her
own otherwise we wouldn't have done it again. How could

it be possible for either of us to love another child as much as we loved Martha? And it wouldn't be fair to have a second baby if we couldn't love it properly. This anxiety, which occupied the whole of the pregnancy, faded away unnoticed the minute I cradled Felix in my arms.

Jenny was 29 and worked part-time in a legal publishing company in Sussex. She and her husband Bruce had a two-year-old son. Jenny had mixed feelings about having a second child, and throughout the pregnancy she too felt ambivalent even though she knew she wanted the baby.

> I think if social pressures and family pressures weren't on me and I didn't think it was bad for James, I don't think I would have had any more. I love James a lot, and I had this strange feeling that it was going to be like telling Bruce, I'm sorry, but I've got another husband and he's moving in at Christmas and you'll only have half my time. I felt like I was letting James down in some way.

## Age Gaps Between Children

But for many, once the toes are in the water, there is no question of only having one child. Lee and Simon from Nottingham had been together for nine years. They married for the specific reason that they were ready to have children: 'We both decided to have two children to replace each of us on this overpopulated planet.'

Nicki, a special needs teacher, had conceived twins – Max and John – by accident 22 months earlier at an awkward time for her and her partner Mike. (She had just finished her MPhil at an American university, and they had planned to travel around South America for four months.) Despite a traumatic birth, Nicki knew that she still wanted to have another child as soon as possible: 'Getting pregnant with Anna was the most selfish thing I've ever done; I just needed to have her; I was desperate for another baby.'

Twenty years ago much was written about the optimum age gap between children. Today there is a growing awareness that the relationships between parents and children and the way older siblings are prepared for new babies are more important. Two Swiss psychologists, Julius Ernst and Cecile Angst, reviewed the cornucopia of research, seeking a correlation between a child's position in the family and achievement. Their results, published in 1982, theorised that although birth order, family size and the age gap between children did affect an individual, other variables were at least as important. For Ernst and Angst 'dethronement' – a Freudian term hijacked by development psychologists – did not necessarily characterise an elder child's perception of the usurping second baby. The biggest study on siblings in Britain, carried out in Cambridgeshire by Professor Judy Dunn and associates, reached the same conclusions.

Dunn, a British psychologist based at Pennsylvania State University, visited forty families who were expecting a second baby, then three times after the birth. The age gaps between the children ranged from 18 to 43 months. She found that, although younger first children were generally more clingy when the new baby arrived, the size of the age gap was less important than the sex of the children, the relationships between children and parents and the temperament of the older child. With the mother often much less available after childbirth, the bond between the elder child and the mother's partner assumed great significance.

Caroline is now 28 and has four children, Emma aged 9, Anthony aged 7, Richard aged 4 and Jessica 2. Despite her husband Malcolm's initial reluctance – 'he didn't object; he did his bit' – she had always wanted a large family. On each occasion the timing of the pregnancy was influenced primarily by her emotions: when she felt broody, she came off the pill. She also admits that her children's characters – how demanding they were – were important. Because her second child had difficulty sleeping she left a longer gap than she really wanted before conceiving her third.

> I gave myself an extra year to recover. But also because
> I felt that Anthony needed to be that bit older since he
> was less mature than Emma was.

Once the decision has been made, consciously or not – whether it is a first or a subsequent child – most women are impatient to be pregnant right away and resent the period of uncertainty we all have to endure. Few of us, though, have much idea of how conception actually occurs and what goes on in those first four weeks when our bodies know we're pregnant even if our minds do not.

# Is it Positive?

## Weeks 1–4

For years I dreamt you
my lost child, a face unpromised.
I gathered you in, gambling,
making maps over your head.
You were the beginning of a wish
    Katherine Gallagher, from 'Firstborn'[1]

The opening sequence in Woody Allen's film *Everything You Always Wanted to Know About Sex But Were Afraid to Ask*, where the white-clad sperm battle their way towards – and into – the poor unsuspecting ovum, is in some ways an accurate representation of the surprisingly haphazard nature of conception.

It was Aristotle who, in the fourth century BC, first suggested that the embryo developed gradually. His misconception was that sperm acted on menstrual blood, a process he christened epigenesis. Five hundred years later, the Greek physician, Galen, suggested that semen was the sole active ingredient. Galen's Christian contemporary, Clement of Alexandria, theologically defined seminal fluid as something that was almost, or about to become, human.

The supposed primacy of the male contribution held sway for many centuries until finally, in 1672, a young Dutch surgeon called Regnier de Graaf discovered the ovum and its peregrination from the ovary to the womb. But even De Graaf reached the wrong conclusion, believing that the ovum contained a tiny model of the parent just waiting to grow, like enlarging a photograph. Supporters of De Graaf's rival, Van Leeuwenhoek, clung to a similar idea except that for them the human blueprint was located in the head of the sperm. This Lilliputian debate rumbled on until the turn of the nineteenth century, when ovulation was discovered by a British physician, John Power, who tentatively suggested that ovulation and menstruation might be connected. Even so, the belief that the fetus was made from menstrual blood remained widespread – despite scientific discoveries in Europe that eggs were ejected spontaneously from the ovaries (in 1845), and proof that neither menstruation nor pregnancy occurred in women whose ovaries had been removed. Gradually over the second half of the century, however, science started to propound more accurate theories of the gradual development of a human fetus over a nine months' gestation.

Most cultures equate sexual intercourse with conception – although even in the 1960s a tribe in North Queensland believed a woman became pregnant because she'd been sitting over a fire on which she'd roasted a fish given to her by the prospective father. In some cultures the number of times a couple makes love is considered the deciding factor. A distinguished headsman of the Sema tribe in post-war India told a European visitor that it was 'ridiculous to suppose that pregnancy would result from coition on one occasion only'.[2] Though in some circumstances this is, perhaps, an expedient argument – even in countries whose populations technically have access to reliable contraception advice – there are many young people who still believe that you can't get pregnant the first time you make love.

## Conception: a Hit and Miss Affair

Human conception is an inefficient business and although different studies suggest different average levels of fertility it seems likely that a fertile couple making love at the most fertile time of a woman's cycle has only a one in four chance of conceiving that month. In every 100 couples, 30 will have conceived within one month, 75 will have conceived within six months and 90 will have conceived within a year. In Britain, couples are generally eligible for professional counselling once they have failed to conceive after trying regularly for one year. However, if you're over 35, it's best to see your GP if you're still trying after six months. Despite their own experiences, most of the women interviewed for this book had that six-month figure fixed in their mind as an average, were surprised if it happened more quickly and worried if it took longer. Eve summed it up:

> I did think I was in for 6 months of totally fun, spontaneous sex, and in fact got pregnant the moment we threw the cap away. So that was a shock, and when actually finding out I'd conceived I felt a bit let down.

But conception is a chance encounter. The fallopian tube has only one chance every month of securing the tumbling egg, no bigger than a grain of salt, as it explodes out of the ovary. (Many women recognise the stabbing pain or cramping sensation, known as *mittelschmerz* – middle pain – as indicating that ovulation has taken place.) As many as four times out of ten the egg misses. In 15 per cent of cases the ovum itself is defective and cannot be fertilised; in 25 per cent of cases fertilisation takes place but for a variety of reasons fails to implant and the egg silently aborts. The massacre of the millions of ejaculated sperm begins the second they reach the hostile environment of the vagina. The surviving sperm rely on the fallopian tubes and the downward contractions of the uterus to guide them towards the egg. White blood cells wait to ambush stragglers, while those who choose the wrong fallopian tube are lost.

For the sperm, timing is all. If they arrive too early, they may die of old age while waiting for the egg; if they are too late, the egg itself will have started to deteriorate. Only in 20 per cent of cases do sperm and egg meet successfully in the right place at the right time.

When the egg appears dozens of vigorous sperm rush up to try to pierce its tough outer coating, by spraying their enzymes on the egg's protective membrane. Only one sperm will break through to force its way into the egg, as the membrane surrounding the egg is instantly sealed, preventing the entry of any more sperm. The nuclei of the two cells fuse, and fertilisation is complete. The cell divides about once every 12 hours during the three-to-four-day passage down the fallopian tube to the uterus.

After 72 hours a small cluster of cells – known as the blastocyst – moves out of the fallopian tube and enters the uterus. By the eleventh day after ovulation the blastocyst has embedded itself in the fertile, blood-thickened walls of the uterus (the endometrium) which have been prepared by the four reproductive hormones.

The luteinising hormone (LH) and the follicle-stimulating hormone (FSH) are collectively known as the gonadotrophins: they stimulate the female hormones, oestrogen and progesterone, not only to ripen and release the egg but also to prepare the endometrium to receive the blastocyst.

Once implanted, the fertilised egg sends out signals to tell the woman's body to carry on producing progesterone (responsible for tender, enlarged breasts before a period), which suppresses menstruation and is the reason why many women mistake the earliest physical feelings of pregnancy for an imminent period. If conception had not taken place the progesterone level would have begun to fall, the endometrium would have been shed and the stored blood would have started to ooze out.

Some women are more aware of their cycles than others and do try to make love around the time of ovulation if they want to conceive. Joanne, a 30-year-old music teacher from Australia, and her 34-year-old partner Georgina have lived together in London for ten years. Joanne had always known that she wanted children – six originally, now revised down to two – but Georgina had been adamant that she would never bear a child and had been less than keen on being a parent at all. But about three years ago, they did decide that they would look for a donor.

Many lesbian couples opt for artificial insemination by an anonymous donor, despite an increasing shortage of sperm donors, not least to avoid the possibility of a distressing custody battle further down the line. But, in the end, however, Joanne and Georgina decided that they wanted their baby to have a flesh-and-blood father, not least because they also wanted to give him or her an extended family, a granny and granddad, aunts and uncles. They set about asking people until a close friend suggested that her brother might be interested. Joanne couldn't steel herself to go to meet him, feeling that it would be a judgement on her if he decided against going ahead. So Georgina undertook what might have been a delicate mission alone, returning some hours later with a hangover and a jar of sperm.

Self-insemination is a straightforward business, often

mistakenly confused with artificial insemination, which is used in cases where couples are having difficulty conceiving. As in heterosexual intercourse the sperm are released as high as possible into the vagina, using a syringe or a pipette.

Joanne had been keeping accurate temperature and ovulation charts and knew it wasn't the right time, but they went ahead anyway. To no avail. Then they gave their donor a list of Joanne's most fertile dates and each repeated her or his contribution on the next appropriate occasion. It was successful first time, and their son Rowan was conceived.

Once Hugo had decided that the time was right to start a family, Debra didn't want to have to leave anything to chance. She made sure she knew exactly when she was ovulating so that she would get pregnant straight away.

> I thought it should all be natural, but I was scientific
> about it. I did it very, very methodically, looking at the
> days on my cycle. I was interested in the medical side
> of it, actually, and I hadn't really known about it before.
> So we did that, and it worked first time.

## Influencing the Sex

Increased knowledge of the process of conception has extended the reach of the issue of sex selection. The phenomenon isn't new, and the tendency has always been to put higher value on the birth of a boy than of a girl. The Ancient Greeks believed that cutting off the left testicle would produce a son since they thought male sperm were produced in the right testicle. During the Middle Ages in Germany couples desiring a boy were encouraged to make love when there was a full moon, a technique likely to render barren women whose cycles did not correspond to the moon and tides. Welsh folklore advises that lying on your right side during intercourse will produce a daughter; others believe that for a boy to be conceived the woman must be the dominant partner in lovemaking. Greek-Cypriot custom still holds that rolling a chubby baby boy up and down the bridal bed will ensure that the marriage is blessed with healthy male offspring.

In 1992 Ron Wells, an Australian doctor with a background in health statistics, published *The Sexual Odds: Can You Choose the Sex of Your Baby?*, a book giving basic recipes and suggestions for those determined to influence the sex of their child. This jostles for bookshop shelf space with Dr Landrum Shettles's bestselling *How to Choose the Sex of Your Baby* which the author claims is 75 per cent effective. In *Boy or Girl? Choosing Your Child Through Diet*, Françoise Labro and Françoise Papa confidently assert that a diet high in sodium and potassium will produce sons and one high in magnesium and calcium will produce daughters, provided the regime is adhered to at least 10 weeks before conception.

The sex of your baby is decided by the individual spermatozoon that fertilises your egg, a fact that hopefully brings some posthumous embarrassment to Henry VIII who ran through three (out of six) wives before he found one, Jane Seymour, who bore him a son. The ovum carries only the X – the female – chromosome, whereas the sperm can carry either X or Y chromosomes. X- and Y-carrying sperm have different properties. Those carrying the male Y chromosome are not only a fraction smaller but also about 3 per cent lighter than Xs. If ejaculated on or as near to ovulation as possible, Ys will outrun the heavier, slower-moving female sperm. On the other hand, female sperm live longer, so ejaculation three or four days before ovulation is more likely to ensure that only X sperm are still around when the egg is released. For every ten sperm carrying X chromosomes there are only nine bearing Y chromosomes yet more boys than girls are conceived on a worldwide ratio of 10 to 9.

Using the sperm separation techniques of an American doctor, Ronald Ericsson, the London Gender Clinic was opened in January 1993. Through his 46 franchised clinics across Europe, Asia and America, Ericsson was claiming a 70 per cent success rate for girls and 80 per cent for boys. Soon after, other gender selection clinics began to pop up around the country.

In 2003, a public consultation carried out by the Human Fertilisation and Embryology Authority (HFEA) found that 69 per cent of the public felt that sex selection should not be available. Even so sex selection using sperm separation techniques is still unregulated and clinics continue to operate around the UK. While most of them claim a success rate of 70–90 per cent, there's still no scientific evidence to suggest that sperm selection is any more effective at producing babies of a particular sex than making love when there's a full moon.

The only sure way to get either a boy or a girl is through a technique called Pre-implantation Genetic Diagnosis (PGD). This involves mixing a couple's sperm and eggs to produce embryos and then removing one cell from each embryo to test it for gender. Embryos of the chosen gender can then be placed in the mother's womb. However, this technique is only available on medical grounds in the UK, for example, if a couple have a life-threatening disease running through their family that only affects one sex.

Child sex preselection raises many ethical and sociological questions about the role of science and its application, as well as about the motivations of parents. It is a complicated issue, beyond the scope of this book. Suffice to say that science is not – and never has been – neutral. According to the Victorian philosopher and doctor Oliver Wendell-Holmes:

The truth is that medicine, professedly founded on observation, is as sensitive to outside influences, political, religious, philosophical, imaginative, as is the barometer to changes of atmospheric density.[3]

None of the women I interviewed tried to influence their baby's sex, even if they had a preference. Many were not even aware that the timing of ejaculation could be decisive, and some were openly sceptical. A lot of the women were confident about their patterns of ovulation, whether they were actively trying to conceive or not. Tessa admitted:

I knew exactly that I was conceivable on that night, and I did suggest that I leave my cap out specifically because I knew that I would conceive if I was ever going to conceive. And I did, that very night.

## Preparing for Pregnancy

Lisa, then a 32-year-old lawyer, had been with her 39-year-old partner Rob for about 20 months. Having been conscientious about contraception during her twenties, using the cap in stable relationships and condoms for flings, they had been relying on the withdrawal method.

I think at the back of my mind there was this lingering feeling that I wasn't fertile, which maybe came from when I was 17 and I had dysentery. My mother took me to a gynaecologist in Harley Street and the stupid man said, 'well, she's infertile', which I obviously was at that particular point. And because of that, and because I've never had to have an abortion despite having taken risks through my sexually active life, and having a sister who'd had problems conceiving,

I found myself in my thirties wondering if I was fertile at all.

Both Lisa and Rob wanted children at some point, but the timing couldn't have been worse and a child just wasn't in their immediate plans.

We went away for the weekend – my birthday weekend – and normally it was part of our lovemaking that one or the other would check if I was safe. It's a bit like getting your cap – instead of going off and putting it in, the question would be asked, 'Is it safe for me to come inside you?' He didn't ask, and I didn't say. As soon as he came I said, 'You know, that was a really bad time, Rob. That was bang midcycle, exactly 14 days . . .' But at the same time I shrugged it off, and said, 'You just don't get pregnant that easily', and, 'If I do, I do . . .', not really thinking that I would.

Most of us are still haunted by miserable teenage memories of the desperate wait for our three-day-late period, where we made bargains with ourselves and deliberately didn't carry tampons, as if the blood being there would compensate for the embarrassment. Then there were those doctors' waiting-rooms where we solemnly waited to be lectured on how there was no safe time of the month. And we all know women who have made love and conceived during their periods, whose spermicidal jelly and diaphragms haven't worked.

In the end, given the odds on fertilisation occurring, it is amazing that any woman ever gets pregnant. So it's luck if you do conceive, luck if you don't, depending on what you want. Jane, who had only been with her new partner Matt for a couple of months, immediately knew that luck had gone against her: 'One night, when we were very pissed, we were careless. I remember lying there afterwards thinking, "that was an incredibly stupid thing to do".'

Back in 1992 – when Greg and I were thinking of having a second child – there was a certain amount of information about pre-conceptual care but it was not a major issue. By 2007, most women *intending* to become pregnant are aware that diet and lifestyle can not only make a difference to their chances of conceiving in the first place, but can also affect the ultimate health of their baby. Some simply feel that they want to be as fit and healthy as possible – for themselves – so as to give themselves an easier time of it. Others just don't want to run the risk: after all, nine months of abstinence isn't so very much to ask . . .

Dr Graham Barton of the Department of Anatomy at Cambridge University has commented that the dangers of smoking should be pointed out before conception, 'because by the time of the first antenatal appointment, the damage to the placenta is already done'.[4]

Debbie came off the pill six months before trying to conceive. She made a conscious decision to cut out junk food, eat as many fruit and vegetables as she could manage, and to exercise to become as fit as possible.

> I'd read a lot about it, and I just think that it's very important that you prepare your body for the pregnancy. I wasn't interested in whether it was a boy or a girl, just to get your body in good shape must be good for the baby as well.

Debra did stop smoking a month before (although her smoking was only at the level of an odd puff at the week-ends), and although she had a pretty healthy diet she had a tendency not to eat enough: 'But I didn't know diet made a difference anyway, that if you'd been eating healthily a few months before that might make a difference to your baby.'

Joanne didn't adopt a special clean-out diet but, as a teetotal, no-caffeine non-smoker with a near vegetarian diet devoid of biscuits and chocolate, she was pretty spotless in the first place. Lee and Simon too felt that their diet was extremely good to start with, and many others did stop drinking or smoking in preparation. With Felix I couldn't have been in a worse physical condition due to stress and general exhaustion. In order to compensate and give my body a boost I took vitamin supplements, until I read that an excess of vitamins A, C and D could have detrimental effects on a growing embryo. I'd also read that research – for example, from the Medical Research Council's Vitamin Study – had cautiously suggested that some congenital disorders of the central nervous system, such as spina bifida and anencephaly, could be prevented by multi-vitamin and folic acid supplements taken around the time of conception. It had never occurred to me that having too many vitamins might actually harm a baby.

In pregnancy most of us are more susceptible to expert advice – especially the written word – than ever before, but much of the official and not-so-official literature is unbelievably contradictory. I remember sitting at the railway station, livid that as an informed layperson I was supposed to be able to assess which scientific advice was valid and which should be rejected. Had I taken my vitamin level up excessively high or not? Many women are wearied by this supposedly impartial advice, exacerbated by the fact that women have been having babies for thousands of years unfettered by such stringent attention to preparatory diets.

The Department of Health puts a great deal of time and effort into producing clear and efficient guidelines for pre-conceptual and antenatal care. All first-time mothers are given a free Pregnancy Book, there are several helplines for diet and well-being in pregnancy and most health authorities produce their own 'what-to-expect-when-you're-expecting' booklet.

Some of the most important advice given to women is that on folic acid. Doctors recommend a 400 mcg dose of folic acid daily before conception and for the first three months of pregnancy to help reduce the risk of spina bifida and other neural tube defects.

Most glossy magazines carry advertisements for supplements such as Pregnacare or Preconceive. There are also naturally folate-rich foods including cooked black-eye beans, Brussels sprouts, yeast extracts, kale, spinach, cooked soya beans, cauliflower, cooked chick peas, oranges, peas, parsnips, wholemeal bread, cabbage, brown rice. Many breakfast cereals are fortified with folic acid too.

Information and support for the decisions we make in pregnancy are clearly important. There is a danger, though, that we will be lulled into believing that we can control everything through what we eat and don't eat. This is taken from one folic acid leaflet:

> So if you take one a day and follow our simple advice on diet and vaccination, you should have nothing to worry about . . . except choosing a name, of course . . . and what colour to paint the bedroom . . . and . . .

It's reassuring, of course – and the word *should* is in there along with good advice on diet and vaccinations – but to me there is still an implication that babies can be designed, that if women only act 'responsibly' and do what they're told, then nothing can go wrong. Is it surprising that many women feel that it is their fault if there is something, however minor, wrong with their baby?

There's also a danger that women's needs as individuals automatically start to take second place to those of her unborn child. In America there have been a few examples of women taken to court for pre-natal neglect. In *Backlash*, Susan Faludi quotes a case in Iowa where a baby was declared a ward of state at birth because the woman had 'paid no attention to the nutritional value of the food she ate during pregnancy'!

There are all sorts of reasons why someone might not change their eating habits in pregnancy, might not take the recommended supplements, might still smoke or drink too much. Judgemental comments, 'it'll-serve-you-right-if-something-goes-wrong' attitudes and pompous self-righteousness are not the most helpful way to support women in pregnancy. Pam, who was pregnant at 41, found that friends and strangers alike would feel they had the right to comment on everything she did:

> I've always been a great one for reading lots of books, and finding the good way of doing things, the right way. I've only realised in retrospect that there isn't any right way and there isn't any good way and there isn't any bad way of doing anything. So I knew all the right diets, the right foods to eat, not to smoke, to get your body healthy before you conceive. I knew everything, but did I do it . . . ?

With Martha I tried to regulate my diet and take more exercise. I completely stopped drinking and smoking, before I was jolted by the realisation that if I didn't get pregnant immediately then I could start to resent the would-be baby and the constraints it was putting on my life. Yet I knew that if I had just one glass of wine in the first month and then there was anything whatsoever wrong with the baby, I would be haunted by that drink for the rest of my life. Publicly I wanted to be seen to be making my own, sensible decisions about how to conduct my pregnancy. Privately, I was both upset with myself for not asserting my own needs and over-concerned about Martha's health.

## When You Can't Conceive

Many women felt indignant when pre-conceptual sacrifices didn't reap immediate rewards. Lynne was 28, a part-time health visitor. Six months before trying to conceive, she and her 31-year-old husband John had cut down on drinking, concentrated on eating a healthy vegetarian diet and John had drastically reduced his nicotine intake. Finally the day arrived; they were prepared, clean, the cap could be thrown away. It took them nine months to conceive ... 'I felt very cheated, totally frustrated and thought, "I'm supposed to know all about this, why isn't it happening after all this preparation?"'

Lynne hadn't expected to get pregnant straight away, but once eight months – and eight regular periods – had elapsed she was worried enough to visit her GP. She had been experiencing what she thought were double periods, having some spotting after ovulation. Her GP diagnosed the secondary bleeding as actually happening before and during ovulation and suggested that – so long as neither of them were squeamish – they could get round the problem by making love a few days earlier. The GP was right and Michelle was conceived.

One woman in her mid-twenties who took two years to conceive her daughter felt confused as well as upset. It had never crossed her mind that she might not be able to conceive and, as the months went by, she started to feel angry too. Tests discovered nothing physically wrong with either her or her partner. They both found not knowing why she wasn't conceiving extremely hard and it drove a wedge between them as they unconsciously blamed each other.

> My mother in particular kept going on about when were we going to have a family, that we didn't want to leave it too late. I just kept saying we'd do it when we were ready, when all the time we were trying and nothing was happening.

She is now a full-time mother of three. She still has no idea why suddenly she became pregnant.

Fertility in women is extraordinary. Lodged in its mother's womb in the earliest weeks and months of a female embryo's gestation, millions of ova are laid down in her minuscule ovaries. At six months' gestation no more than a million or so are left. The number continues to drop through birth and childhood until by puberty only about 300,000 immature eggs remain, ready to be released on the cyclical monthly countdown of a woman's fertile life. Only about 400 ova – just 0.13 per cent of those present at puberty – will mature fully and be set free from the ovaries. An even tinier proportion will survive the hazardous process of release, fertilisation and implantation. At the menopause only about 300 ova remain, by which time most are defective and incapable of being fertilised.

The pattern of male fertility is linear, not cyclical; once it is turned on and the pituitary gland begins pouring follicle-stimulating hormone into the bloodstream only extreme old age can shut it down. In the 1950s two American scientists analysed the sperm of 1000 new fathers for number, motility (movement) and morphology (shape). As a result they defined a normal sperm count as around 125 million sperm per ejaculation (only 2 to 5 per cent of semen is actually sperm). Some men produce more – up to 300 million – but, depending on sperm quality, as little as 3 million may be necessary to cause pregnancy, the quantity present in a virtually invisible drop of seminal fluid. Maximum normal survival time in the vagina is thought to be about six hours because of the acidity of the vagina, but for sperm that battle through into the protective environment of the cervix, uterus and fallopian tubes, survival can be as long as 6–7 days although the average is nearer 3–4 days.

An infertility epidemic now seems to be stalking the USA and Western Europe. Around 12 per cent of couples in the USA are infertile, while in European countries this figure is about 14 per cent. Infertility is also known to increase with age, affecting 5.5 per cent of people aged 25–29, 9.4 per cent of people aged 30–34 and nearly 20 per cent of those in the 35–39 age group.[5] But for those unsuccessfully trying to conceive, statistics are meaningless, empty ciphers with no relation to their feelings of frustration, failure and pain.

One woman in her mid-thirties had been trying to get pregnant for seven years, before she was diagnosed by a fertility clinic as having a hormone imbalance and her husband as having a low sperm count. 'I can't describe the feelings of grief and loss when my periods started. I came to hate the sight of my own blood.'

History documents a plethora of infertility cures, the majority aimed at women. The Ancient Greeks baked bread in phallic shapes to aid conception; the herb bryony was popular in sixteenth-century Europe, and in the Book of Genesis the childless Rachel asks Leah for mandrake to help her conceive. Surprisingly commonplace foods have been considered to have aphrodisiac qualities, from potatoes in the seventeenth century to tomatoes in the Victorian period (perhaps because of the corruption of the Italian *pomo d'oro* – golden apple – to the French *pomme d'amour* – love apple). In Asia powdered rhino horn is still considered to be a powerful aid to conception: in 1915 the Indian government had to establish a rhino sanctuary to prevent the species' extinction. The word 'honeymoon' comes from the old northern European custom of drinking honeyed wine or mead during the first month of marriage as an aphrodisiac and to aid conception.

## Reasons for Infertility

Science takes a different view. The problem lies with the man in 30 to 40 per cent of infertility cases. Poor sperm motility, frequent abnormal forms, the presence of antibodies, low sperm count perhaps due to excessive drinking or smoking may all affect fertility, as can pollution. In 2005, a team of researchers led by Rome-based scientist Marcello Spano found that DNA damage in the sperm of 700 men rose in relation to their exposure to common environmental pollutants called PCBs. The effect was seen in all ethnic groups studied apart from Inuit men. Men who had had the highest exposure had 60 per cent more DNA damage than average:

> PCB exposure might negatively impact reproductive capabilities especially for men who, for other reasons, already have a higher fraction of defective sperm.[6]

As with most medical research, particularly in the area of human fertility, there are those urging caution. Commenting on the research, Dr Allan Pacey, secretary of the British Fertility Society, said: 'We still have a lot to learn about how man-made chemicals interact with the male reproductive system.'[7]

Smoking affects women's fertility too. One major American research project suggested that 38 per cent of non-smokers conceived in their first cycle compared with 28 per cent of smokers and that smokers were 3.4 times more likely to have taken more than a year to conceive. Now, links between infertility and smoking are assumed in most pregnancy handbooks and official literature.

Being extremely underweight or clinically overweight will reduce fertility, as can emotional distress. Depression, bereavement, persistent low-level illness, redundancy, may very well all act as short-term barriers to pregnancy. Science writer and broadcaster Vivienne Parry includes stress as a factor affecting fertility:

> When you're having a difficult time, your periods are disturbed. It's an easily recognised sign of how emotions affect the hormones of your reproductive cycle. But while it's common knowledge among women, scientific evidence has been unavailable.[8]

The single most important identifiable cause of infertility in women is pelvic inflammatory disease (PID), which can be the result of contracting a sexually-transmitted disease. The most common sexually-transmitted infection in the UK is chlamydia, which research suggests is the cause of 39 per cent of all PID cases. In 2004, more than one per cent of young women aged 16–19 were diagnosed with it, although since at least 70 per cent of women have no symptoms, the real figure is thought to be much higher. On infection of the membranes surrounding the embryo (chorio amionitis), affected women run a higher risk of stillbirth and prematurity and about 60 to 70 per cent of babies born to infected women contract the disease during delivery, resulting principally in infant conjunctivitis and pneumonia. After one PID attack a woman has a 15 per cent risk of becoming infertile; two attacks and the odds rise to 30 per cent; after three attacks, 45 per cent of women can no longer conceive.

Polycystic ovary syndrome (PCOS) is the most common cause of infertility in women who have irregular or no periods, where the ovaries are usually, although not necessarily, slightly larger, smoother and thicker than normal, with tiny follicles on the outside. Each follicle contains an egg that doesn't reach maturity. Sufferers may have skin problems, including acne, have a tendency to be overweight, suffer from hirsutism (excessive body hair) or even hair loss, and have higher than average levels of insulin in the bloodstream. The main hormonal abnormality is increased LH levels with normal or low FSH levels. As yet no one knows what causes PCOS.

Many women who seek fertility counselling do so because they experience depressing and confusing secondary infertility; about five per cent of couples, having conceived once, find they cannot conceive again, according to Infertility Network UK. The cause may be PID, or that some women suddenly stop ovulating altogether. Others develop antibodies to their partner's sperm that kill them off.

If you – or someone close to you – is having trouble conceiving, the most important thing is that they should not to be afraid to ask for help. Most chemists sell over-the-counter ovulation kits, to help you work out when you are at your most fertile. If, after all your best efforts, you still have not become pregnant, don't be embarrassed to go to your GP and ask for advice.

## The First Signs of Pregnancy

But let's say that the miracle has occurred and conception has taken place. We left the blastocyst implanted in the blood-rich walls of the uterus seven or eight days after conception. There it is kept alive by the corpus luteum which produces progesterone to prevent menstruation and enough human chorionic gonadotrophin (hCG) to maintain the pregnancy. A blood test done just seven days after conception will be able to detect a high enough level of hCG to confirm pregnancy. By the fourth week the pregnancy can be seen by a trained naked eye.

Pregnancy – or gestational age – is dated from the first day of the last menstrual period rather than from the date of conception; if you have an average 28-day cycle, fertilisation is counted as taking place at around day 14 after the first day of one's last period and not day 1 of the pregnancy. This timescale allows that an average pregnancy, which actually lasts some 266 days from conception (280 from the first day of your last period), continues for 40 weeks, although two weeks either side is considered normal. This of course means that the second week after conception is actually considered week 4 of the pregnancy by the medical profession. This is part of the reason why doctors, midwives and women so often disagree about exactly when a baby is due: the woman knows when she made love, and counts from there. And not surprisingly only 2 per cent of babies do arrive on their estimated date of delivery (EDD).

Some women, like Siân, just know that they are pregnant in those first four weeks, before a home test would be reliable: 'I was pretty certain within days that something had happened. Physically I just felt, I don't know, as if the world had shifted.'

Frequency of urination can be a telltale sign, sometimes occurring as soon as one week after conception, possibly because of the hormonal changes or even the early swelling of the uterus starting to exert pressure on the bladder. Some women even become constipated straight away. Uncontrollable tiredness and fatigue can also start within days of conception. (Although doctors cannot agree why this affects some women and not others, progesterone – a sedative in human beings that possesses powerful tranquillising and hypnotic effects – is believed to be its cause, with the raised levels experienced by newly pregnant women simply taking some getting used to.) Every woman I talked to said that her breasts had changed within days of conception, some noticing a mass of blue veins like rivers on a map, although many dismissed it as exaggerated premenstrual symptoms.

Tessa had an immediate thickening of the waist: 'I lost my waist, I'm sure, the night I conceived. Well, I didn't ever have much of a waist, let's be frank, but I'm sure.' Fran's husband Jim noticed the veins on her breasts ten days before she did a pregnancy test at 5 weeks. Lynne was astounded and – she admits – rather pleased:

> My bust went berserk, there's no other word for it. Having been a very modest 34A, by 4 weeks and 3 days when I measured myself I was a 36B.

With Martha I was suspicious in what turned out to be the fourth week of my pregnancy. Although my breasts felt sore and hard, as if I was about to start menstruating, it all felt somehow different and my armpits ached. Since we had made love only three days after my period had finished I dismissed my physical symptoms as descendants of poor Mary Tudor's phantom pregnancies – all in the hopeful mind. With Felix I trusted my instincts. I knew within hours that I had conceived and by the time I was able to do a home pregnancy test a week after my period should have started, I had already told several people that I was pregnant. I wrote this in my diary at three weeks:

> 22 FEBRUARY 1992: I feel heavier, pulled down, although this could of course be due to an increased winter appetite and no exercise. Add to this sore, granite

breasts, crampy pains, queasiness over the smell of coffee and an unattractive bloated look, well it all just seems too specific.

Obviously women who have been pregnant before are more likely to recognise the signs. Sharon was 24 and working as a secretary when she conceived her twin daughters Charlotte and Katie. She'd had a 16-week abortion at the age of 15, followed by a traumatic 13-week miscarriage with complications when she was 22. Both times she'd had sore aching breasts, so with the twins she knew immediately that she was pregnant: 'I recognised the symptoms much more; whether they were stronger or whether I just accepted them, I wouldn't like to say.'

Having not known until a pregnancy test was positive first time round, Sarah, a full-time mother from London, knew she was pregnant with Abigail much earlier because of the physical signs.

> I had a hangover that lasted one day, then it was still there the second day. I thought this wasn't really right, I felt odd and funny and then I suddenly realised – I call it the 'need to burp' feeling.

But even when privately convinced, most women wait, like Pam, until they have had a positive test before allowing themselves to start being a different person, a pregnant woman.

> It was only then I allowed myself to believe, and it was a great feeling, a wonderful feeling.

# I Feel Sick

## Weeks 4–8

I'd made up my mind that if the sickness didn't stop by
the end of the next week, I'd have to leave work. I
couldn't keep it up. Although I fed myself religiously
with all the right, digestible, nourishing foods I could
think of whenever I felt they'd stay where I put them,
the constant repetition of throwing up every morning,
followed by the titanic effort involved in getting myself
to work afterwards, was telling on me. I felt perpetually
feeble and weepy.

Lynne Reid Banks, *The L-Shaped Room*[1]

### The Baby

Weeks 4 to 8 are the most crucial to a baby's healthy development, which is one of the reasons that doctors urge women
who *might* be pregnant to avoid smoking, drinking or taking
drugs that could be harmful. By 5 weeks the blastocyst, now
an embryo, is 2mm long (less than a sixteenth of an inch),

and the spine, nervous system, head and trunk are just starting to take shape. By week 6, the head is formed, the abdomen, brain and spinal cord complete and the limb buds appear. Seven days later, the heart begins to pulse.

The placenta is developing, although it is not yet ready to take on its nourishing and sustaining role. During week 7 the limbs, like little paddles, start to move and the baby's own blood cells start to circulate throughout its tiny, half-inch (13mm) body. Its intestines have grown, but they are not yet in their proper place. By week 8 all the internal organs, including the lungs, are formed and growth of the ears and eyes is now taking place. The baby-to-be is now nearly an inch long (22mm).

## Doing the Pregnancy Test

Unless a woman is successfully suppressing the signs, or is experiencing breakthrough bleeding that she's mistaking for a light period, suspicion sends her hurtling to the chemist or GP at about 5 or 6 weeks. However confidently she has read her pregnant body's signals, rare indeed is the woman who does not use some form of test for confirmation.

Pregnancy testing has been around for thousands of years: an Egyptian doctor would have recommended putting wheat and barley seeds into separate cloth purses for a woman to urinate on every day; if both sprouted, she was pregnant. Today's home tests are claimed to be so accurate that many can be done as soon as a woman's period is even a day late. Most tests trumpet a 98 per cent reliability rate, although many women would query this figure.

Caroline felt that a positive test result was a mere formality; her menstrual cycle is completely regular. She followed the instructions to the letter despite being, as the mother of three, a bit of a dab hand. She was mystified – and disappointed –

when the test was negative. A test at the doctor's the following week was positive.

Tessa and Mark had made love on the fourteenth day of her regular cycle. As soon as her period was late she bought a test – negative. Four days later she did the second test – negative again. Bemused, she invested another £9 in a second kit of a different brand – still negative.

> I thought 'this is ridiculous, I can't believe this is possible. I've done it on the right night and the right time and I thought I knew I was; how could I be so wrong about my own body?'

With Felix I was completely sure and I tried the day after my period was due, a Friday:

> 31 JANUARY 1992: Woke at 3am trying to decide whether or not to do the test this morning, after all my period's only a day late. Spurred on by the size of my breasts, 7 o'clock found me in the bathroom, Martha on my left hip, trying to piss into a cup. Didn't feel nervous. First I realised the cup wasn't full enough; second, because I'd been to the loo I thought it might not be concentrated enough, so when it wasn't positive I didn't feel devastated. But immediately I felt less pregnant and didn't want any breakfast, even though at the bottom of my heart I'm still sure that it's the test that's wrong ...

For the next week I brooded on phantom pregnancies and silent abortions, waiting for a week to pass. I was continually in the loo checking for any telltale signs of bleeding. At the same time I was nauseous and developed a heavy, white and sticky discharge. I felt there was something

pulling inside my breasts, gathering in the veins like strands
of cotton.

> 7 FEBRUARY 1992: Woke up at 5.45 desperate to do the
> test. Tried to talk myself out of it – how would I feel if
> it was negative, better not to set myself up for disap-
> pointment etc. – but couldn't go back to sleep. 6.35
> finally crept along to the bathroom, still saying I wasn't
> going to do it, but turned the bathroom light on which
> made it clear that I was. Cleaned glass, got out kit –
> urine looked perfect, concentrated and golden – then to
> pass those endless five minutes washed *and* conditioned
> hair, put on socks, made a bottle of Ribena for Martha,
> all trying not to look at the little window. Caught a
> glimpse of the marker upside down, saw the right box
> had a smudge in it and felt a flash of confirmation. But
> still when I went back upstairs to look at the allotted
> time I felt sick with nerves. Then, a strong pink blob
> (which, stupidly, made me think that everything was
> especially healthy) and a wave of pure joy and excite-
> ment, very different from last time. As I sit here writing
> this at 7.03, I'm already pondering about midwives.

Lots of women talk about how the thought of doing the
test takes over their mind; how they mentally set a day to
do the test, then sneak it in earlier; how they pretend to
themselves right up until the point where they open the
box that they aren't really going to do it. Regardless of
whether the pregnancy was planned or not, almost everyone
has appalling exam-like nerves as they struggle through
the 5-minute, 20-minute, half-hour waiting time. Desperate
for a positive result, Caroline found the waiting almost
unbearable, as she recorded in her diary.

Still have no sign of a period, but I only have to wait until this afternoon to go to the clinic. Then a miracle coincidence – a friend has found her un-needed second test and brings it round – but horror I have to wait half an hour. I can't bear it. Start to think I'd rather not know one way or the other rather than know I'm not. One and a half minutes to go – I can't wait – I must go and see if it's changing. Yes, it's blue!'*

## Ectopic Pregnancy

One of the distressing reasons that a woman might feel pregnant but have repeated negative tests is that the pregnancy is ectopic. From the Greek *ektopos*, literally 'out of place', it occurs when the fertilised ovum takes too long to travel down the fallopian tube and on the seventh day, instead of reaching the uterus and implanting itself there, it embeds itself in the fallopian tube instead. Occasionally it implants in the ovary itself or, even more rarely, in the abdomen or cervix. Ectopic pregnancy was first described in AD 936, and operated on successfully in 1759.

Because hormone levels are lower with an ectopic pregnancy, pregnancy tests are less likely to prove positive. Sufferers are also marginally less likely to experience the nausea associated with early pregnancy. On the other hand enlarged breasts, slight spotting of very dark blood, low abdominal cramping possibly on one side, dizziness or shoulder-tip pain are all warning signs. Medical help should be sought immediately since a rupture of the tube can be life-threatening or dangerous to future fertility.

Ectopic pregnancy is on the increase: in northern Europe

---

* The colour is nothing to do with indicating the sex of the baby: different tests just use different colour base dyes, usually pink or blue.

the rate of ectopic pregnancies rose from 11.2 to 18.8 per 1,000 pregnancies between 1976 and 1993, while in the USA the number of admissions to hospital for ectopic pregnancy rose from 17,800 in 1970 to 88,400 in 1989. In the UK, the number of ectopic pregnancies is static at about 11,000 cases a year, but the number of related deaths has risen from three deaths per year in 1991 to four per year in 2004.[2]

A number of factors are linked with an increased probability of ectopic pregnancy: having suffered from pelvic inflammatory disease or having a history of excessive abnormal vaginal discharge; previous pelvic infection following either miscarriage, abortion or childbirth; any kind of tubal surgery or reversal of sterilisation; previous ectopic pregnancy; infertility treatment; and major abdominal surgery such as an appendectomy.

In 1989, an American case control study was published showing that women who reported smoking during pregnancy were found to have more than double the risk of ectopic pregnancy. Another more recent study found that women's risk of ectopic pregnancy rose according to how many cigarettes per day they smoked.[3]

If detected early enough, non-surgical treatments for ectopic pregnancy offer a 70 to 80 per cent chance of a woman conceiving again normally. Many women now have an intramuscular injection of a drug called methotrexate rather than surgery. Fifteen per cent of women need more than one dose. Methotrexate devitalises the cells surrounding the embryo, causing it and its sac to wither within four to five days then disappear altogether over a period of four to six weeks. Dr Essam Dimitry of the Heatherwood and Wexham Park NHS Trust says:

The greatest advantages of the method are that it is done on an out-patient basis and, because it eliminates the risk of scarring, the chances of the woman going on to conceive successfully are greatly increased.[4]

The treatment is successful in more than 90 per cent of cases, but one woman in a hundred will need additional surgery. In cases where the ectopic pregnancy is not diagnosed quickly enough and irreversible damage has been sustained, the fallopian tube itself might also need to be removed. Sixty five per cent of women go on to conceive again following an ectopic pregnancy, regardless of whether they have lost a fallopian tube or not.

I'd been sure that I would be able to keep my worrying under control second time round, having had one successful pregnancy. But despite the nausea and strong positive signs of pregnancy, I worried about Felix being ectopic. At 8 weeks I had a few days of spotting dark, rusty blood and a persistent low stitch in my groin. I was conscious that stitch scarcely qualified as 'severe abdominal pain' – listed as the strongest symptom of ectopic pregnancy – but I still moulded my symptoms to fit the diagnosis in my medical handbook.

Though Tessa was convinced she was pregnant, her persistent negative test results unsettled her. Then at about 5 weeks she was struck with severe abdominal pain, like extremely bad, stabbing period pains. She'd had similar pains 18 months earlier, which had turned out to be due to chlamydia. The infection had been treated successfully – as she'd thought – by antibiotics. But when she went for a preliminary check, she was sent straight away to Glasgow Royal Infirmary for a scan since the GP suspected that the pregnancy might be ectopic.

Because I'd thought about chlamydia I could have coped with chlamydia, but to be told that there was possibly something even worse wrong just seemed horrific.

After a blood test confirming that she was pregnant, she was admitted to the general ward. Her husband Mark was driving a van full of furniture down the M1 from Glasgow to London so couldn't be contacted. Tessa lay alone and terrified that she might never have children. At five the following morning she was pumped full of water in preparation for the scan. She was then kept waiting – with another sixteen women – until ten o'clock when an extremely pompous radiologist waltzed in.

> 'What are you wriggling for?' 'I'm going to piss all over your table . . .' – silence – then: 'Well, there's nothing wrong with you, a perfectly normal pregnancy, get off.' And I could see it, it was a teeny little bag with a little dot in it.

Tessa and Mark were ecstatic, despite the hospital warning that the pain could be a threatened miscarriage: a miscarriage is only a miscarriage, they thought, whereas an ectopic pregnancy . . . Tessa went home and slept almost solidly for the next four weeks, at which point the pain and the nausea lifted and the pregnancy progressed without a hitch. Ironically, Tessa did in fact have an ectopic pregnancy a couple of years later. It did not affect her ability to conceive and their third child, Louis, was born in July 1996 . . .

## A Positive Result

Many women feel nothing but pleasure and satisfaction when the test proves positive. Lee experienced no early physical symptoms of pregnancy, so only went to her doctor for a test once her period was late. 'I felt warm from the toes upwards, and I thought I'm going to be a Mum and everything's going to change.'

Lynne, who'd been trying to conceive for nine months, did the test when her husband was away. They had huddled together dejectedly in the bathroom too many times in the past to make this time a special occasion. But at last the test was positive and she leapt around the flat for joy 'like a lunatic'. When John came home they did a second test together, just so he too could have the pleasure of watching the colour in the little window change: 'It was a lovely, lovely feeling – we started talking to the poor little blob almost immediately.'

Caroline was thrilled every time, and found it disappointing that so few people congratulated her on her fourth pregnancy because they assumed that it had been an accident: 'I didn't get the phone book out and ring everybody I knew. But I was always really, really pleased.'

But many women are surprised by their own mixed reactions to a positive test. Those for whom it was an accident are often amazed to feel excitement along with the panic; those who thought they wanted it are often confused to feel upset. Sasha, who was 38, had committed herself to pregnancy by having her coil removed, but emotionally she was still ambivalent about motherhood. For her, the first indication of how much she wanted to become pregnant was her pleasure and unreserved excitement at the positive test result.

First of all it made me into a normal woman. Here I was trying so hard not to be a normal woman, in the sense that whether I'd had any sort of innate maternal feelings and had blocked them off, or whether it wasn't OK to have them because if you did have them then you weren't a professional, I don't know. But it kind of obliterated everything; the shift in my attitude from what my life had been was absolutely instant.

Greg and I had not been using contraception, but when Martha's test was positive our reaction was more shock than celebration. Sharon had very much been trying to conceive for six months, worrying that her previous abortion and miscarriage had damaged her. But she dreaded the idea of the window turning blue as much as she was disappointed at it staying resolutely white:

> Every month I was horrified about perhaps being pregnant, I was horrified about having a baby, I was horrified about all that goes with it. But I wanted it as well. It delighted and terrified me, and the thought of actual childbirth itself has always terrified me since being a young girl myself.

## Unplanned Pregnancy

Lisa – who had not intended to conceive and who knew that the timing could hardly be worse in terms of her career, Rob's career, their domestic and financial situation, everything – was feeling very premenstrual and did not believe that she could be pregnant. Once her period was five days late, she thought she might as well do a test to put her mind at rest.

> To my absolute astonishment, it didn't just come out pink it came out bright pink – no doubt whatsoever. I phoned Rob at work. I knew it was a selfish, horrible thing to have done, to catch him on the hop – he had his work voice on – but I knew that if I didn't tell him I'd have to tell someone; I just couldn't wait until the evening. Because what I discovered was that I was so excited, so there was no way that I could last all day.

Nicki knew she was pregnant with the twins but, because it was such an ill-timed accident, didn't want to mention it to her husband until it had been confirmed. She went for a test at the student medical centre at the campus of her American university. They told her what she'd expected to hear, then she phoned Mike who said 'congratulations' in a stunned voice, 'as if it was nothing to do with him'. But she knew she wanted to go ahead, despite all the problems the decision would bring.

Sue, a 22-year-old freelance journalist, had just moved to London to live with her boyfriend of three months' standing. One night of unprotected sex found Sue with a late period and fluctuating emotions, as she wrote in her diary.

> I felt really sick this morning and began to panic because it was like confirmation of everything I have been worried about. I'm still not sure if I am pregnant as both the home tests I've done have come up negative, but I'm eleven days late and so have to accept the possibility that I may well be.
>
> This period of waiting is very hard for both of us and is playing havoc with our emotions. During the day, when I'm on my own, being pregnant is the last thing I want because I can't stand the thought of having to be cooped up with a baby. But once Max comes home my feelings change and I want to be pregnant with his child. There are just so many practical issues involved, like not having anywhere sensible to live and not having any money – it's so difficult.

She too decided to do the third test on her own. It was positive, so she rang Max at work: to her delight, he turned up with a bunch of flowers and took her out to lunch.

Many women talked about feeling selfish, believing it was their responsibility for not having been more careful in the first place. Jenny and Bruce were living in South Africa, having been married a month. Abortion was illegal there except in cases of danger to the woman's health and for extreme fetal deformity. 'But anyway I didn't have any excuse to have one really; we were married, we knew we wanted children one day.' [Abortion was made legal in South Africa in 1996].

## Ending an Unwanted Pregnancy

Pregnancy is one area where there is no compromise: you either are or you aren't. You either choose abortion or you don't. One of the hardest situations to resolve is when one partner feels strongly that abortion would be the most sensible decision and the other feels equally strongly that it wouldn't. They may both feel that it is – or should be – the woman's decision, but at the same time love and plans for the future as a couple, rather than as two footloose individuals, can complicate the issue.

Abortion has been common throughout history. In Assyria in 2000 BC the punishment for abortion, whether or not the woman was still alive, was 'to be impaled and not to be given burial'. Women in every culture have taken abortifacients: herbal remedies such as black hellebore, seneca snakeroot, oil of penny-royal, ergot, rue, tansy oil and savin or oil of juniper – even arsenic and quinine* – to encourage the body to expel the fetus.

The early Christian Church tolerated abortion in the first 40 days after conception (namely, before the fetus had acquired its human soul) but by the twelfth century enough abortions were being procured in Britain for it to be made an offence under canon law. By the thirteenth century abortion had become illegal under common law, although at the

---

* Tonic waters and some other fizzy mixers have to state on their packaging if they contain quinine.

same time there were efforts to distinguish between early and late attempts to induce a miscarriage. Until 1803 abortion was grudgingly tolerated in Britain provided 'quickening' (fetal movement) had not occurred, and it stayed legal in America until 1880. But after 1803 the British legislature declared it illegal at any stage of pregnancy, although there is strong evidence that it continued to be a commonly used form of birth control.

Hundreds of thousands of women have died of the abortionist's ministrations. Methods vary from knitting needles to knives and pieces of wire which were inserted into the uterus. By 1850 rubber catheters were being used by abortionists to puncture the amniotic sac; the catheter was then rotated to dislodge the fetus. Herbal and chemical remedies also continued to be employed, to the degree that in the Offences Against the Person Act of 1861 it became a criminal offence for a woman to 'administer to herself poison or any other noxious thing' as well as 'to use an instrument or other means' to try to abort an unwanted child.

The contemporary synthetic alternative to those 'noxious things' is the abortion pill. Originally pioneered under the brand name RU-486 in the early 1980s by Professor Etienne Emile Baulieu, the pill contains a drug called mifepristone. This works by blocking the hormone that helps the lining of the womb to hang on to the embryo, and can be used up to 20 weeks of pregnancy. The procedure involves taking a mifepristone pill followed a couple of days later by a pessary inserted into the vagina to encourage the uterus to contract and expel its contents. Once the uterus starts to contract, the abortion is usually complete within 12 hours.

One of the mothers I interviewed had taken the pill when she was 8 weeks pregnant. Physically she continued to feel odd, but put it down to stress, overwork and side-effects of the drug. At 16 weeks a scan revealed that she was still pregnant.

There were 186,400 abortions in England and Wales in 2005, with the highest rate, at 32 per thousand, among women aged 20–24.[5] In 2000 a quarter of young women aged 16–19 said they had first had sex before their sixteenth birthday[6], yet in 2005 only 3.7 per thousand abortions were carried out on girls under 16.[7]

Rightly, abortion continues to be an issue the world cares passionately about. Wrongly, the arguments are too often inflammatory, aggressive and attempt to deny people the right to disagree. Abortion is still illegal in both the Republic and Northern Ireland and it was only in 1996 that Jersey, Guernsey and the Isle of Man reviewed their laws to allow limited abortion rights. Meanwhile a 2001 MORI poll reported that 65 per cent of people believed that a woman had the right to choose whether or not to continue with her pregnancy.

Contrary to the impression often given, Britain does not in fact have abortion on demand under the terms of the 1967 Abortion Act. Legally, a woman can only have a termination if two doctors agree that her pregnancy involves greater risk to her physical or mental health, or to her existing children, than if it were to be terminated.

In 1990, the Human Fertilisation and Embryology Act reduced the upper time limit from 28 weeks to 24, except in cases of severe fetal abnormality or grave risk to the life of the mother. In fact, nearly 90 per cent of abortions are carried out before the 13 week mark. The current sophistication of testing procedures meant that in 2005, only 137 abortions were carried out after 24 weeks.[8]

Despite the subjective assertions of some GPs and Pro-Lifers, no woman wants to go through the traumatic experience of abortion. For most women, caught between a rock and hard place, it is a question of the lesser of two evils; a human decision, not a political one. They have to decide whether or not abortion is the only responsible course of action given their individual circumstances. As the journalist Angela Neustatter wrote:

> Although I have always marched and campaigned for a woman's right to choose, along with so many of my contemporaries, when it came to deciding to end a pregnancy, I was shocked by the distress and confusion I felt. I did not like having to take personal responsibility for ending a life, even though I believe that women have to make this choice when the odds make a child seem intolerable . . .
>
> For several months afterwards I experienced a curious upheaval of the emotions; an unaccustomed sense of nihilism; a turbulence in my private life which I felt unable to control. The feelings subsided and passed. I still regret not having been able to have the third child. I still think about it, but I am sure it was not the wrong decision, just a sad one.[9]

## Making a Decision

Jane had promised herself that she would never again go through the experience of abortion, having been forced into one some 18 months earlier. She and Matt had known each other for just three months, and had only made the decision to live together a matter of days before Jane realised that she had become pregnant. 'One, I felt absolute horror and distress; and then there was another part of me that was quite pleased, because I wanted a child.' Matt was ten years older, a freelance journalist who enjoyed his bachelor lifestyle. He had never wanted children. Equally, he was aware of her feelings about abortion and therefore the nature of the choice he was being asked to make.

I bullied him into it, because basically he had the choice of either saying yes and staying with me; or no, and the likelihood is I would have gone ahead anyway and we would have split up.

One woman interviewed had been with her partner for several years, married for four, when she became pregnant by accident. They wanted children in the future, but only when their domestic and professional situations allowed it. Her periods are regular, so when she was three days late and working at home because of an office move, she did a test. The positive result numbed her.

I was completely in a state of shock. I went and got two videos, then lay on the floor at home watching them and waiting for my husband to come home from work.

She had nothing but negative feelings and she expected at least a mixed reaction from him since the timing couldn't have been worse: he had just started a year's training course, she was about to start a new high-powered job and they lived in a small, one-bedroomed flat. But he was unequivocally delighted, and so upset when she said that she was considering an abortion that he couldn't talk to her about it at all.

I knew that the responsibility for all of this would be mine, regardless that he felt so positive and was thrilled. I was the one who was going to have to continue to work, mine was the only salary and it left me feeling shaky. I realised that part of being a feminist and working hard meant that I'd lost the support my mother had, in terms of someone taking over the financial side and giving you a breathing space when you had your children.

For the next five days she tried to come to a decision alone.

> I felt pressure because I felt if I decided to have an abortion I would really be jeopardising our relationship for the future. That he wouldn't love me any more.

In retrospect she believes that her conscious, practical feelings were completely at odds with her subconscious, emotional wishes anyway. She decided to go ahead with the pregnancy, and from that point on never regretted the decision.

## Physical Changes

Alongside these emotional decisions and readjustments, weeks 5 to 8 bring substantial physical changes. An internal examination would reveal a slightly swollen and enlarged uterus and a vagina and cervix that have softened and taken on a blue hue. Some women notice that their labia are swollen, and may even develop varicose veins, which will shrink after birth. Oestrogen and progesterone hormones have already enlarged the breasts; now the areola, the area surrounding the nipples, generally becomes darker and develops little nodules called Montgomery's tubercles. This is not always noticeable, though, as Eve mused with regret:

> I kept waiting for my nipples to get darker, because everyone told me they would. I thought this would be wonderful and I was looking forward to having these sensuous big brown splodges on my breasts. But nothing ever happened.

For many the most welcome physical symptom of pregnancy is amenorrhoea – missed periods – although implantation (breakthrough) bleeding at the time menstruation would have happened is not uncommon. One of the reasons that Sharon didn't have her abortion until 16 weeks was that she thought she was menstruating as normal.

Jenny, who took the mini-pill, developed what she thought was a stomach upset and went to a doctor, who diagnosed a strain of gastric flu and prescribed antibiotics. She duly took them, but still felt no better. Finally a pregnant friend reinterpreted her so-called flu symptoms. Even then, Jenny pointed out that she had just had a period and had had another four weeks previously. She wondered: 'I'm feeling sick in the evenings, so I can't be pregnant. The funniest thing is, though, I can't stand alcohol any more.' When the test was done at the local doctor's surgery, she proved to be about 11 weeks pregnant.

## Morning Sickness

There is a folk theory that no nausea or 'morning sickness' indicates a less entrenched pregnancy and that the woman is more likely to miscarry. But even though it is the build-up of pregnancy hormones that causes the nausea, only about 50 per cent of women have to put up with it. Many who don't feel sick have perfectly healthy pregnancies, just as some women who feel dreadful miscarry.

Maggie Profet of the University of California at Berkeley believes morning sickness is 'the embryo's canary', a way of avoiding toxic food. But no scientist has yet come up with a satisfactory explanation of why it affects some women and not others.

The phrase 'morning sickness' is rather misleading. After a night without food when blood sugar levels are low and stomach acids have had the chance to accumulate, the odds are that those women who do feel sick will suffer most in the morning. But it can – and does – strike at any time.

Most handbooks are encouraging and claim that nausea, perhaps accompanied by bouts of vomiting, will generally start at 6 weeks and go on until about 12 weeks.

This might statistically be true, but the women in this book who experienced either no nausea or textbook nausea that stopped at 12 weeks were in the minority. And, as is so often the case, those of us who continued to feel nauseous or throw up all the way through our pregnancies sometimes thought that we were somehow not being successfully pregnant: after all, if we were, surely we wouldn't be so out of kilter with the medical advice books.

Eve was one of the lucky ones, only having textbook nausea between weeks 6 and 10.

> Queasy is exactly the right word for it, a sort of pit in the stomach, a slight rolling, just feeling a bit delicate, almost a bit hangover-ish where you've eaten the wrong food the night before and you feel a bit off-colour.

Lisa was unlucky, throwing up several times a day between 7 and 18 weeks.

> Motion was terrible, even walking was terrible, so I had to change my form of transport to work. I used to go on the bus, just get off the bus in time at Oxford Street, throw up into the first green bin. I got to know every single green dustbin from Oxford Circus to my office.

Sue felt nauseous from week 6 to week 16; Joanne threw up throughout her pregnancy and labour; Nicki felt queasy until week 14, with a funny metallic taste in her mouth; Sarah had

only felt queasy from week 6 until week 12 in her first pregnancy, but with Abigail it lasted until week 20 and she was
sick from week 6 to week 9.

> One day I was at this friend's house who I hadn't been
> planning to tell. I was just feeling so awful, and she'd
> cooked this lunch. I knew I couldn't physically get
> through the day without her knowing, so she would
> understand my behaviour.

At 6 weeks Sasha started to be violently and explosively sick
at least twice a day: it lasted for the entire pregnancy, which
was particularly difficult because she didn't want anyone at
work to know for as long as possible.

> I was so devious. I would do things like carry a poly-
> thene bag up my sleeve, then when I started retching
> excuse myself, puke in the bag, run to the loo, put it in,
> then carry on the conversation. And the number of times
> Lou just sat there eating while I had to puke in the
> kitchen sink . . .

Rachel too felt wretched for five weeks from 6 weeks into
her pregnancy but, like Sasha, had to try to hide it from
colleagues at work: 'I'd throw up in a bucket at work, then
take people out to lunch.'

But because most women expect to feel sick in pregnancy,
their attitude was often that they felt well despite the nausea.
Some even said that they had no health problems at all, having
just told me about week after week of vomiting and nausea.

Women seem prepared to tolerate an extraordinary level
of physical discomfort when pregnant. About 1 in every 500
pregnant women experience *hyperemesis gravidarum*, severe
and intractable vomiting which leads to serious dehydration

from the loss of body minerals and chemicals. Specialised treatment might have to be given in hospital but, if treated, it does not alter or increase a woman's chance of miscarrying, or of giving birth to an underweight or deformed baby. Many of the women interviewed did feel that the nausea signified a healthy pregnancy, so were able to be stoical.

## Remedies for Nausea

Medical attempts to moderate nausea and sickness have had tragic consequences in the past. In 1961 the drug thalidomide, successful in eradicating the symptoms of morning sickness in early pregnancy, was withdrawn in the UK after babies whose mothers had taken the drug had been born with phocomelia (stunted limbs). Over the years many British women have taken Debendox (an antispasmodic and anti-histamine with vitamin B6) to relieve vomiting and nausea: it was marketed as Bendectin in the United States and Lenotan in other countries. Despite the lack of scientific proof to suggest that the drug was unsafe, it was withdrawn in June 1983 as a direct result of litigation brought against the manu-facturers. Given the history, it is hardly surprising that many women suspect that any drug solely for the use of pregnant women may have been less rigorously tested before being put on the market than those for society in general.

Most women prefer to resort to their own ways of coping with the nausea and vomiting. In Ancient Rome a drink of lime juice and cinnamon water every morning was recom-mended. Women in eighteenth- and nineteenth-century England took infusions of spearmint, rose and cinnamon water and, in extreme cases, belladonna. Today's recom-mended herbal remedies include camomile and wild yam root, false unicorn root (since it helps to balance hormone levels), balm and meadowsweet. Homoeopaths might prescribe ipecacuanha 6X three times daily for five days. Many women talked about pasta and rice helping (perhaps because they are digested so slowly and evenly), bicarbonate of soda, fizzy drinks (I found low-calorie – non-quinine – watered-down tonic water pretty good), ginger biscuits, dried fruit and nuts, Vitamin B6, porridge, Rice Krispies and Cornflakes. A teaspoon of cider vinegar in a cup of warm water first thing might help, if you can swallow it in the first place. Alternatively, two heaped teaspoonfuls of brewer's yeast in milk and mashed banana calmed some people's rolling stomachs.

Despite nausea, one's thirst and appetite can also increase dramatically. I was ravenous from the minute I conceived. At the same time I felt extremely nauseous and very bloated, as if I'd just eaten a steamed sponge pudding. The only time I didn't feel sick was when I was eating, and snacking little and often seemed one of the best ways of keeping it under control.

## Aversions and Cravings

There is a range of foods that many women go off immediately, most of them not particularly good for you in pregnancy, such as coffee and tea, alcohol, anything fried. Certain foods appeared time after time on women's craving lists – cereals, apples, anything salty, chocolate. Tessa, despite being Jewish and vegetarian, lusted after sausages and bacon. Nicki could only cope with white foods. Sharon and Lee walked around with fruit in their pockets and Lee also confessed to a short-lived fancy for Mr Kipling's almond slices. In her third and fourth pregnancies Caroline ate up to ten packets of Polos a day: 'I had to crunch them though; it was the crunchiness I wanted.'

Pica – the desire for bizarre or unusual things to eat, such as kippers with jam, coal, chalk, pickles with ice-cream – seems to be less common than in our mothers' day. Perhaps this is because in our age of freezers and worldwide food production it is possible to eat most foods at most times of the year. There are many theories as to why pregnant women have unpalatable, even bizarre, cravings. They may be our body's way of asking for extra iron or extra calcium, however unacceptable the required culinary combinations might be. Some feel that cravings are born from a subconscious desire to give our unborn baby what we think it would most like, such as sweets for a treat. Some homoeopaths think it is the baby's preferences that are being satisfied.

A few women also admitted to craving specific smells. Caroline had a fetish for Pine Flash, or Dettol if no Flash was available:

> It made me go all tingly in the throat, and I had to clean the bath a lot because it doesn't smell the same when it's in the bottle.

Discovery, sickness, adjustment; elation, fear, ambivalence. You and your baby have made it through to week 8.

# I Didn't Expect to Feel Like This

## Weeks 8–12

> A body cupping a body
> does not make two
> that would be error
> too grave to be borne
> given your season.
>> Meena Alexander, from 'Young Snail'[1]

These can be the hardest weeks to cope with. The excitement of finding out has passed; you have been trying to adjust emotionally and physically to being a different sort of woman, a pregnant woman; you might well have told close friends and family, enjoying seeing their reactions and feeling that in some way you are being applauded. Then what? Although you are settling into a new rhythm and feel differently, you don't look different. You just don't look obviously pregnant and that can be an anti-climax.

Greg, Martha and I were away on a two-month trip at the beginning of March. Although already I didn't feel too good,

I reckoned I could cope with the nausea better on a sun-drenched antipodean beach than in rain-sodden Lewisham. But the first four weeks away were the most miserable and depressing that I can remember. Physically I was decrepit, constantly sick and eternally weary, unable to sleep and obliged to pitch camp overnight in the loo rather than trudge backwards and forwards from the bedroom five times between midnight and 7 a.m. I experienced a total loss of confidence and became convinced that it was madness to think we could cope with another child. My character was slipping away from me. Vague, suppressed memories of lying wanly on the sofa when 10 weeks pregnant with Martha assailed me, a time when I truly felt that parenthood was not for me. But I couldn't remember being afflicted with such an overwhelming sense of blackness. Worst of all was the isolation. Even though I was excited to be travelling I also felt that I was somehow running away from my real life. My jet-lagged body-clock gave up trying to work out which end was up, and gave me morning sickness 24 hours a day for a month.

> 6 MARCH 1992: yet again up at 6 in the morning, while everyone else carries on sleeping. As usual I feel queasy, and as usual I'll spend the next half an hour deciding on what to eat as I get Martha's toast. Whatever I have I know will make me feel bloated, although it will briefly banish the sick-feeling. I hate these early mornings. I feel resentful that it's me not Greg who's sitting here watching *Sesame Street* on the video. I just have to keep convincing myself that once the nausea goes I'll feel less miserable.

That one's physical condition is likely to have an effect on one's mental condition is undeniable, and in retrospect I think that the despondency was partly caused by worry. The day before we were due to leave England I started spotting dark, rusty blood. There was just enough to stain my pants and it was accompanied by gentle lower back pain. Despite my ambivalence about having another child, I desperately didn't want to miscarry. Sporadic visions of haemorrhaging on a Qantas flight over Malaysia shattered my faith in the pregnancy.

## Early Warning Signs

The most common physical signs of miscarriage are bleeding, discharge and spotting, and low abdominal pain like period cramps and backache. The most common mental signs are a sense of unease and just not feeling pregnant any more. Estimates of the number of women who experience bleeding or spotting in pregnancy without ill-effect vary between 10 and 15 per cent. Caroline spotted at about eight weeks in her first and fourth pregnancies without problem. And Sharon had dark brown discharge at about 10 weeks, which she took as a sign that she was threatening to miscarry again. Nothing else happened and the doctor could give no reason for the discharge at the time: she later learned that this sort of spotting was common with multiple pregnancies.

When I saw the blood, I immediately phoned Becky Reed, one of my midwives. She said that if I really wanted to take some action I could rest, but confirmed that if my body was going to expel the fetus then expel it it would. Recognising my distress, she suggested doing another home test in a week's time. If I had miscarried, my hormones would have settled down and the test would be negative; if it was positive then I was still pregnant.

There is nothing distinctive to see in an early miscarriage, it's just like a heavy period. This makes it extremely hard to come to terms with. Not knowing, being powerless to influence events, led me to strike bargains with myself. Up to this point I'd actively been following a healthy diet. So now I punished myself for taking too much for granted by eating foods previously designated *non grata*, such as chips, biscuits, chocolate and coffee. The rationale was that if I stopped taking care of my body then Sod's Law would ensure that I was still pregnant. What's more, in my twisted rationalisations I could then feel guilty about having bombarded the baby with additives and refined sugar. Psychologically I was trading outrage about not being *able* to control my body for guilt about having *chosen* not to control my body.

For the next three weeks I clocked every physical symptom as proof of pregnancy or miscarriage. I had lower back pain on and off, slight cramping, was convinced that my breasts had shrunk back to their pre-pregnant size, and didn't feel nauseous. On the other hand, blowing my nose when I was 9 weeks pregnant and bursting a blood vessel was a good sign, as the extra blood pregnant women have to pump around makes this a frequent complaint. Fainting is also common, so I interpreted my dizziness as another good sign.

Usually a woman threatening to miscarry is checked by an ultrasound scan, since in borderline cases an internal examination could trigger off a miscarriage. Despite this risk, at 12 weeks I felt I had to have confirmation that I was still pregnant, so visited a doctor in Melbourne. She assured me that my cervix was tightly closed and that the blood had not come from my uterus. She put forward two theories as to why I might be spotting: first, that over-enthusiastic sex had led to grazed vaginal blood vessels; second, that constipation had led to straining and bursting a few capillaries.

## Miscarriage

Since 1992, when the upper time limit was reduced by four weeks, miscarriage has been legally defined as 'the expulsion of a fetus from the womb before 24 weeks' gestation'. The change was partly initiated by the Stillbirth and Neonatal Death Society (SANDS) who – supported by the Miscarriage Association and the National Childbirth Trust – wrote to the Secretary of State for Health requesting that the legal definition of stillbirth be revised.

Technological advances in the care of premature babies were beginning to create potentially distressing anomalies. For example, a 26-week baby might survive with the help of a special care baby unit but if it lived for only a few hours it would have to be classified as a miscarriage. The baby would not be registered and would therefore not even have the right to a burial in a municipal cemetery. If only for consistency, the law had to be amended to take account of the shifting parameters of science so that babies were not lost in this modern-day limbo.

A conservative estimate is that between 10 and 30 per cent of pregnancies end in miscarriage in Britain per year – as against 645,835 live births in 2005[2] – of which the majority (60 per cent) occur during the first trimester. Medical science now divides women who miscarry into two groups: primary miscarriers, women who've never had a live birth; and secondary miscarriers, those who've had at least one successful live birth.

The NHS rarely investigates the reasons for miscarriage until a woman has suffered three in a row, and for many women not knowing *why* things went wrong has serious emotional consequences. Some people talk about feeling guilt – conscious and in retrospect subconscious – at their body's failure to hold on to the baby, despite overwhelming medical evidence that the majority of miscarriages occur because of an unavoidable natural process. Many women lose confidence in their ability to be pregnant at all.

There are three common identifiable reasons for a pregnancy failing to progress: a defective embryo or fetus, of which 98 per cent will abort before the end of the fourth month (60 per cent of fetuses with chromosomal abnormalities abort, as do 75 per cent of those with Down's syndrome and 95 per cent of those missing a sex chromosome); faulty implantation of fertilised ovum in the uterus, or other physical problems associated with the uterus or cervix; and hormonal deficiencies.

Even though most women are at least aware of these statistics, many still attribute their miscarriage to events within their control, and so speculation as to why it happened can haunt subsequent pregnancies. Hippocrates was advising women in the fifth century BC to avoid unnecessary 'psychic stress', and many people still cite overwork and stress as a contributing factor. Some women feel that illness in early pregnancy is responsible, and others castigate themselves for having exercised too vigorously. It would be unwise for a woman who has suffered a previous miscarriage or who has had bleeding or slight cramping to embark on a challenging sports programme in early pregnancy over and above her usual limits. But if fatigue is taken as a guide – since you could be depriving the growing fetus of oxygen if you overdo things – and respond to pain as a signal to slow down or even stop, exercise is essential for a healthy pregnancy. Women also attribute miscarriage to having taken drugs, whether prescribed or not. Clearly the body of a long-term addict of some biodegenerative drug is less likely to cope with the physical strain of pregnancy. At the other end of the scale some women blame readily available but contraindicated medication, such as flu antibiotics, anti-malarial drugs, anti-epilepsy drugs or soft drugs, such as nicotine, alcohol and marijuana. And they are possibly right. The truth is that doctors can rarely do more than speculate on the reason for a miscarriage.

## Feelings of Loss

Many women of course miscarry without even knowing they were pregnant, although perhaps with hindsight they may harbour suspicions. But the psychological trauma of those who miscarry in the first few months is often underestimated. Advice such as 'you can always have another one', or 'I expect there was something wrong so it's for the best', or 'but it wasn't really a baby yet, was it?' can be extremely hurtful to a woman who has lost her child. And, if the miscarriage happens when she still feels uncertain about motherhood, the woman's sense of guilt can be reinforced, as if the thought had become mother to the deed. As one woman put it:

> I know it is better to lose an abnormal baby – but the loss coincides with the ambivalent feelings you have at the start of the pregnancy. Half-feeling it was a bad idea – even if the pregnancy was planned – just makes you feel guilty when you do miscarry.

Sharon's first reaction to her positive pregnancy test was to hedge her bets. Having lost a baby before, she suppressed her excitement and mentally prepared herself for loss by focusing on those elements of pregnancy and parenthood that she was least happy with.

> Oh God, am I going to have another miscarriage, do I really want this baby, how would I cope with a baby, do I really have to go through childbirth?

Sasha was unlucky enough to suffer two early miscarriages before successfully conceiving Freddy. In common with many women, she had read that most miscarriages happen in the first 12 weeks, so they hadn't told anyone that she was pregnant first time round. At the same time, she hadn't expected anything to go wrong: 'Having gone through the pregnancy barrier I thought everything was going to be OK.'

At 8 weeks she developed backache one night, then the next morning there was a little old blood, which was followed by new, bright red bleeding. Her GP sent her to the hospital where she was given a scan. They found a heartbeat, but told her that she was threatening to miscarry and that it might become inevitable whatever she did. In their opinion, there was no more than a 50 per cent chance that the fetus would stay put. The bleeding continued, and her baby miscarried.

> I really felt the world had come to an end. In eight weeks my attitude had changed so much that it really, really mattered. I was devastated, and although Lou and friends were supportive, I don't think anyone understood.

Doctors and midwives often advise waiting for at least one month after a miscarriage before trying to conceive again. Physically, it is important that no traces remain of the previous pregnancy. Jenny, for example, had an unexplained miscarriage at about 8 weeks, and had to have a dilation and curettage (colloquially known as a D & C, opening the cervix and scraping the inner walls of the womb). She successfully conceived three months later.

Leaving a time period between pregnancies helps to avoid associating the two too closely. Trying for another baby immediately can also lead to the feeling that you are trying to replace the miscarried fetus rather than allowing the new baby to exist in its own right. Sasha and Lou heeded this advice. They cleaned out, stopped smoking and Sasha started taking special pregnancy vitamin pills. Three months later she conceived. But she never recaptured the same sense of excitement and was haunted by a feeling that failure was inevitable. When she again miscarried at about 8 weeks she started to worry that there was something wrong with her. (Lou, who already had two teenage children, seemed to be in the clear.) They even had blood tests to see if there was some sort of incompatibility between them: 'I felt utterly pessimistic, a terrible sense of disappointment and anger and loss of confidence.'

After waiting another three months, Sasha and Lou suffered a six-month wait before conceiving Freddy. The worry that she was jinxed never lifted even when she made it through the 8-week barrier. 'Every time I went to the loo I thought I was going to be bleeding, every time for nine months . . .'

Many women feel that meeting others who've miscarried then gone on to have healthy pregnancies greatly boosted their confidence.

When I was pregnant again I went to NCT. It was a huge relief to find that three other women there had had miscarriages too, and one of them had had a child since. Now I could talk about it, but it was a bit late in a way. We all felt that we should have been given more help at the time. Apart from my husband, there wasn't anyone I could talk to and the doctor kept saying that there was no reason why it wouldn't be all right next time, but since she couldn't tell me why it had happened in the first place, that wasn't really very comforting.

## VDUs

The scientific consensus now is that the very low levels of radiation emitted by VDUs are not dangerous to expectant mothers. Nonetheless, all users, pregnant or not, should avoid working for more than 50 minutes without a break anyway, and should take that break away from the screen.

## Listeria

Caroline had a 6-week miscarriage between her third and fourth pregnancies. Since she had eaten virtually nothing but pâté, with hindsight she is convinced that it was listeriosis that lost her the baby.

The *listeria monocytogenes* bacteria first came to public attention in 1988. Diagnosed by a blood test or urine analysis, it can be treated with antibiotics and, except in severe cases, is not usually serious in healthy adults and children. But suspicions arose that miscarriage or stillbirth could result if pregnant women ate contaminated food, and by 1990 the British Department of Health was advising all women in the first trimester of pregnancy not to eat chilled pre-cooked foods (particularly chicken) unless piping hot, even if supplied by reputable supermarkets and eaten before the expiry date. Soft cheeses such as Brie and Camembert were also to be avoided (especially if made from unpasteurised milk), as were blue cheeses and products made from goats' or ewes' milk. (Cottage cheese is not a carrier of listeria.) In tests, prepared salads, salamis, pork sausages, meat pies, pre-cooked poultry and other prepared foods such as pizza had all shown high levels of the bacteria. Raw eggs were to be avoided at all costs and yolks should always be hard not runny.

Alarmed women – particularly those who'd been living on prepared salads, Brie and pâté – scoured pregnancy books for descriptions of the characteristics of listeria infection. Few books published before 1990 even mention it. The British Medical Association's *Complete Family Health Encyclopedia* published in 1990 has the following entry:

> The only symptoms in most affected adults are fever and generalised aches and pains. There may also be sore throat, conjunctivitis, diarrhoea and abdominal pain. Listeriosis can be life-threatening, particularly in the elderly, in people whose immune system is suppressed, in pregnant women and in the newborn. An unborn child that is infected through its mother's blood may be stillborn. Listeriosis may be a cause of recurrent miscarriages.[3]

It was a peculiarly British obsession and one that, for the most part, was shortlived. There were only 108 reported cases of listeria in 1992, of which 25 were pregnancy-related and led to three miscarriages, yet almost every woman I interviewed was worried about listeria. Now most of the advice – such as heating pre-cooked meals thoroughly, avoiding pâté and 'mouldy', cheeses, such as Camembert, not eating food that has passed its sell-by date, washing all vegetables and fruit thoroughly – has passed into general good health advice. If you are worried about listeria in particular, though, do talk to your GP or midwife.

## Toxoplasmosis

With the increasing problems of food contamination, it was not only listeria that ruled out certain foods for pregnant women. Toxoplasmosis first came to public attention in Britain in 1989, through a series of television documentaries and features. Caused by the organism *toxoplasma gondii*, which may live in uncooked meat and in the intestines of cats and dogs and is excreted in their faeces, toxoplasmosis usually produces no ill-effects except in those suffering an immuno-deficiency disorder such as AIDS or when transmitted by a pregnant woman to her unborn child at about the time of conception or during the formation of the internal organs (organogenesis). It may also cause miscarriage and stillbirth.

Of the 0.2 per cent of pregnant women who do contract toxoplasmosis in the first trimester, only 15 per cent are likely to pass it on to the embryo or fetus. If the infection is caught in the second trimester, the risk of a baby being infected is 25 per cent, and the risk of transmission in the third trimester is 65 per cent.[4] The point at which the woman becomes infected makes a great deal of difference to the outcome. Severe disease – enlargement of the liver or spleen, hydro-cephalus, blindness and neurological damage – occurred in 14 per cent of first trimester cases: no one suffered such devas-tating consequences when the disease was contracted during the last trimester. Women looking for guidance in non-specialist British and American pregnancy handbooks published before 1990 were unlikely to find any reference to toxoplasmosis whatsoever. Now all pregnant women are advised by their health clinics, GPs and midwives to avoid handling cat litter trays, to ensure that hands are thoroughly washed after playing with cats and kittens, and to ensure that all meats – especially lamb and pork – are cooked prop-erly and not stored raw alongside cooked meats. (An esti-mated 25 per cent of pork and 15 per cent of lamb eaten by humans contains toxoplasma organisms, and most human infection comes from eating undercooked meat.)

Although there are no more than about 700 to 800 cases a year in the UK leading to recognised illness or effects on the fetus, infection worldwide is extremely common and in many other European countries such as France all pregnant women are routinely screened. There are often no physical symptoms. For those who do exhibit outward signs – a feverish illness, retinitis (inflammation of the retina), choroiditis (inflammation of the blood vessels behind the retina), vague abdominal pains and swollen lymph glands in 10 to 20 per cent of cases – the diagnosis can be confirmed by a blood test and the sufferer treated with anti-malarial drugs, such as pyrimethamine combined with a sulphonamide drug. Most women I talked to did reluctantly take the toxoplasmosis warnings to heart, even if they had ignored advice about liver, listeria, alcohol and nicotine. It seems at this time that there's virtually nothing you can do or eat that's not potentially dangerous. As one woman put it,

> It's pressure that you can determine your baby's health, just like that, but there are lots of things that can go wrong and they're not necessarily the woman's fault. It's just one more thing to worry about, one more thing to feel guilty about.

### Eating for a Healthy Baby?

For all sorts of reasons most women I interviewed tried not to have caffeine. Excessive caffeine can lead to high blood pressure, insomnia, irritability and headaches, but most women were more concerned that it would have the same effect on the baby as on them – make it over-lively! Some cut down their regular intakes to levels suggested in pregnancy handbooks: no more than three caffeinated drinks a day. Others took to drinking decaffeinated coffee and tea, and several cut out coffee and tea altogether, one because she had read that the tannic acid in tea drunk with a meal could render the iron in the food unabsorbable. Some even banned all refined sugars, additives and foods that had little or no nutritional value. Others felt that altogether too much fuss was being made, and that so long as they ate sensibly – protein, carbohydrate, fibre, fluid, vitamins, minerals, calcium, iron, folic acid, salt – then it wouldn't matter if they had digestive biscuits, crisps and croissants too.

Despite feeling obliged to take the advice seriously, many women felt resentful at the intrusion into their pregnancy. Not only did it stir up anxiety about problems that affected a tiny proportion of pregnant women, but the awareness that the medical establishment could in any case be working on a false premise meant that so-called expert advice seemed more like scaremongering. Several women commented that lack of firm knowledge meant that the advisory leaflets given out routinely by many antenatal clinics and doctors' surgeries were often childish or vague. In one leaflet the advice was:

> There are certain precautions women should take during pregnancy, for instance avoiding certain foods and being careful about contact with animals.

Whether the leaflet is referring to live or dead animals is not altogether clear . . . And they were often contradictory: in one you would be advised to eat a healthy diet of poultry, cheese and salads; in another to avoid poultry, certain sorts of pre-prepared cheese and certain – unspecified – pre-packaged salads.

In the end, most women felt that the information provided served little purpose other than to alarm, as Lisa commented:

> I was given all those leaflets and I did read them, and sort of vaguely took them in, but I sort of forgot about them as well. I remember coming out of one antenatal and I was absolutely ravenous, so I went and got a

smoked salmon and cream cheese bagel. I was munching away and had almost finished the whole thing when I suddenly thought . . . aagh . . . cream cheese. But actually I realise now that cream cheese was OK, and there was a certain amount of confusion anyway.

## Weight

For many of us, of course, what we eat during pregnancy is influenced by something altogether more personal. In the weight-obsessed West, most women – and increasing numbers of men – have an uncomfortable relationship with food. Weight Watchers has nearly one million members in the UK. Severe eating disorders such as anorexia and bulimia affect children as young as eight while the diet industry continues to grow. Despite this, we are all apparently getting fatter: according to the latest government figures, more than half the British population is overweight, with 23 per cent of women and 22 of men clinically obese.

From superwaif child-models on catwalks to the pages of all the glossy magazines, girls are taught that thin is desirable. It is a hard lesson to unlearn and even at this early stage of pregnancy, it was something that preoccupied several of the women I interviewed. Tessa, for example, had hoped that being pregnant would change how she thought about herself. It didn't:

My attitude to weight has always been fairly stupid, because I've always been about the same weight – give or take half a stone – and I'm probably thinner now than I've ever been. But for the first 16 weeks I immediately thought 'I'm an ugly fat blob', mostly because my bosoms were so big. So that wonderful feeling of losing them again after your period has started, when you feel normal again . . . well they just kept blowing up. I felt so distorted, because I'm so short.

And Sue, at 10 weeks pregnant, wrote in her diary about how her dissatisfaction with her appearance was making her miserable.

I went out looking for a dress or a suit for our wedding and got really depressed. It's quite a problem because I don't know what to wear. I don't want to wear bridal stuff – that would look stupid and ridiculous – but I do want to look good. The other problem is that I don't really want to look pregnant or, even worse, fat. I'm getting to the stage where my waist is going and my belly is bigger. It doesn't make me look pregnant yet, but I don't look my best. I look as if I have about half a stone to lose, and it's not fair because I haven't even put on any weight yet – I'm too sick to eat most of the time.

## Not Feeling As You'd Expected

It seems as if the presence or lack of problems is, to a degree, less important than how one feels about oneself. Lee is convinced that her positive state of mind ensured that she felt extremely well throughout her pregnancy. Pam also thinks that it was a question of mind over matter.

I didn't feel pregnant at all other than the bulge growing. It worried me that I was avoiding feeling. I've never used illness to get attention, and I knew that I wasn't feeling the normal things of pregnancy because I didn't let them get in.

If one's expectations are not being met, either for better or worse, that in itself can be undermining. Debra yearned for the physical signs of pregnancy so as to have something concrete to focus on.

> You hope that you will feel something as well. I wasn't ever sick, I just felt a bit funny for three months. But I was tired, almost more emotionally than physically. I felt more worried and apprehensive then – it seemed like it was very soon that it was going to happen and I hadn't done anything or thought about it, and Hugo didn't know anything about it either. I kept saying, 'why aren't you making plans, doing something?'

Sarah had sailed through her first pregnancy, so her shock at feeling so bad the second time round cast a shadow over the early part of the pregnancy.

> I think that my physical condition meant that it took a long time for me to mentally come to terms with being pregnant again. As well as feeling ill, I was pretty miserable (and miserable company) for most of the first 16 weeks.

Sue was surprised at how emotionally vulnerable her physical state made her feel, writing in her diary:

> I'm fed up these days now I seem to spend all my time either falling asleep or being sick. I'm now nine weeks pregnant – not very much at all – but I can't stand the thought of another 31 weeks of this. If only the sickness would stop I might be able to cope with the tiredness.

## Physical Changes

As well as my worries about miscarriage, I felt much worse than I'd expected with Felix. On top of the tiredness, nausea and painful breasts, I started to look yellow around the lips (as if nicotine stained), suffered shooting pains behind my eyes, developed a permanently blocked nose with a corresponding sniff to match and tingling, restless legs. Since most of these debilitations hadn't started until at least 28 weeks with Martha, I felt cheated and hard done by. By this time I was also convinced that everyone around me thought I was malingering anyway. In week 10 I even got heartburn, which all the books list as a 'later in pregnancy' problem.

Almost everyone interviewed needed to pee more often since the baby is so low down at this stage. Once it moves up, it should stop using your bladder as a trampoline, but several women – Joanne, Debbie, Tessa, me – all complained that these first 12 weeks established the pattern for the entire pregnancy. And once the uterine muscles have been stretched by childbirth, many women find that they need to urinate more frequently ever afterwards. Stress incontinence – where women leak a small amount of urine whenever they laugh, cry, sneeze, play sport – actually affects a third of all women who have given birth: as Tessa put it, 'when I cough I wee'. The only sensible remedy is regularly doing pelvic floor exercises – tightening and relaxing the pelvic muscles – during and after pregnancy.

Constipation also affected most women at some point or another during their pregnancy. The bowel starts to work even less quickly from about week 11 and food passes more slowly through the digestive system. Those who were prescribed iron supplements found their constipation increased: some persevered with the tablets, others stopped, and most commented that they would have appreciated their doctors telling them that constipation, along with queasiness and one's faeces going black, were 'normal' side-effects.

In these fibre-conscious days, most people know that high-fibre diets will help the bowel to work efficiently and that refined sugars will help to clog it up. But in extreme cases, squatting daily, massaging your abdomen or consulting a homoeopath about prescribed remedies, such as nux vomica 6X three times daily for up to a week, might succeed where bran breakfast cereals and bananas have failed. Floradix, available from whole-food shops and some chemists in liquid or tablet form, is a natural dietary food supplement with iron, vitamins, yeast and herb extracts which can help boost a flagging haemoglobin count. And it doesn't have the same unpleasant side-effects as synthetic iron supplements.

Heavy vaginal discharge is common. This is one way in which your body prevents infection travelling up your vagina to your womb. Headache sufferers often find that pregnancy increases the number and severity of attacks. Sharon, for example, was so desperate that she went to her GP, who prescribed paracetamol:

> I thought, 'Two paracetamol are not going to do an awful lot of harm'. I allowed myself two a day, because the headaches were so, so painful.

Nicki and Eve noticed a funny, metallic taste in their mouths during the first trimester, and slightly bad breath; I brushed my teeth several times a day in an effort to feel more comfortable. Hair can transform from greasy to dry, wavy to straight, or even fall out. Lynne's hair grew long and lusciously during her pregnancy, as did Fran's. But in the end, however well a woman knows her own body, it is impossible to assess exactly how it will react physically to being pregnant.

**The Baby**

But what of the baby? At the end of the eighth week the embryo becomes a fetus. It weighs about as much as a teaspoonful of sugar and is very vulnerable. This is the very worst time to get German measles because the ears and the eyes are forming: it can also cause congenital heart disease. In the worldwide rubella epidemic of 1964, over 20,000 children were born with serious birth defects, and since 1969 rubella vaccines, with a success rate of 95 per cent, have been available. The natural disease has an almost permanent protective effect against recurrence. In Britain children are offered the MMR vaccine (measles, mumps and rubella) at around 13 months of age then again at the age of three.

A blood test before pregnancy will confirm rubella immunity, but if you do need to be vaccinated then it is very important that you don't conceive for the following three months. Figures released by the Department of Health in 2005 showed that 81.7 per cent of UK children were having their first dose of the MMR. However, the World Health Organisation says that more than 90-per-cent coverage will be needed before congenital infection due to rubella during pregnancy becomes a thing of the past.

By the end of week 9 the now-lively fetus will be about the size of a paper-clip – about 1.25 in (3 cm) – and by week 10 (2 in long), the umbilical cord will have formed, although there is still no placenta. The fetus will have doubled its body weight and developed webbed fingers and toes. By week 11 the fetus is recognisable as a human being: its eyes are completely formed, it is now 2.25 in long (5.5 cm) – about the size of a Yale key – and it weighs just over a quarter of an ounce (10g). Tooth buds are forming and the vocal cords are beginning to develop.

Also at this stage the fetus begins to pass urine into the amniotic fluid (enriched salt water) which fills the space around it in the womb. Nutrients are absorbed through the fetus's skin, which is only a few cells thick. The last week of the first trimester – week 12 – takes the fetus to 3 inches (7.5 cm) and a staggering five-eighths of an ounce (18g). Your baby has a face, it becomes stronger as its muscles develop, and its sex is starting to become evident as the external genital organs grow.

The period of organogenesis – when the fundamental forming of all the internal organs takes place – is over and from now on major congenital catastrophes, other than those brought about by environmental hazards and prematurity, should not be able to occur.

Women need to ensure that they are physically able to cope with the demands of pregnancy. But to what extent should they sacrifice their personal desires for the assumed good of their unborn child? Often the needs of both parties can be met together: a healthy diet will provide the mother with an appropriate level of energy to nurture herself and the baby. But sometimes the frontiers of responsibility become blurred if a woman's psychological strength is supported by things potentially harmful to the baby.

**No Smoking!**

For the healthiest possible pregnancy most midwives and doctors will advise women to give up smoking. Smoking-related disease, including lung cancer, is the biggest single killer in Britain each year. The anti-smoking lobby won a substantial victory when in August 1992 the British Medical Association and the Department of Health agreed to classify smoking as a cause of death. This meant that doctors could put smoking on a death certificate without recourse to a coroner. It will also mean that more accurate figures for death due to smoking should be able to be compiled.

In the past few years, a consensus has been reached about smoking. Don't do it if you're expecting a baby. Tobacco companies, by law, now have to state the dangers, all official pregnancy advice recommends not smoking. The grim figures are these: babies of smokers are, on average, 200–250g lighter at birth; there is a third greater risk of stillbirth and perinatal death and a 25 per cent higher chance of miscarriage.[5]

The Back to Sleep Campaign was launched in 1992 and has been extremely successful in reducing the rate of cot death in Britain. Babies of smokers are not only twice as likely to be born prematurely but are also three times more likely to succumb to sudden infant death syndrome (SIDS), as cot death is officially known.

The problems do not stop at birth. Babies of women who smoke are twice as likely to suffer from serious respiratory infections. Smoking during pregnancy can also increase the risk of asthma, and hospital admissions for asthma in children under four have more than doubled since 1979.[6] Professor Jean Golding, professor of paediatrics at Bristol University, believes that smoking during pregnancy is one of the factors causing this asthma epidemic.

> Our research shows that smoking in pregnancy has a major impact on the development of babies, making them more likely to suffer from wheeziness and to develop asthma.[7]

The chemicals absorbed from cigarette smoke directly limit fetal growth by reducing the number of cells produced in both the baby's body and brain. Nicotine makes blood vessels constrict, so reduces the blood supply to the placenta, interfering with the baby's nourishment. Some sources suggest that babies of smokers are more likely to have a cleft lip or palate as well as disorders of the limbs, genitals and urinary system. Babies are particularly vulnerable to smoking during the first three months of pregnancy, so if a woman can give up during this time, she will have a better chance of producing a healthy child. Cutting down does not seem to have the same beneficial effect.

Studies show that, if you give up during the first three months of pregnancy, your risk of placenta problems, such as placenta praevia, goes down significantly and so does your risk of stillbirth and having a low-birthweight baby. Stopping smoking also lowers your baby's chances of being ill after the birth: in one study, only 8.8 per cent of babies whose mothers had stopped smoking in pregnancy needed hospital attention during the first month of life compared with 11.4 per cent of babies whose mothers had carried on smoking.

In 2000, 35 per cent of women smoked before becoming pregnant and 20 per cent continued to smoke throughout their pregnancy. Of pregnant women who stopped smoking, 20 per cent gave up before conceiving, 73 per cent gave up once their pregnancies were confirmed and seven per cent gave up later in pregnancy.[8] All the women I interviewed who continued to smoke did feel guilty about the effect it might be having, but at the same time they protested, like Pam, that cigarettes were part of their characters, emotional supports that they were unwilling to forgo. Pam found that even though the midwives and doctors didn't actually tell her to stop, peer group pressure was persistent. She was smoking no more than five cigarettes a day, but friends considered they had the right to express their disapproval. Because Pam was 41 and it was her first pregnancy, she felt the unspoken comment 'at your age' lay behind the criticism.

That outsiders have no right to criticise a woman's choices

for her own body, regardless of whether it is harbouring a baby or not, was undisputed by those who continued to smoke. The arguments are less straightforward when a partner – who will also be assuming parental responsibility after the birth – objects. Pam's partner Gérard was particularly vocal on the subject of her giving up:

> I kept maintaining, 'The more you go on at me the less I am likely to do it', which was stupid because I knew I should do it. 'But in retaliation for you trying to dictate to me what I should and shouldn't do, I'm going to do what I want.'

Rachel was desperately worried during her entire pregnancy. Doctors asked her if she knew the dangers of smoking: when she replied 'yes', they left it at that.

> The desire to smoke was almost overwhelming. It was as if I was masochistically torturing myself. I worried terribly. It was bonkers looking back on it; I can't really believe I did it. But in all honesty although I lied to the doctor and to everyone else around me at the time, I probably smoked in excess of 20 a day.

Caroline continued to smoke about ten a day during her first pregnancy, the only advice she received being that smoking was 'bad for baby' and that it could lead to low birthweight. Her first child, Emma, weighed 7lb 12oz at birth so she didn't take the warnings very seriously after that. She maintains that her smoking increased over her four pregnancies, as did the weight of her babies. Tessa and Jane cut down to the odd puff in the evening. Some women, like Sharon, are helped by their bodies making the decision for them.

It was the same with drink. I didn't make a conscious decision to stop drinking, but drink just made me feel ill. Coffee I couldn't drink any more, it made me feel ill, and tea I don't drink anyway. I lived on milkshakes, strawberry milkshakes.

Sue – writing in her diary – found her body dictating to her.

Had to go to the doctor this morning to get the result of the hospital test. It was positive, so now there is no doubt. The next three months are going to be vital. I have already given up smoking and now I'm cutting out alcohol. Luckily, it has all been quite easy because I feel so rotten that I don't feel like smoking or drinking.

## No Drinking!

Continuing to do something potentially harmful to your child and choosing to do something that will not do it good are different issues. Medical opinion is unanimous that smoking when pregnant is potentially dangerous, but experts cannot agree on whether or not there are safe levels of alcohol. Does a limited amount do any harm, or does it simply not do any good? At the top end of the scale there is little medical doubt that children born to alcoholics are likely to suffer a range of mental and physical abnormalities.

Dr Ann Striessgarth, a leading researcher into fetal alcohol syndrome (FAS) at the University of Washington, has listed the main risks as being mental retardation, retarded growth, abnormalities of the central nervous system, malformations and death *in utero*.

A study in Dundee of nearly 1000 first-time pregnancies suggested that babies of pregnant women who drank less than 100g of alcohol a week (equivalent to about ten standard drinks) would suffer no ill-effects. And although many hand-books written by medical practitioners recommend complete avoidance – since some of the alcohol from every drink reaches the baby's bloodstream – they also recognise that there is no conclusive evidence that an occasional drink does any harm to an unborn baby. 'Safe' estimates vary from one or two drinks once or twice a week to no more than one unit a day, usually with the caveat that if possible all alcohol consumption be avoided in the first trimester, the crucial development time for the fetus.

Certainly in the UK attitudes to alcohol in pregnancy are more liberal than in the USA where any drinking at all in pregnancy is frowned on. And in September 1996 a study of 15,000 pregnant women conducted by Professor Jean Golding at Bristol University actually came up with surprising results.

> We found a U-shaped curve where women who had
> never drunk alcohol during pregnancy were more likely
> to have a low birth weight baby than those who drank
> occasionally.[9]

Those women who had cleaned out in order to conceive did not drink at all; many others stopped as soon as they knew they were pregnant, feeling that seven or eight months of abstinence was not too much to commit themselves to. Lisa found herself irritated by what she saw as the excessively purist approach to pregnancy. She was confident that the odd drink or joint would be harmless so, although she rarely drank or smoked anyway, she didn't attempt to stop during the early weeks. It was only later in the pregnancy that she realised that part of her confidence had come from ignorance.

> I was very anti about reading anything or doing anything
> about it until I was ready to. I was quite stubborn, and

there were periods when I read pregnancy books and
other periods when I didn't read anything at all. At the
beginning I wasn't very curious.

Several women who had gone off the smell – let alone the
taste – of alcohol in the first 12 weeks did allow themselves
the occasional watered-down glass of wine after that point,
particularly those who had already had one successful pregnancy. For Fran the smell of lager (and curry) during her first
pregnancy had been enough to send her hurtling from the
room. Carrying Rowan, she found she needed a drink after
a hard day's teaching. Paradoxically, she became almost
addicted to lager:

> There was the feeling at the back of my mind that I was
> doing something wrong, particularly with Rowan when
> I was drinking alcohol. While I needed my glass of wine
> in the evening, I also thought 'Oh my God, I could be
> damaging her.'

Sarah had felt a little guilty about drinking red wine during
her first pregnancy, but was more confident about making
her own decisions second time round: 'I'd read enough to
know what sorts of levels of drinking would be harmful, plus
having done it once you feel well, Kirsty was all right, so . . .'

## Other Drugs

Drugs were a bigger issue, in that advice varied from place
to place as to what level of basic over-the-counter drugs such
as paracetamol or Lemsip were safe for the fetus. Some doctors
and midwives consider limited standard pain relievers safe,
others advise avoiding all medication. Paracetamol is considered safe at the usual recommended dosage, but aspirin is

now considered unsafe during pregnancy (unless prescribed
by a doctor) due to the effects it has on your blood circula-
tion. Again, some doctors and midwives suggest Gaviscon to
cope with indigestion and heartburn, while others say that all
but natural remedies (such as milk) should be shunned. The
safest rule of thumb is to go easy on any drug in the first 12
weeks, however innocuous it seems, and ask your doctor or
midwife for help if in doubt.

Several women confessed that they were interested in
knowing if having smoked marijuana or grass once they were
pregnant was likely to have any ill-effect on the baby. Most
felt awkward asking their GPs, and found that many books
only discussed so-called 'social drugs' in general terms of
disapprobation and that medical – not moral – advice was
hard to come by. There is no research to show that moderate
– as opposed to chronic or constant daily – smoking of marijuana will cause fetal malformation, although there is obviously a risk to the baby from tobacco, if used. The chemicals
in marijuana and grass have not been thoroughly tested, so
it's probably sensible to cut down as much as possible but
not worry unduly about that odd Saturday-night puff before
you knew you were pregnant.

With hard drugs – cocaine, crack, heroin, Ecstasy – the
amount and the point in the pregnancy at which the drugs
were taken will make the crucial difference as to the effect,
if any, on the baby. Always contact a doctor or midwife if
worried – they are bound to keep your confidence.

A couple of women were unlucky enough to have taken
contraindicated medication in the weeks before their un-
intentional pregnancies had been confirmed. Research
suggests that women who have inadvertently taken the pill
have a slightly increased risk of complications such as ectopic
pregnancy. Jenny, who did not discover she was pregnant
until week 12, continued taking the mini-pill throughout that

time. When she asked the doctor if this might have been dangerous for the fetus, he simply replied that she shouldn't worry about it. Her son James was fine.

Caroline had taken strong antibiotics for flu during the early weeks of her fourth pregnancy.

> I was annoyed because all the books said you shouldn't have antibiotics and stuff like that when you were pregnant, that it could cause birth defects. But when at first I said I was worried they simply said I shouldn't worry. They were good in the end, though, and gave me my scan early so I could see the baby was all there. I think it was because I'd got three children already and they didn't think I was the type to make a fuss over nothing.

Lisa had been taking a strong Chinese herbal medicine which is specifically listed as off-limits during pregnancy. The herbalist tried to be reassuring, but as it had been made so clear in the first place that it was never to be taken in pregnancy, she couldn't help feeling anxious. It was also frustrating not to be able to do anything about it. However careful she was for the rest of the pregnancy, damage might have been done in the deciding few weeks.

> I did what I could do, which was stop taking it. I wasn't so worried that I thought I should contemplate abortion or anything. It's more later in the pregnancy when I looked back.

After Harry was born, Lisa's midwife commented that she had rarely seen such a healthy – or large – placenta!

As with most things during pregnancy, it is a case of balance. If self-denial will be more undermining than the worry about the effects on your baby of drinking, smoking, whatever, then you should set limits that you are comfortable with. And if you are confident that the occasional drink will be fine, then go ahead. But if your subsequent self-reproach could outweigh the enjoyment of your glass of wine then plainly you are better off abstaining.

## Food, Glorious Food

But what of food itself? After all, there is a world of difference in not having non-essential things and in actively trying to influence things for the better. Leaving aside cravings and aversions, women were surprised by their appetites during pregnancy. Feeling sick, some expected not to want to eat at all yet found they were ravenous. Others just couldn't face anything. Firm decisions might well be taken about eating certain foods, but sometimes changing tastes mean that a healthy, balanced diet is hard to follow. And the pace of twenty-first-century life means that we don't always have the time to ensure that there are handfuls of dried fruit and nuts nesting in our office desk drawers rather than cheese and onion crisps.

Despite the pressure to eat for the baby more than for yourself, a good diet in pregnancy is sensible – though not essential – if only to meet the physical demands. The same is true of exercise. Our body is designed to move towards stability, with all its functions in balance. This process is known as homoeostasis and guides such complementary medical theories as the Alexander technique, where the aim is to rid the body of bad habits and restore it to a natural equilibrium. To this end, most pregnancy handbooks have comprehensive sections on what constitutes a healthy and balanced diet. A rough guide is: one third fruit and veg, one third starchy foods like bread and pasta, 12–15 per cent protein, 12–15 per cent dairy and five per cent food high in sugar, fat or salt.

Debbie was advised by her GP to have a daily intake of the four Fs – fruit, fibre, fluid, fowl – and to avoid meat from any four-footed animals. Caroline continued to eat no fruit and vegetables (except potatoes) and to have regular cups of coffee, because she wasn't prepared to force herself to eat things that she couldn't stand: 'I didn't eat anything that's good for you, that's for sure, and certainly nothing green.' Nicki, too, couldn't bear anything green although she did get vitamins from her favourite concoction: a baked potato with beetroot.

Like Debra, Lynne, Debbie and Joanne tried to have the right balance of foods every day.

> I just thought I've got to eat something, and it's got to be good. In one of the books I read it said you had to have some protein and some green vegetables and something this and something that every day, so I did that.

Several women were vegetarian, and although iron supplements were routinely offered in some places – for example Northern Ireland, Sussex, Hampshire, Glasgow, Manchester, certain parts of London – most found that it was the handbooks that tended to be more alarmist about a pregnant vegetarian's struggling iron levels than the obstetricians, who took more notice of the woman's general state of health than her haemoglobin level. As a vegetarian, who had an extremely low haemoglobin level towards the end of Martha's pregnancy, I did take special care to eat all the old favourites like spinach, nuts, dried apricots and bananas, the occasional drop of red wine and – the most enjoyable way of taking in extra iron – plain, dark chocolate. Another excellent source is liquorice, but I just couldn't quite bring myself to eat that . . .

Once this first 12-week trimester is over, most women have

adjusted to being pregnant and are able to enjoy their changing attitudes. With Felix my self-pity finally lifted at about 11 weeks when I felt a small hard lump at the bottom of my uterus as I lay in bed, as if I was balancing on a grapefruit. The baby was there, and as soon as I started to think of myself as pregnant rather than ill the excitement of the first couple of weeks came back and the nausea and everything else suddenly seemed less important. My physical symptoms didn't actually change much, but they no longer ruled me.

# A Safe Pair of Hands

## Weeks 12–16

Fast Forward to 1941. I was living in Seminary Hill, Virginia, a community near Washington, DC, with Clifford and Virginia Durr, to whose teeming household I was shortly to add yet another member. Virginia, herself the mother of four, insisted that I should go to the hospital for the birth of my second baby. I hated that idea – why not have it at home? Absolutely not, said Virginia. All one needs is a quantity of stout brown paper, boiling water, and a competent doctor, I pleaded – but to no avail. She chased me off to a highly touted, fashionable 'obstetrician', a word I'd never heard before. I soon had a dramatic falling-out with him.

Jessica Mitford, *The American Way of Birth*[1]

Much of the advice about lifestyle and diet will have come from official leaflets handed out by doctors and clinics. But emotional adjustment to the idea of being a mother can dominate to the exclusion of everything else at this stage, and many women cannot think about the practical details until the demanding psychological and physical changes have been assimilated. This can mean that a woman receives no ante-natal care until she is at least 12 weeks pregnant. Unless a woman has personal knowledge of the options available she must rely on professional advice, while also digesting local rumour and hearsay. Some make up their own minds about the sort of antenatal care and birth they would like, waiting until they are sure in their own minds before even approaching a doctor or midwife. But since the choices offered will largely depend on where you live and the opinions of the people with whom you come into contact, making a deci-sion in isolation can lead to disappointment.

## The Doctor Will See You Now

Many women, particularly those who have moved away from the area in which they grew up, don't have a local GP who can advise them and see them through their pregnancy. Finding a good GP is very much the luck of the draw. Some GPs and obstetricians are co-operative, well informed and flexible; others are obstructive and give inappropriate, even inaccurate, advice.

By the time I was six weeks pregnant with Martha, Greg and I still hadn't got round to registering ourselves with a local practice. We hadn't ever stayed long enough in one place in London to make it worth it. I simply asked a local woman with children which local female doctor she would recom-mend, and struck lucky.

Although most pregnancy handbooks say that the doctor will confirm your pregnancy at this first meeting, this isn't always the case. Of those interviewed, only women who specifically asked for a urine or blood test to confirm the pregnancy were actually given one. In all other cases – and to the surprise of many – GPs simply accepted the pregnancy as fact. As Sarah said, 'She basically took my word for it, as they seem to these days, and set the paperwork going.' Some found they were in and out in a matter of minutes, having been given a booking appointment for several weeks later; others were talked through the options available.

When we went along to register, I was still pretty astounded at being pregnant in the first place. I hadn't thought about antenatal care at all and certainly hadn't considered anything other than being clocked into the standard NHS system with a hospital birth at the end of it. I felt so insecure and so unconvinced of my own ability to carry a baby to term and give birth to it, that I would have moved into the hospital there and then if I had thought it would be safer!

Having taken Greg's and my full medical histories, and my gynaecological background, Dr Parker gave me general advice on healthy pregnancy care, handed out the leaflets and briefly outlined the available tests. She then ran through the relative pros and cons of the three hospitals servicing our area, explaining that I could have shared care with her practice and the hospital or have all my antenatal care at the hospital.

Next came a short discussion on the relative disadvantages and advantages of being booked into the hospital for the minimum of two days or the maximum of five. After a productive question-and-answer session, I felt able to make a choice about what would suit me best. I was then officially assigned to the system and a hospital booking appointment was arranged for six weeks later.

## Giving Birth in Hospital

Ninety-eight per cent of women in Britain give birth in hospital (99.6 per cent in NHS hospitals, 0.4 per cent in private ones)[2] and most feel reassured by the presence of the latest life-saving equipment. The sense of being part of a system can, in itself, be comforting, especially for those who still feel that pregnancy is the most peculiar thing they've ever done. The bureaucratic solidity of printed antenatal cards and a set hospital routine can reinforce the idea that women successfully have babies every day of the week, every week of every year. With Martha, I found that the smell of the hospital, the smell of it being normal, convinced me that everything was going to be all right.

In major cities there is often more than one hospital within a local health authority's catchment area, so a woman can choose which might suit her best. Jane had worked as a nurse, so was aware of the vagaries of the huge National Health Service system. Her sister had been delighted with the antenatal care she had been given, so Jane felt confident about choosing to give birth at the same hospital in west London. Ironically, while her sister had nothing but praise, Jane's experience was appalling.

Lynne was a part-time health visitor, so knew many of the people involved in antenatal services in her area. She was able to arrange to have Michelle at the hospital with which she worked, even though she and her husband lived outside its catchment area.

Sue didn't know exactly what sort of care she did want. But local gossip was that their nearest hospital in east London was incredibly busy, so she chose to go to St Bartholomew's instead. She was happy with the care she received, so went back for the birth of her second baby, Hannah.

Other mothers-to-be are simply booked into the hospital which serves their area. Debra went to her local medical centre when she was about 8 weeks pregnant. They made an appointment for a booking visit at her local hospital five weeks later.

They said 'unless you're really confident about being at home, since it's your first one we'd rather you came into hospital.' I must say I felt quite pleased that I didn't have to choose. Because a lot of people had been telling me things, and there seems to be quite a lot of – not pressure, exactly – but onus on active birth and non-medical intervention and everything. And as much as I'd like to think that I could do that, I'm glad that they said it would just be better if I was in hospital.

Tessa was confident about her pregnancy, but because her mother had had four miscarriages both of her parents were anxious. They offered to pay for antenatal care under the Harley Street gynaecologist who had delivered both Tessa and her brother, with delivery booked privately. Tessa did register with a local GP at the same time, thinking it would be sensible to have a local family doctor once Joe had been born. When Tessa told the GP what arrangements they had made for antenatal care, the doctor's response to hearing that she wouldn't be using the local hospital was: '"Jolly good, because it's crap." And I thought "Thank God for that!" Who wants to go somewhere if even the doctor thinks it's bad?'

Siân had her son Alexander in hospital after a speedy drug-free, stitch-free labour. She was pleased with the care she received and had felt able to give birth without unwanted intervention. So even though they had moved to another part of London in the interim, she happily opted for a second hospital birth with Katherine. They barely made it, the labour was so short, and again she had no drugs and no stitches: she nearly became one of those 0.1 per cent of women whose births are recorded under the heading 'elsewhere' . . .

Home birth never really appealed, to be honest. I couldn't be bothered with thinking about the mess.

There wasn't a room in the house where I thought I'd like to have a baby. I'd be worried about getting blood on the carpet in the front room; the back room is a bit uncomfortable because it's bare boards; any of the bedrooms upstairs there'd be the feeling that you'd have to have the curtains drawn unless you wanted the whole of the neighbourhood looking in. So there was just this feeling that I'd rather be able to go away and have the mess somewhere else, then come home as quickly as possible afterwards.

## Worries About Hospitals

The majority of the 630,000-odd women who give birth in hospitals in Britain each year are attended by caring, concerned and experienced professionals who have their well-being – as well as their baby's – at heart.

But a surprising number of women interviewed admitted to being intimidated by hospitals and doctors in general. Most women and their partners think that it is safer to give birth in hospital, particularly with one's first child. They want to have life-saving equipment on hand just in case anything goes wrong, and feel that if there are any problems during or after the birth, their child will be safer in hospital. The health service hierarchy is also persuasive in suggesting that a doctor or consultant obstetrician has a safer pair of hands than a midwife. In fact, 36 per cent of babies are now delivered by hospital doctors compared with 24 per cent in 1989–90.

Although most parents-to-be want the security and safety of the hospital – just in case – many women still worry that their wishes during labour will be overruled. The options for specialised institutions are declining. In June 2006, campaigners won a temporary reprieve for Stroud Maternity Hospital when it was threatened with closure after 53 years of providing maternity services to the women of Stroud in Gloucestershire. And with growing concerns over the shortage of NHS midwives, and falling confidence in the ability of the NHS to cope, some women suspect that they will be anonymous in a major hospital.

One hospital in Kent admitted that a midwife who had worked for them for a period of 13 months had AIDS. They set up an advice line for all mothers who had been attended by the midwife, whilst giving reassurances that only eight women were at even minimal risk. In September 2006, a national newspaper carried the story of Miriam Grice who was left alone for three hours after giving birth in a large maternity unit. In the end, she was forced to phone to ask her own mother to come and help her.

The trauma experienced by parents in these situations is incalculable. Unlikely though they are to stop women going into hospital to have their babies, incidents such as these obviously do affect the level of confidence people have about the care they might receive.

Even in hospitals with progressive reputations, hospital care can vary from visit to visit, depending on the opinions of the person who happens to be on duty that night. Lee knew she'd wanted to give birth to her first baby in hospital, and was happy to be booked into her local hospital in Nottingham. At the same time, she knew exactly what sort of birth she wanted to have. At her 14-week booking visit, Lee and her husband Simon explained to the senior midwife that they would like a water birth. The midwife was interested and supportive, despite having no first-hand experience. But the male obstetrician had strong, ill-informed, prejudices.

It was one of those mornings when you just know this one doctor is going to be a problem right from the beginning. You go in, you're lying there with your legs in the air, and some person breezes in, doesn't look at you, he's got his white coat on, goes straight to your notes and mutters '. . . er, it's Mrs . . .' So I said, 'Who are you, the milkman, you could be anybody.'

He rudely commented that his wife was a midwife and that he wouldn't 'let' her give birth at home, never mind have a water birth. Lee feels that it was only because she and Simon were so determined that they weren't beaten down.

## Giving Birth in Your Own Home

In theory every woman has a right to have her baby at home, whether it's her first, second or fifteenth. Sadly, some women interviewed who asked about home births first time round encountered such opposition that they abandoned the idea. They felt cajoled into having a hospital birth they did not want, but couldn't face the disapprobation of their doctors and the implication that they would be putting their baby's life at risk by not going into hospital. Few women want the stress of such disagreements during the early weeks of their pregnancy.

One woman, who was training to be a National Childbirth Trust teacher, decided she would like to have a home birth for her second baby. She had not enjoyed her first delivery in hospital, although it had all been straightforward, so she asked her GP for information. Because of her NCT training she was aware of the relative safety of home versus hospital birth. Her GP was not.

She said 'Do you really want to do that? It's terribly dangerous, you know.' She then told me about a woman who lived in the next street who, only the week before, had to be rushed off in the middle of the night because her home birth had gone wrong.

There are a few midwife-led hospital units and independent birth centres although the latter are increasingly threatened with closure as health services become more centralised. In some – technically all – areas, the NHS runs teams of community midwives who will happily attend home or hospital births. You stand a good chance of being accompanied in labour by women you know and who have overseen at least part of your antenatal care.

Attitudes towards home birth have been slowly changing since the publication of the government's *Changing Childbirth* in 1993. It supported what maternity campaigners and mothers had been saying for years – that women themselves should be able to choose their care, with the support and advice of health professionals.

Even so, it has been hard to shift some of the prejudices against home birth. The report makes it clear that

> GPs who feel unable to offer care or support to a woman who wishes to have a home birth should refer the woman directly to a midwife.[3]

Yet the figure for home birth stands at just over 2 per cent, only slightly higher than it was in the 1990s when I was first researching material for this book.[4]

In October 1996, a campaign was launched by the *Changing Childbirth* team and the National Childbirth Trust to help make women more aware of their choices. As the NCT's Head of Research, Mary Newburn, said:

> Our research shows many first-time mothers, especially, aren't aware of what questions to ask when discussing

maternity care and to find out about getting what they want. After the birth, they say 'if only' . . .[5]

Ten years on their work finally seems to be paying off and home birth rates are creeping up in some areas of the country: 5.8 per cent of women in Devon now give birth at home and 5.3 per cent of women in East Sussex.

## But Are Home Births Safe?

Until the 1930s some 85 per cent of women in Britain gave birth at home. Doctors were expensive, and usually called in only in an emergency. One woman, speaking on a BBC documentary in early 1993, *A Labour of Love*, remembered having to put £2 on the table outside the bedroom before the doctor would even come in. One child in six died before its first birthday, and maternal infection and death as a result of childbirth were still widespread.

The National Health Service Act of 1946 aimed to provide free, professional health care for all. More and more women started to go into hospital as a matter of course to give birth, where they were able to rest – usually for ten days – after their babies had been born rather than rush straight back to their domestic duties. Maternal and neonatal mortality figures started to drop.

Women with problem pregnancies plainly did need constant hospital monitoring, but NHS policy tended towards encouraging all women with straightforward pregnancies into hospital too. Pregnant women as a group came to be treated as patients and the Victorian concept of pregnancy as a sickness gained ground once more. By the 1950s, official NHS policy was that first births should be in hospital, with second and third births at home for women with straightforward pregnancies, then back to the hospital for fourth and subsequent deliveries. By 1965, 66 per cent of all births in Britain took place in hospital.

In 1970, when the rate for home births had dropped even further, to 13 per cent, a British government committee published the Peel Report, which stated that hospital beds must be provided for all women giving birth. Sheila Kitzinger thinks that the Report was one of the key factors in almost eliminating home births in Britain:

> This was accepted as the basis of policy without any evidence, and the maternity services were reorganised around that premise. The views of the women who were using the service were ignored.[6]

Today over half a million women die every year as a result of pregnancy or childbirth. However, 99 per cent of these deaths are in the developing world where, in some areas, childbirth is still the leading cause of death among women of childbearing age. But general levels of health, fertility, malnutrition and anaemia are hardly comparable to those in the West. In parts of sub-Saharan Africa a woman has a 1 in 16 lifetime chance of dying during pregnancy or as a result of pregnancy and childbirth. For a British woman the probability is 1 in 3,800. The quality of antenatal care in the developed world means that few serious problems should go undetected, and those that are discovered can be dealt with by an efficient referral system. (In the United States, the quality of care depends on the cheque book to a far greater degree.)

Current statistics suggest that planned home births are the safest of all. They have the lowest rate of perinatal mortality stillbirth or death within the first six days, 3.4 per cent per 1000 births as opposed to the national rate of 8.5 per cent.[7]

The Albany Midwifery Practice in Peckham, south-east London (formerly the South East London Midwifery Group

Practice), has a home-birth rate of 57 per cent, despite being situated in an area of high social deprivation and looking after an all-risk caseload of women generated by the local GPs. The midwives, who are based in a local health and leisure centre, provide continuity of care throughout pregnancy, birth and up to 28 days postnatally. About 70 per cent of the women they look after need no pain relief during labour, the caesarean section rate is 13.5 per cent – significantly lower than the national average of 23 per cent – and 79 per cent of mothers are still breastfeeding 28 days after birth compared with less than 50 per cent nationally.[8]

Arguments about where to give birth actually mask the real issue. Women want different sorts of things in labour. A highly-technological birth will be perfect for one person, whereas leaning over a beanbag in the sitting room will be right for another. Unless there are genuine medical complications, we should each be free to make our choices for each and every pregnancy.

Few of the women I interviewed had political motivations for wanting to give birth at home rather than in hospital. It was rather that they felt they would be more relaxed and confident in their own everyday environment. Many women were frightened by the idea of being transplanted to clinical, alien surroundings at the onset of labour, and were reluctant to submit themselves to somebody else's rules and regulations (such as restrictive visiting hours). Most thought that at home they were more likely to be able to control their own labours without being pressurised.

## Independent Midwives

In order to ensure that they were delivered by familiar faces, some women took themselves outside the system altogether and hired independent midwives. Women booked for a hospital delivery commented that they often saw different faces at every antenatal visit. They were unlikely to know the doctors or midwives in attendance at the birth, and sometimes felt that they knew nothing – or very little – about the progress of their pregnancy. I wrote this in my diary when I only suspected that I might be pregnant, before even missing a period.

> 18 JANUARY 1992: I want to have a relationship with midwives this time. I feel that someone who'd mothered me all the way through would care more and take more care. It would matter to them too if there was something wrong, we wouldn't just be a statistic. That's the issue.

NHS community midwives work in teams, and aim for a woman to have met every member of the team before she is due to go into labour. But teams vary in size, and there is obviously no guarantee that those with whom you have the closest relationship will be on duty when you call.

Pam knew that, as a 41-year-old first-time mother, the NHS would categorise her as high risk. She had never been in hospital in her life, and felt confident in electing to have the baby at home. Rather than fight the system, she hired independent midwives and arranged to have her scans at a private maternity hospital in London. Although extremely expensive, it had a good reputation for a non-interventionist approach to childbirth and for giving so-called 'high-risk' patients the right to choose the sort of labour they wanted.

Joanne also knew she didn't want to get embroiled in the system and couldn't see any reason not to have her first baby at home. She booked herself in for a home birth with local independent midwives, and although some friends did ask her whether it was wise – 'you don't know what it's going to be like' – she always felt it was the right decision for her.

Lisa hated hospitals, and put off entering the system. In a way she feels she was avoiding the issue as week by week she grew bigger and bigger. She was aware that her partner was worried about the idea of a home birth for a first baby, but gradually her confidence rubbed off on him. Finally, when she was approaching 30 weeks, she took the plunge and booked with independent midwives. Like Joanne, Lisa immediately knew that it was the only decision that would have suited her.

There are several teams of independent midwives operating in London. The fee is usually between £3000 and £3500, depending on an individual's situation, to cover all your antenatal care, delivery and postnatal services in your own home. Most have worked in the NHS, but enjoy having the freedom to offer truly woman-centred care that practising independently allows.

Since *Changing Childbirth* many of the principles of independent midwifery have been incorporated back into the NHS system. Ask your GP or ring the NCT to ask if there are any teams in your local area. Ironically, hand-in-glove with some of these improvements have come revisions to insurance requirements. One independent midwife, faced with an annual individual insurance bill of £7100, said she could barely afford to keep working . . .

## Doing It Differently Second/Third/Fourth Time Round

Most women who were happy with the delivery of their first child went through the same procedure the next time, whether they'd had their baby at home or in hospital. The births in hospital of Nick and then Hannah had been good experiences for Sue, but by the time she was pregnant with Lottie they had moved to another part of London. So rather than be booked into a new hospital, she decided to go for a home birth instead.

> I was attracted by the idea of being at home in an informal setting, with the kids just next door. And, to tell you the truth, I thought Max and I would have a good laugh. He'd seen two of his children delivered, and I reckoned he could deliver the third himself!

I was astounded that I wanted to give birth at home the second time round. With Martha I had had a highly managed induced hospital birth with an epidural, a fetal scalp monitor, drip, the lot . . . and enjoyed every minute of it. My care had been excellent, my wishes were respected, and even though the rather nervous midwife did muck up the suturing – I had to go back three months later to be recut and resewn – I didn't feel that things could have gone any better. The atmosphere in the postnatal ward was supportive, not to mention informative, and I had enjoyed almost every minute of my five-day hospital stay.

Broadly speaking I have always been – and still am – a supporter of hospitals, not to mention the technological advances of medicine and variety of pain relief available. More than that, I felt that the phrase 'natural childbirth' had been hijacked by the anti-hospital lobby to mean birth without pain relief. I strongly felt that women should be able to choose whether or not they wanted pain relief, yet there seemed to be increasing pressure on women to give birth unaided.

## Natural Childbirth

In the 1940s a British obstetrician, Grantley Dick-Reed, developed a delivery technique which he called natural childbirth. It minimised medical intervention and concentrated on the mother's conscious effort to give birth to her child. His premise was that childbirth need not be accompanied by excessive pain and that many labour pains result from unnatural physical tension caused by fear. He constructed a pre-natal instruction course which helped women to relax, strengthened the muscles most used during labour, gave guidance for breathing and aimed to enable women to use their endorphins (the body's natural painkillers) effectively.

Dick-Reed's ideas were opposed by many physicians, who countered that it denied the progress of modern medicine and needlessly primitivised the process of birth. But by the late 1950s the method had gradually become accepted and was used by a growing minority of women, especially in the United States and Britain.

The objective of giving women power over their own labours is a good one. But in practice it sometimes means that women feel inadequate if they do want to take advantage of the sophisticated medical technology available. By 1989, when I was pregnant with Martha, the phrase natural childbirth was bandied around rather indiscriminately, implying, so far as I could see, that medical intervention was always wrong and suggesting that it was almost always undertaken for specious reasons. Much of the home birth material I read propagated a sort of macho – and mystic – competitive attitude to birth, as if feeling pain somehow made the experience more real, more valid. As Tessa put it:

> There's something terribly intellectual about a lot of women going through it which I don't understand, because it feels to me very basic really. And the one thing we all know about pain is that it's not very pleasant. Of course women have babies in the forest, have babies everywhere, but God Almighty, we live in

incredibly civilised times when if you have a tooth pulled you have an anaesthetic.

The inference was that if suffering pain was natural, then choosing not to feel contractions must be unnatural. Assuming that all women want to be in hospital with an epidural is a denial of a woman's right to govern her own labour; by the same token, postulating that no women want to be in hospital and implying that all pain relief is unnatural is just as bad. As one antenatal teacher said to her class: 'Natural childbirth is what we're all going to do; active birth is when you don't have any drugs.'

But despite my very positive feelings about Martha's birth, and my rather negative ones about much of the culture surrounding home birth, within days of knowing that I was pregnant with Felix, Greg and I found ourselves discussing the 'what ifs' of doing it at home. I knew little about it in practice, although four months earlier I had been present at my niece's birth at home. Although I shuddered at my sister's pain as I rubbed her back during her brief, three-hour labour, the atmosphere itself must have had a strong effect on my subconscious. Five minutes after Jessica had been born, Caroline's three older children, our mother, Greg and Martha were all in the bedroom with Caroline's husband and the two midwives, munching toast and drinking tea. It just all seemed so normal.

I also wanted to do something different for Felix, so that his birth wasn't simply a re-run of Martha's. I felt that already he got everything second-hand, so here was a way of ensuring that his birth was as special and unique a memory as Martha's birth was.

I was influenced by my GP's reaction too. Having congratulated us, she asked me if I wanted to do things differently second time round, a home birth perhaps? Since I'd had forceps, had needed stitching and had lost a fair amount of blood, I hadn't cast myself as an obvious candidate for the so-called natural approach. But her confidence boosted mine and by the end of the half-hour appointment I almost thought that I would go for a home birth. Over the next few days the decision gradually took shape, although once it had been taken I felt both extremely excited and extremely nervous, as if I was about to go into an exam. What had I let myself – us – in for? My worries about doing it at home didn't subside until I was crouched on all fours at the top of our stairs . . . in labour.

## The Booking Visit

Whatever decisions have been made or postponed, by 12 weeks most women are ready to be booked. Whether you have opted in or out of the system, antenatal care in Britain follows a pattern. As a first-time mother, you are checked about once a month up to 28 weeks, then every three weeks until 34 weeks and then every fortnight. If you go over 40 weeks you will be monitored more often just in case the placenta starts to show signs of weakening and to check that your baby is OK. Obviously if you already have a relationship with a GP or a midwife, or are on a second or subsequent pregnancy, the booking visit is likely to be less detailed.

Most pregnancy handbooks have comprehensive sections explaining what checks are done, and why, and run through the terms used in your notes. Short for hand-held maternity record, you are likely to be given your notes on your first antenatal visit and they detail the results of the routine tests and the progress of your pregnancy: blood pressure, urine, fetal movements, and so forth.

Independent midwives tend to keep different sorts of records. With Felix, I had a book in which my midwives summarised each visit: they concentrated on the social and emotional aspects of the visit, rather than just recording physical progress. It can be a pleasurable memento to have of pregnancy.

## Family Medical Background

At the booking visit for a first pregnancy a midwife or doctor will take down your full family medical history and that of your partner, in an attempt to assess hereditary factors such as heart disease, asthma, multiple births, genetic or chromosomal disorders. This background information can influence the sorts of screening test you will be offered. It is surprising how little most of us know about our families; several women commented that they wished they'd known that they'd be asked if their paternal grandmother had suffered from diabetes because they could have done a little research and found out . . .

For some, obtaining background biological information that might be relevant to the course of the pregnancy is difficult, if not impossible: for single parents where the male partner is not available to ask; for couples who have used anonymous sperm donations; and for women or men who are adopted, since although adoption agencies will give basic information if they have it, it is rare for them to have detailed medical backgrounds for both the mother and the father.

## Adopted Children

Two women interviewed were adopted. Caroline didn't worry about hereditary problems, although she had always thought she would trace her biological parents when she reached the age of 18. In the event she didn't set things in motion until her first daughter, Emma, was about a year old. It was the reality of being a mother herself that was the catalyst.

It was just to see what they looked like really, nothing else. I know it sounds stupid – because you don't always look like your parents do – but I wanted to know what I'd look like when I was older.

Lynne, on the other hand, became interested in finding out as much as possible about her biological parents when she and John were having difficulty conceiving. As a health worker, she knew from first-hand experience how many genetic and chromosomal disorders do run in families. She was counselled, given her real birth certificate and a couple of addresses to follow up. Sadly, the agency records could only tell her that there was no known history of TB or epilepsy on either side of the family, which didn't allay her fears: 'It was such a disappointment and so worrying to find out so little, and such contradictory information.'

**Just a Few Questions ...**

Once you have given as much family medical history as you can, the midwife or doctor will turn to your – and your partner's – general medical history: how much you drink and smoke, allergies, kidney problems, surgical operations, contraceptive and menstrual history, any previous births, what sort of professional and social life you lead. You will then be given a full medical examination, partly to determine how healthy you are in general and partly to have a point of reference against which weight gain, appetite and so forth can be measured. Your height – and shoe size – may sometimes be useful indicators of pelvic size, although in the developed world there are relatively few women who are genuinely unable to give birth to their own babies because their pelvic outlet is too small.

### I'm Not Fat, I'm Pregnant

As recently as 1990 everyone was weighed at an NHS booking visit and at all subsequent antenatal appointments. But the value of regular weighing has been challenged and in many parts of the country it is already no longer routine. Poor weight gain can indicate interuterine growth retardation (IUGR), that the baby is not flourishing; sudden weight gain in the final trimester can indicate the onset of a serious condition, pre-eclampsia. But in most cases the mother's weight does not really reveal how healthy the baby is. Furthermore, in March 1992 the *British Medical Journal* ran a report suggesting that, except for teenagers or women with eating disorders, routine monitoring often did more harm than good because women were continually measuring themselves against standardised guidelines.

> Other researchers say that since different women gain weight at different rates, it is impossible to be dogmatic about how much any one individual should weigh. If a woman starts her pregnancy underweight, she and her baby may benefit from a bigger weight gain than the woman who begins pregnancy already overweight. It is 'normal' to put on between 9 to 13.5 kilograms in pregnancy, but some women gain more with no ill effect.[9]

More often than not the precise level of weight gain is to do with appetite, exercise and the woman's feelings about her size in a world where to be skinny is to be beautiful. A woman who feels too awful to exercise or to eat anything but iced buns during her first 12 weeks is obviously likely to put on more weight at the beginning than the woman who eats nothing but fruit and continues to play tennis every day. Experts estimate that most women can expect to put on something between 20 and 40 lb in the nine months (9 to 18 kg). Most women are likely to gain more in the second half of their pregnancy, something in the region of just over 1 lb (0.5 kg) per week from about 20 weeks on. The weight, by rough rule of thumb, is made up of:

Baby: 6 to 10 lb
Placenta: 1 to 2 lb
Uterus: 2 lb
Amniotic fluid: 2 lb
Breasts: 1 to 3 lb
Blood: 2.5 to 4 lb
Fat: 5 to 8 lb
Tissue and fluid: 4 to 7 lb

Regular weighing can encourage competitiveness, either in putting on too little weight or too much. There is also a mistaken equation of healthiness with thinness. But a woman who gives her body what it needs is likely to be healthier than one who starves herself in an attempt to achieve a weight inappropriate for her build and height.

Except in extreme circumstances the baby's health is unlikely to be affected. Sue put on most of her extra weight at the end of her first pregnancy, going from 9st 4lb to 11st 4lb; but with her second child, Hannah, it all went on in the first few weeks: 'So I worried I was going to put on 4st in all which would take at least five years to lose . . .'

Many women, like Rachel, felt resentful that it was an issue at all.

The limits they give you in pregnancy books are very low – most people I know put on twice that much – so I just thought I was going to be one of those people

who was going to get enormous. And I was starving all
the time.

Several women, such as Siân and Tessa, said that pregnancy
was the one time when they felt they were allowed to eat
what they wanted and not feel judged about getting bigger.

> I allowed myself to eat more, I allowed myself to
> completely satisfy my appetite, which is different from
> it getting bigger, because I tend not to eat very much
> usually.

Joanne is nearly 5ft 10in and went from 16st to 17st 10lb,
having had an extremely healthy pregnancy and a quick,
drug-free home birth. In Caroline's four pregnancies – where
she put on between 2st and 3st 12lb – she did find that there
was a correlation between how much weight she put on and
the baby's birthweight, but the differences were really very
slight. Pam was, in her own opinion, two stone overweight
when she conceived so she couldn't be bothered to worry
about how much more she was putting on; Sarah also felt
she was overweight before she became pregnant with Abigail,
so although she did try not to put on too much – since she
had found the additional weight difficult to lose after Kirsty's
birth – she didn't consciously count calories. As Caroline said,
'I wasn't thin to start with, so when you've got a fair old
wobbly bit over the top, you don't really notice the bump
growing.'

Eve had always been especially proud of her flat stomach,
so didn't like trousers feeling tight around the waist
before she'd even done the pregnancy test. Yet she too felt
that she should follow her appetite and worry about weight
gain after Annie's birth.

I also had this idea that because I was going to breast-feed – and that was the main thing I was looking forward to anyway – it would all go away, so there wouldn't be any worry.

Lee, on the other hand, is 5ft 6in and only went from 8st to 9st 7lb. Sasha, who is one inch taller, put on exactly a stone, partly because she was so violently sick throughout her pregnancy. Jenny, too, put on less weight than recommended in her pregnancy handbooks first time round – going from 8st 4lb to 9st 5lb – and was worried by it.

Some women never really enjoy eating throughout their pregnancies. Jenny was pleased that she wasn't enormous, but was upset by other people's insensitive comments. At 5lb 6oz, her son James was only fractionally lighter than Eve's daughter Annie, and Eve had gone from 8st 7lb to 11st 6lb. They are both 5ft 4in tall, and both returned to their pre-pregnancy weights within six months of giving birth. Jenny commented:

> Other people made remarks like 'where is it?', which rather upset me, so I felt that there must be something wrong. And every time I went to the doctor they said it was fine, but they didn't give me any statistics or tell me why it was fine. I feel a bit of a failure for having produced a 5lb baby, and that in some way it's my fault for not having eaten the right things. So second time I tried to produce a bigger baby . . .

Douglas was born on his due date, weighing in at 7lb 15oz.

## You're As Attractive As You Feel

Self-image obviously plays a large part in how good a woman feels about herself throughout pregnancy. Interestingly, at this stage when few women are visibly pregnant in their clothes, those who felt most uncomfortable about constant weight monitoring tended to be those who were – or who had made great efforts to be – slim.

Lisa is 5ft 7in and had never weighed more than 8st 7lb. She had spent most of her adolescence and adult life being encouraged to put on weight rather than to lose it, so thought she would enjoy being bigger. Her pre-conception weight was 8st 2lb. It was a surprise to her to find the first 20 weeks so undermining: she felt fat, and didn't like it. Jane, too, was surprised at how badly her self-confidence was affected: 'That period before you have a pregnant bump, I felt fat, I felt heavy and I felt unattractive.' I am 5ft 3in and was 9st 8lb when I conceived Martha, which was about average for me at the time. By the time she was born I'd eaten my way up to 11st 7lb, due in no small part to having treacle sponge and custard for breakfast for much of my pregnancy. I only realised that my increased size was not wholly due to the baby when a pair of baggy trousers felt tight on the legs rather than the stomach. But I felt comfortable being big. Afterwards the whole business of being pregnant and giving birth seemed to change my metabolism entirely, and by six months after Martha's birth – having cut out the chocolate and stodge – I'd shrunk to just under 8st.

Second time around I was 8st exactly when I conceived Felix. I knew I didn't want to be quite so heavy again, but I didn't expect to fret about calorie intake or about when clothes started to feel tight. But, having been thin, I was depressed about – and undermined by – my weight gain throughout the whole pregnancy. It obsessed me. I felt ashamed of being preoccupied by something so trivial in the first place, especially because in the early days I had a desperate urge to tell people that I was pregnant so that they wouldn't think I was fat. I used judgemental, emotive words like fat and overweight, which were an accurate indicator of my state of mind. Many women, like Sue and Tessa, admitted rounding up their dates for this reason.

> And I met women who were six foot [Tessa is 5ft 1 in], who didn't look pregnant at all, who said to me 'I'm eight and a half months pregnant' and I'd say 'oh yes, me too' when I was in fact only six . . .

## The Baby

This booking visit is the first time that the baby itself joins the system's ranks, as its position is checked and its heartbeat listened to with a Sonicaid. This can be a fantastic moment, to hear that incredibly fast and robust thumping and to know that there really is someone inside. A baby's heart beats roughly twice as fast as an adult's, between 120 and 160 beats per minute.

Between weeks 12 and 16 the placenta takes over from the corpus luteum in nourishing and helping the fetus to grow. The baby is completely formed by now and from this period on grows in size rather than complexity; it is consequently less likely to be harmed by drugs, infections or poisons. By week 14 its neck has lengthened and its head is not so bent on its chest. The abdominal wall closes, concealing the intestines, which until this point have been on the outside. By the beginning of week 16 all the baby's joints are moving, fingernails and toenails are grown, and a fine hair – lanugo – covers its little body. It is now 6in (16cm) long and weighs nearly 5oz (about 130g). The amniotic fluid, which replenishes itself completely every six hours and maintains a constant warm temperature, cushions it from bumps. Your baby can suck and swallow, yawn and stretch, even frown.

**The First Kicks**

In most handbooks, the estimate is that identifiable fetal movements will begin between 18 and 22 weeks, and that they are more likely to be felt later in first pregnancies. Several of my interviewees were aware of their babies moving much earlier, even though the sensations had no pattern to them. A woman will not necessarily feel a second or third child moving earlier than her first, and it seems probable that the position of the baby is the most relevant factor.

According to Aboriginal belief, the spirit of the child picks its parents. At some time during the pregnancy, usually at the time the first movements are felt, it is accepted that the spirit has chosen and entered the woman's body.

Lynne felt her first kick just before 15 weeks, 'a really gentle tickle', at the bottom of the right side of her pelvis. She was standing on the Underground, holding on to one of those dangling straps, and she knew it was Michelle. At about ten o'clock one night I was walking with Greg and Martha around a hideous shopping centre on the last stages of our two-month holiday, eating ice-cream. Then low down in the centre of my pelvis I distinctly felt Felix shift position: the sensation was like a key turning in a lock. I too was 15 weeks pregnant, and didn't feel any other movements until about 19 weeks. But it was exciting and, like Lynne, I knew that it was the baby, not another unknown muscle twinge.

Caroline's first baby, Emma, moved at 18 weeks; number two, Anthony, wriggled at 16 weeks and her third, Richard, at 14 weeks. Jessica, her youngest child, didn't move until she was nearly 19 weeks pregnant. It was this lack of early movement – coupled with the flu antibiotics she had taken before she knew she was pregnant and the pleurisy she had contracted at 11 weeks – that prompted her to ask for an early scan. Everything was fine.

## Kicking for Two

Despite it being her first pregnancy, Nicki actually felt movement at 9 weeks, although there wasn't a regular pattern until she was about 20 weeks: 'It was a sort of rolling, fluttering feeling.' Because she and Mike were travelling and because they didn't know any other pregnant women and hadn't read any pregnancy books, they didn't realise then that this was extraordinarily early to be feeling anything.

Sharon remembers walking home through the park at about 15 weeks and suddenly having to sit down because of this odd, low-down rolling sensation. Both Nicki and Sharon were carrying twins, although neither was aware of it at the time. They subsequently discovered that it is common for twins' movements to be felt earlier. They both also commented that this was the first time they became aware of the lack of practical experience most doctors have of multiple births. Sharon found her advisers generally didn't know how to adapt the usual guidelines to the specifics of her situation. What's more, most handbooks and leaflets frequently fail to mention twins at all.

> You go to all these hospital antenatal classes and appointments and get told all these things, then the person would turn to me and say 'Of course, it will be different for you' – but nobody tells you how or why.

## Physical Changes

Physical changes can be relatively slight between weeks 12 and 16. The sickness and nausea passes for some, leaving partners and women alike astounded at the new-found energy levels. As Fran said, 'I'd been incredibly sleepy for the first few weeks, then I sort of got a second wind.'

Some women started to be plagued by heartburn, which worsened as the pregnancy progressed. The hormones released during pregnancy soften the valve between the oesophagus and stomach. As a result, foods and gastric acids may reflux back up, irritating the lining of the oesophagus and causing a burning sensation in the upper chest. I had never had heartburn before being pregnant with Martha. Unfortunately now, if I eat too quickly or too late, I still get that stinging sensation in my throat, as if I'd knocked back a double whisky without pausing for breath. Certain stimulants, such as tea and coffee, often exacerbate heartburn: some women find that alcohol and spicy, greasy and fatty foods bring on an attack. Traditional herbal remedies include one teaspoon of slippery elm powder mixed with water or milk, and fennel infusions.* Homoeopaths might recommend remedies such as natrum phosphoricum 6C three times daily or mercurius solubilis 6C.

Sharon was unlucky enough to develop haemorrhoids, which she occasionally still suffers from eight years on. They are surprisingly common during pregnancy.

> Nobody tells you about the haemorrhoids and they are painful. My friend's just had a baby, and she's a really intelligent woman, and she said 'I didn't know what these things were, I thought they'd left the stitches hanging out'.

Haemorrhoids are varicose veins around the anus caused by pressure on relaxed blood vessels. Commonly known as piles, they usually start with irritation and itching around and inside the anal area and, exacerbated by straining when

---

* Fennel is one of the active ingredients in gripe water, used for treating babies with colic.

constipated, sometimes protrude. There are ointments, such as Anusol or Nelson's Ointment for Haemorrhoids, to be used every time you have a bowel movement. Herbalists would suggest cold compresses soaked in witch hazel or pilewort, or inserting a clove of garlic into the rectum at night . . .

One or two people mentioned their legs getting restless at about this point. With Martha I'd had this in the last month, but was plagued between weeks 13 and 16 of my pregnancy with Felix. Jane summed up the feeling graphically; for her it lasted until after delivery:

> I called it itchy bones, which just used to drive me absolutely wild. I felt like I wanted to take the layer of fat off, take the layer of muscle off and really have a good scratch.

Many people notice their skin changing in general ways when they're pregnant, for example becoming less spotty than usual or more greasy. At about 14 weeks the linea nigra may start to appear. A dark line that stands out against the rest of your skin, this can be up to an inch wide and stretches up from the pubic bone to the navel, or even to the breastbone. It usually disappears within six months of delivery: after Felix, I still had a faint line ten months later.

Birthmarks, moles, freckles and recent scars might darken and, surprisingly, they tend to be more noticeable in women whose skins are darker to start with. I was spotty and pale throughout my pregnancy with Martha; with Felix, however, I looked as if I had a permanent suntan, particularly on my chin and nose. Fran developed a small chloasma patch on her face in Matthew's pregnancy, which disappeared completely a week after he'd been born: 'It looked as if I'd dribbled gravy down my chin.'

Chloasma – sometimes known colloquially as 'the mask of pregnancy' – are brown patches that can appear on the face or throat. They are caused by a skin pigment called melanin and are often noticeable in women taking oral contraceptives too. They can be aggravated by sunlight, but they are not dangerous and will disappear within three months of delivery. Black women may find they develop patches of white skin on their face and neck, which will also fade away once the baby has been born.

## Braxton Hicks

This stage in pregnancy also witnesses the beginning of Braxton Hicks contractions. This involuntary tightening and relaxing of the uterus can be frightening the first time it happens, and women who have had difficult pregnancies often say that their initial response was fear of going into premature labour.

Named after the obstetrician who first discovered their purpose in pregnancy, Braxton Hicks contractions actually happen throughout your life just as other organs – such as the heart, intestines and blood vessels – regularly contract and relax. During pregnancy, the enlarged uterus makes the sensation more noticeable. They ensure a good blood supply, fostering uterine growth. Most books estimate that women won't be aware of them until 20 weeks at the earliest, and some put it as late as the eighth month.

Siân never experienced Braxton Hicks in either of her two pregnancies, but women on second or subsequent pregnancies are often aware of them early. At about 13 weeks I noticed with Felix that whenever I swam in cold water I could feel my uterus harden. From that point on, I experienced a tightening at least once a day, particularly after exercising.

## Emotional Changes

Emotionally, those who were ambivalent about their pregnancies didn't find this time very enjoyable. For one woman these miserable second pregnancy weeks were especially disappointing as she'd been so happy first time round.

> I thought, I wish I wasn't pregnant; I've got x weeks of this to go, how am I going to get through them; I don't want another baby – although I don't think I came out and said that I didn't want the baby to anyone, it would have seemed somehow disloyal.

Jenny, too, found that her equanimity was more strained the second time round:

> I think I'd thought pregnancy was a one-off experience and I'd done that; yet there I was again, so there wasn't even the excitement of thinking 'What's going to happen next?' I wanted the baby, I just didn't want to be pregnant.

But the majority of women, like Tessa, talked about relaxing into their pregnancies at this point. Emotionally and physically it felt as if it was all at last falling into place.

> I'd been very emotional, furiously angry, nasty and aggressive for 14 weeks, very weepy. Then suddenly I was totally placid and calm.

Debra, who had found the first 12 weeks mentally daunting, was surprised how the world of pregnancy took over her mind so completely. Approaching the time when tests and scans would be done, where stretchier clothes would become

the only comfortable alternative, the halfway mark was
suddenly in sight:

> At first there had seemed too much to take in, and I felt
> guilty for working and not doing enough. You want to
> know what every feeling is as it happens, but there are
> just too many opinions. But after that, feeling preoccu-
> pied was the most unlikely thing. Not minding about
> other things or people. It was harder to carry on as
> normal, and I felt great admiration for other women in
> harder situations, alone and working.

As the worries about miscarriage disappear, many women
start to allow themselves to think about actually cuddling
their baby in their arms. The mental adjustment to the idea
of being a parent has begun, and this can lead to reorganising
one's life in anticipation, both emotionally and practically. For
many professional women it means weighing up their working
agenda for the next few months, and starting to think about
how they will manage once the baby has been born. Equally
common is refusing to think about finishing work and having
a baby at all, since the idea is still too challenging. For others
it is a question of logistics, of moving house or reorganising
existing space to make room for another person.

For some, planning for the future takes the form of formal-
ising their relationship. For many couples, wanting children
is the catalyst. Both Debra and Lee had been with their respective partners for a long time and married for the express
reason that they wanted to start families. For Sarah and Sue,
it was simply a matter of bringing existing plans forward.
However, these couples were bucking a growing trend for
couples to have babies while cohabiting. There were only
308,600 marriages in 2003, a drop of two-fifths since 1992.[10]
In 2004, 42 per cent of births were outside marriage.[11]

For other women and men I interviewed, marriage was simply a question of rethinking their commitment to one another, a way of announcing to the world that they were both changing their lives by becoming parents.

Although completely supportive, Matt found it difficult in the first 12 weeks or so of Jane's pregnancy to come to terms with the idea of being a father. From 13 weeks onwards, however, he started to feel very positive. And at the same time Jane, who had never wanted to be married, acknowledged that some form of official, public commitment was important to her. So they started planning, with a view to getting married about six months into the pregnancy.

> He rather fancied the idea of not getting married until after she was born; where my viewpoint was that if we didn't get married until after she was born then what was the point of getting married.

Sasha and Lou, who had been together for over ten years, had never seen any reason to marry. Lou has two children by a previous relationship, and Sasha feels that this might have affected their decision to marry once they were contemplating a family. It was a sort of public acknowledgement of the pregnancy, a signal that they felt happy about relinquishing the fast lane and settling down as parents.

> I'd always thought I'd never get married, whatever, so it was kind of like a fanfare, a celebration, as if I was saying, OK, this is my present to Freddy.

## Tests, Tests, Tests

### Weeks 16–20

> How the days went
> While you were blooming within me
> I remember each upon each –
> the swelling changed planes of my body
> and how you first fluttered, then jumped
> and I thought it was my heart
> Audre Lorde, from<br>'Now That I Am Forever With Child'[1]

Many of the tests offered in pregnancy are done during this period. There are two kinds: screening tests – which tell you whether your baby has a higher than average chance of disability – and diagnostic tests which give specific information about the individual baby. In recent years, the range and sophistication of tests has increased amazingly. Not only are there some procedures that we were not offered fifteen years ago, but many of the tests that were around can now be done earlier in pregnancy.

Some – and not just those who oppose abortion in any shape or form – are increasingly worried about the ethics of testing. Do they perhaps encourage an attitude where anyone who is not mentally or physically 'perfect' has no place? In India and China the cases of amniocentesis being used to determine sex has led to obscene numbers of girls being aborted and a distorted social balance. What if a homosexual gene, for example, was discovered?

Some midwives and doctors feel that routine testing of all pregnant women is unnecessary; that the long-term safety of ultrasound scanning has not been proved; that tests are an interference that encourages women not to trust their own bodies without the medical all-clear; and that, too often, appropriate counselling and discussion of the purpose of the test is not given.

Most women and men, however, feel reassured by being offered a chance to check up on their baby's health. Some couples might feel they could cope with any mental or physical disability, however upsetting. Others question the morality of allowing a severely mentally disabled child to be born in the first place. Some know they could cope with a physically handicapped child, whereas they do not want to hand over their lives to caring for a brain-damaged child. Many do not even try to imagine how they would feel.

Several of the arguments for and against termination on the grounds of abnormality are similar to those surrounding abortion, not least because it is usually the woman who will bear the burden, both emotionally and practically. Family and friends may also feel they have a right to give their opinions, which can cause a great deal of conflict. One woman said:

> I had the tests, because I knew I couldn't cope with a badly handicapped child. But my sister, who's against abortion, made it clear that she would never forgive me

if I 'killed my baby', as she put it. It was a big pressure and I was really upset by her attitude. But it was us who would have had to cope, not her.

An assumption is often made by doctors that any woman who elects to have screening tests would automatically choose a termination if a severe disability were discovered. But some women who have the tests do so in order to be able to prepare themselves for life with a disabled child. There are several groups for parents who discover that their baby is mentally or physically disabled, such as the Antenatal Results and Choices (ARC), the In-Touch Trust, Contact a Family and the Down's Syndrome Association. These groups can be particularly helpful when the mother-to-be and her partner do not agree.

But for most the range of tests is reassuring. There are psychological and medical aspects to the personal choices a woman makes: many like the security of being tested and feel that their pregnancy is being monitored with care; others resent the intrusion and challenge the value of routine testing. In both cases, the emotional reasons for choosing or rejecting screening or diagnostic tests are as important as the medical implications.

### Roll Up Your Sleeve

Just about all women will have a blood test at some point during their pregnancy, despite the fact that Caroline's attitude – about needles in general – is shared by a large number of women:

> I like everything about being pregnant really, apart from
> the blood tests. I like feeling it move, I feel special, I
> like having to go to the doctor's and hospital a lot,

because it makes you feel different having to go and be checked.

Most have had blood taken from them at their booking visit to check for various things (including their haemoglobin count to make sure they aren't anaemic; their immunity to rubella; and for syphilis and hepatitis B). Blood taken at booking will also disclose blood group – surprisingly few women knew their blood groups – which is important in cases where the mother is found to be rhesus negative. If a rhesus negative woman has a partner with a positive blood group, there is a chance that the baby will also have rhesus positive blood: she may therefore start to build up antibodies and reject the fetus. This is a particular risk in second and subsequent pregnancies.

Fran already knew that she was rhesus negative when she conceived a baby by accident only three months into her relationship. Jim's blood group turned out to be positive, so after her abortion she was given an injection of antibodies so that her body wouldn't reject her next baby. The same procedure was followed after Matthew's birth.

My local hospital actually does a rhesus clinic, and I met women there who were having to have interuterine blood transfusions for the baby. But I didn't need anything.

At the same time as what seem like pints of blood are being drawn from your arm, you might also be asked what – if any – other screening tests you would like. What procedures are routinely offered to women depends to a degree on where you live, but you will almost certainly be offered some sort of blood test and possibly a scan to screen for Down's syndrome.

**HIV/AIDS**

Early on in your pregnancy, your doctor or midwife will ask if you want to be tested for HIV. You do not have to have this test and, if you do decide to go ahead, it is important to make sure that you have thought through the implications of a positive result beforehand. Without intervention, about 15–20 per cent of those babies born to HIV-positive mothers will pick up the virus either in the womb, during the birth or via breastfeeding.[2] This risk can be dramatically reduced by taking anti-HIV drugs during pregnancy, having a caesarean rather than a vaginal birth and by not breastfeeding, as the virus is known to be passed through the mother's milk to the baby.

**The Ultrasound Scan**

Nowadays, it is standard to offer all pregnant women in Britain, Australia and parts of the United States an ultrasound scan. Also known as an anomalies scan, it is usually carried out at about 20 weeks. Again depending on where you live and the facilities available locally, additional scans may be offered. If, for example, you have a history of miscarriage, you may be offered an early scan at about eight weeks to check all is well. If you have irregular periods and aren't sure how many weeks pregnant you are, you may be offered a dating scan at about 10 to 13 weeks. And more and more women are now offered a nuchal scan at 11–14 weeks to screen for Down's syndrome. This measures the amount of fluid at the back of the baby's neck. A high measurement can indicate a greater risk of Down's, although only a diagnostic test, such as chorionic villus sampling (CVS), can tell you for certain whether or not your baby is affected.

The ultrasound scan is a simple and – when carried out on up-to-date equipment by an experienced member of staff –

technologically astonishing procedure. A warm (sometimes . . .) sound-conductive jelly is squidged on to the woman's abdomen and a device rather like a truncated table-tennis bat is pressed against the uterus. The instrument pulses high-frequency sound waves (emitted from a transducer in the ultrasound machine). As the sound waves pass through human tissue, they rebound at each surface and return to the machine to create an image which is a cross-section of the growing baby. A thrilling close-up scan of Felix enabled us to pick out all four chambers of his heart with the blood surging through and pushing open the valves.

A few women worry about possible negative effects of ultrasound on the fetus, especially on the baby's hearing. Since the machine is not running continuously and – unlike X-ray devices – it emits no ionising radiation, there is no official recognition of any potential risk. Nor is there currently any proof that there are no long-term damaging consequences either. Because widespread and systematic scanning is a relatively recent development in obstetrics, it is likely that a definitive judgement on the presence or lack of side-effects will become apparent only when the babies who were scanned in the womb are adults.

With the exception of Joanne, who didn't feel any need to see her baby to know that it existed and who did have reservations about safety, everyone interviewed had at least one ultrasound scan. The radiographer who carries out the scan is looking for specific signs of the baby's well-being: the amount of amniotic fluid and its concentration; if the baby is the right size for dates; the position of the placenta; and that all the baby's limbs and organs are in place and working efficiently. It can reveal problems which might otherwise go undetected until labour or birth: if discovered at this stage they can at least be monitored, perhaps even treated. Some hospitals offer you the choice of being told the baby's sex.

Now and then very experienced radiographers also feel confident in detecting the physical signs of Down's syndrome, spina bifida and genetic disorders such as cystic fibrosis which – to the highly trained eye – have visible symptoms. What a scan cannot do is guarantee that there is nothing whatsoever wrong with your baby.

With Martha I expected something to be wrong, and Greg and I left the hospital in tears after the 19-week scan, clutching our fetal photographs (at a cost of £1), delighted and relieved to be told that everything seemed to be in the right place. To me the image looked like a satellite photograph of storm clouds over a grey North Sea. Felix wriggled round from breech presentation (bottom down) to cephalic presentation (bottom up) during the course of his scan and made robust attempts to kick off the monitor. At this point I did not have much sense of Felix's character and was feeling second-baby guilt on his behalf. The scan helped to cement my relationship with him.

Debra found her scan very reassuring, saying that she got more useful information from the radiographer than anybody else. She felt that the way in which the operator routinely measured everything and pointed things out convinced her that there couldn't be anything wrong. Lynne, who had strong fears about having a disabled child, was also relieved to see Michelle alive and kicking on the screen. Caroline enjoyed her scans in all four pregnancies. Debbie also found the scans comforting – and moving – in both of her pregnancies: 'It's lovely to see the baby alive, and see the heart beating and all the rest of it.'

Several women, like Lisa, talked about liking the way it gave their partner a chance to be involved.

> One of the reasons the scan was so terribly exciting for me was the way Rob reacted. He had been terribly

distanced from it, so he was lovely, so proud of me, so proud of the baby.

In one survey of new fathers, many men commented on how the scan made them feel for the first time as if they were going to be fathers.[3] Some people have challenged routine scanning for the benefit of partners, feeling it should only be carried out for medical reasons. They criticise the use of technological techniques to bolster partners' interest in a pregnancy. But because so few men are prepared to take even limited responsibility for their children in their early months, I think that anything that helps partners to begin to adjust to the idea of parenthood is probably worthwhile. The sociological benefits of medical science can, in certain circumstances, be as important as the diagnostic uses.

## Twins and More

Of course the scan can be a shock. Sharon and her then-husband Gary went along for a routine scan at 16 weeks. Out of the blue the radiographer announced that not only were there two babies, but there might even be three.

It was lucky I was lying down. I just could not believe it. Even now I find it difficult to believe sometimes. I think I went around in a daze for a little while, for a few days certainly.

Sharon and Gary were given no counselling or advice beyond the address of the problem pregnancy and multiple births clinic where Sharon was to book herself in. Her feelings, she admits, were mixed. On the one hand she was terrified, on the other she did feel rather special. But most of all she just wanted someone to sit her down and explain what a multiple pregnancy would be like. (For example, she wanted to know if having two placentas would mean that the twins weren't identical, but no one answered this question and even at a 24-week scan they couldn't actually tell her how many placentas there were.) The only specific information given was that one of the twins – Katie, she suspects – was breech and was likely to stay that way. She would have appreciated being told that there were groups for women expecting more than one baby – such as TAMBA, the Twins and Multiple Births Association – so that she could have asked questions of knowledgeable, supportive people.

The funniest thing was how friends and family didn't believe her at first, although she comes from a close-knit community where everything to do with childbirth and pregnancy is celebrated. They soon came round to it, though: 'I come from a very working class background where all the women have children. It was expected that I would have a child, so two was even better.' In the end Sharon's sister, sick of people ringing up and asking if it was true, stuck a note on her front door saying, 'Yes, it's twins . . .'

The number of multiple births in the UK has reached record levels. In 2004, nearly 10,400 pairs of twins, 162 sets of triplets and five sets of quadruplets were born.[4] Two-thirds of these were the result of fertility treatment. Britain also boasts three of the world's sets of sextuplets – the Waltons (yes, really), the Colemans and the Vinces.

Identical (monozygotic or uniovular) twins are not linked to maternal age, will always be of the same sex and will have similar palm and finger prints. Non-identical (dizygotic or biovular) twins – when two eggs are released in a cycle by an ovary and both are fertilised – are more likely to be born to older women. Also known as fraternal twins, they may be of the opposite or the same sex, they will look no more or less alike than ordinary siblings, and there will always be two placentas. Siamese (or conjoined) twins occur when a single fertilised ovum fails to divide completely.

In the UK roughly one in 34 babies are twins or triplets, up from one in 52 in 1980. Japanese women have fewer twins or triplets than anyone else, while women in rural Nigeria hold the record for twins at 1 in every 19 pregnancies. Without fertility treatment, triplets occur naturally just once in every 10,000 births. Medical history was made at King's College Hospital, London, in 1996 when Evelyn Menseh and Wendy Coppin both gave birth to triplets six days apart: three girls each!

Nicki had a similar experience to Sharon's. Because she and her husband had been travelling round South America and hadn't come into contact with other pregnant women, she didn't realise that she was unusually large for 16 weeks. There was no history of multiple births in either family and the possibility of twins simply hadn't crossed their minds. Mike was 'deeply, deeply shocked'. Nicki, although partly excited, was initially convinced that they'd accidentally measured everything twice. It was only when she heard the two heartbeats that she believed that there were two distinct babies.

Nicki too received no counselling and with hindsight felt that she was given a lot of misleading information. For example, she had two placentas and was told categorically that the twins were therefore non-identical: in fact, she gave birth to identical twin boys, and delivered two placentas too.

The Multiple Births Foundation produces information for health professionals on the specialist care of twins, triplets and quads.[5] One of the most important emotional issues addressed is the damage a negative reaction can do to the mother's confidence about a multiple pregnancy. Nicki's radiographer gave them the news with the words, 'I'm afraid it's twins', and from that point onwards all those caring for her talked as if there would automatically be awful physical problems. Even friends, when told the news, tended to ask how Nicki and Mike felt about it before giving their congratulations. It's a far cry from Caroline's attitude: she was always disappointed when the scan revealed that she was not carrying twins or even triplets!

On the other hand Rachel, who has an identical twin sister, was delighted when the monitor showed only one baby. And Debbie wouldn't have been bowled over either, for practical reasons: 'I was worried about having twins or triplets, because there's twins on both sides and there's triplets on my side.' Yet she was a little disappointed, and subconsciously felt that it would be special to be carrying two babies.

An eighteenth-century Russian woman holds the record for the largest number of children. Between 1725 and 1765 she gave birth to 16 sets of twins, 7 sets of triplets and four sets of quadruplets, adding up to 69 children in all.

## When the Scan Reveals a Problem

Eve, Pam and Jane had to cope with shocks of a more upsetting nature. Eve was looking forward to her routine scan at 16 weeks, and she and Stephen enjoyed seeing Annie on the screen and having the photos to take home. Everything seemed fine. But when they got back from the hospital there was a message flashing on their answerphone asking them to come back for another scan because the radiographer hadn't been able to see the baby's spine. Only twenty minutes had elapsed. Eve was 'totally freaked out', imagining a child with no spine, and immediately rang the hospital. The duty sister knew nothing about it, then after several clunks and clicks through the telephone exchange, a senior midwife apologised that all they'd meant was that they hadn't got an accurate spinal measurement. Eve went back a week later and was reassured that Annie's spine was completely normal.

At this same visit the radiographer commented that Eve's placenta was very low in the uterus and that they would like her to come back at 30 weeks to check its position again. Placenta praevia, where the placenta stays low and blocks the baby's way out, can be dangerous in labour. From her extensive reading, Eve knew that this was a relatively common complaint in the second trimester, so felt that the hospital was being unnecessarily – if understandably – cautious. And she was outraged that such a potentially distressing message about her baby's spine had been left on her answering machine. The combination of the two 'problems' introduced worry into a pregnancy that had been physically straightforward: 'It all made me very angry and it made me very mistrustful of the hospital from then on.'

Pam was also looking forward to her scan at the private Garden Hospital. She had booked for a home birth with independent midwives, but because it was her first pregnancy and she was 41 years old, her midwives had suggested that she should at least have one visit to her local NHS hospital just in case she needed treatment that couldn't be provided at home. The hospital consultant kept her and her partner Gérard waiting for hours, and then made it clear that he disliked independent midwives and resented his time and facilities being taken up by women who were not intending to deliver their babies in his hospital. It was from this hostile and opinionated man that Pam learnt the results of her scan. Pulling a form across his desk, he brusquely said:

I see you've got a fibroid and it's grown, so that will mean that you'll have to have a caesarean, so you'll have to come into the hospital, and I hope you don't want any more children because we're going to have to

cut you up here. It's not very nice not having any choice
in life, is it?

Pam stood up, threw the papers all over his desk, and walked
out crying. She resolved that, if it was impossible to have her
baby at home, she would find the money to go into the Garden
Hospital. She knew that she couldn't submit to being under
the 'care' of a doctor like that.

Jane was already having health problems when she went
for an 18-week scan. At 8 weeks she'd had a urinary infection,
then at 16 weeks she developed vaginal warts. They had to be
treated every two weeks at Charing Cross VD clinic, because
there was a slim chance that the baby could contract laryngeal
warts at delivery. It was an extremely unpleasant process and
one that lasted until 36 weeks, when a friendly doctor told her
that vaginal warts were not uncommon in pregnancy and that,
in his opinion, they would clear up after delivery with no ill-
effect to either her or the baby. He was right.

At the same time as the warts developed, Jane suddenly
came up in big red lumps all over her legs and ankles. No
one knew what they were or whether they had any connection with the pregnancy. Although they disappeared two
months later, it was a frighteningly inscrutable experience.

I was incredibly worried. I didn't like the idea of having
something wrong with my body when there was another
body inside.

The result of these twin stresses was that by the time Jane
and Matt were sitting in the darkened room awaiting a
radiographer, apprehension, not excitement, was the dominant emotion. The scan then revealed that Jane's baby Sophie
had abnormal kidneys, too large for the rest of her body. The
radiographer was unable to say what this might signify, but

felt that Sophie should be monitored. Jane's first reaction was of guilt: 'I thought it was my fault, because I'd been abusing my body to such a degree.'

Jane had repeat scans at 22 and 35 weeks, and on each occasion Sophie appeared to be growing healthily. She has had no kidney problems whatsoever, even though she was on a daily dose of antibiotics for the first year of her life just in case anything developed. (Jane had worked as a nurse in a special care baby unit looking after severely disabled children, so she wasn't intimidated by hospital procedures or staff. Even though the scan caused a lot of unnecessary worry, she did feel that she would rather have known about any potential problems *in utero* than discover them at birth.)

## Testing for Down's syndrome

The most well-known chromosomal disorder is Trisomy 21, or Down's syndrome, where an extra chromosome number 21 leads to there being an overall count of 47 rather than 46 chromosomes. The incidence is 1 in 1,000 pregnancies, and it was only in 1959 that this scientific reason for what was then known as 'Mongolism' was discovered. Most people associate Down's with the age of the mother and, although it is true that trisomy abnormalities do increase with maternal age, there is now a certain amount of evidence to suggest that paternal age is also a factor. This is one reason why men over 45 are not accepted by sperm donation programmes in this country.

In October 2003, the National Institute for Health and Clinical Excellence (NICE) recommended that all pregnant women should be offered screening for Down's with a test that is accurate enough to pick up at least 60 per cent of Down's babies. For many women, this means having something known as the Triple test, originally known as the Bart's test because St Bartholomew's Hospital in London was one of the first hospitals to offer it to all pregnant women within its catchment area.

The Triple test is a blood test that can be done any time between 14 and 20 weeks of pregnancy. It measures the levels of three substances in the woman's blood: alphafetoprotein (AFP), unconjugated oestriol (uE3) and human chorionic gonadotrophin (hCG). The results are used along with the mother's age to calculate her risk of having a baby with Down's syndrome and any woman with a risk higher than 1 in 250 is said to screen positive.

Debra was worried about Down's syndrome. At 34, the probability of her having a child suffering from this disorder was 1 in 465. Her Triple test result gave her a chance of 1 in 1400, although her GP unreassuringly added – as she is bound to do – 'You could be the one . . .'

It is important to stress that the Triple test is not a diagnostic test. Its aim is to identify women with an increased risk rather than tell you whether or not the actual baby you are carrying has Down's. It only detects about two out of three cases of Down's syndrome and 9 per cent of women will screen positive when, in fact, they aren't – what's known as a 'false positive'. Most of these women will go on to have a diagnostic test, such as chorionic villus sampling (CVS), which confirms that their baby is perfectly normal.

Several women opted for the Triple test, particularly if they were not categorised as high risk. There was no medical reason why their children should be disabled, but usually there was no reason why they shouldn't. Their anxiety had an emotional source, not a physical cause, and they felt that the Triple test could reassure them and enable them to make informed choices. (Since virtually all chromosomal disorders can be detected through pre-natal screening, some added that it seemed irresponsible not to take advantage of the tests available.)

In some areas, women are now being offered the Quadruple Test. As you might imagine, this is similar to the Triple test but measures four markers in the blood rather than three and has a slightly higher detection rate.

## Neural Tube Defects

As well as Down's syndrome, the Triple test can detect neural tube defects. This is the collective name for congenital disorders of the central nervous system such as spina bifida, anencephaly or hydrocephalus. When an embryo is 20 days old, a groove deepens and its edges curl over above it to form the neural tube: the front part expands to form the brain, the back part becomes the spinal cord.

Spina bifida is a defect in the part of the bony spine that helps protect the spinal cord. The nerves are left exposed, usually the nerves in the lower spine, which leads to lack of muscle control of the legs, bladder and bowels. But spina bifida varies hugely in its severity; a small mole at the bottom of the spine would actually be classified as a neural tube defect. Anencephaly is the absence of the brain and cranial vault (top of the skull). The incidence is approximately 1 per 1000 pregnancies. Hydrocephalus is when the cerebro-spinal fluid, which is secreted into the space around the brain, cannot be absorbed as it should be and therefore accumulates. A couple with one child affected by a neural tube defect has approximately a 4 per cent risk of having a second affected child, although this risk can be drastically reduced by taking a higher-than-usual dose of folic acid. Nationally the incidence of neural tube defects is about 2 per 1000 pregnancies, but around 90 per cent of these end in termination.

The Triple test is particularly effective at picking up neural tube defects when done between weeks 16 and 18 of pregnancy. As with Down's it is possible to get false positives, usually because the woman is not as far along in her pregnancy as she thought (or is further advanced), or because she is carrying more than one baby. However, the test does pick up about 85 per cent of affected babies.

### Nuchal Translucency (NT) Scan

The Nuchal Translucency, or NT, scan is fast overtaking the Triple test as the definitive screening test for Down's syndrome, although not all hospitals offer it yet. Using ultrasound to measure the amount of fluid at the back of the baby's neck, it has a slightly higher detection rate for Down's than the Triple test – about 75 per cent. Another huge advantage is that it can be done between 11 and 14 weeks of pregnancy, which allows more thinking time should you screen positive.

### Other Tests for Down's

In selected hospitals, the NT scan is used in conjunction with a blood test to give a high detection rate for Down's – about 79 per cent with a false positive rate of 2.3 per cent.[6] This is known as the combined test and, like the NT scan, it can be done between 11 and 14 weeks of pregnancy. There is also the integrated test, which combines an NT scan with two blood tests that measure five markers in the blood. Doctors at Barts, where the test has been pioneered, claim an average detection rate for Down's of 86 per cent with a false positive rate of just 1 per cent.[7]

Unfortunately, these tests are only available in certain parts of the UK and you will almost certainly have to pay to have them done privately.

# CVS

Amniocentesis and chorionic villus sampling (CVS) are the only definite ways to get a diagnosis of Down's.

For the CVS test an instrument is inserted through the woman's abdomen or vagina and a tiny sample taken from the chorionic villi. These are the minute protrusions on the outside of the fertilised egg which enable the ovum to implant itself in the mother's womb and which later form the placenta. Detailed laboratory analysis can detect abnormality. The main advantage of this test over amniocentesis is that it can detect Down's as early as 10 weeks and the results only take two weeks, sometimes only 48 hours. If the woman decides to have a termination, the procedure is much less traumatic at this stage, both physically and mentally, than it would be at 20 or 21 weeks after a positive amniocentesis result.

The CVS test has some disadvantages too. There is a risk of miscarriage of between 2 and 4 per cent, as opposed to 0.5 per cent with amniocentesis; it is not always possible to get a result; and there is a 1 in 1000 chance that you will get a serious infection. There have also been suggestions that if the procedure is carried out too early – before 10 weeks – it can result in missing limbs, limb abnormalities and facial deformities.[8] There is often light bleeding or spotting afterwards and it can be painful. One study also found that women who did miscarry after CVS experienced an extremely high level of guilt and felt responsible for having pushed for an 'early' result.[9] Perhaps this underlines the importance of counselling *before* tests are done, not just if something goes wrong.

## Amniocentesis

An amniocentesis is rarely carried out before 14 weeks, the point at which there is considered to be sufficient fluid in the amniotic sac. After a scan to determine the position of the fetus and placenta, a small area of the abdomen is treated with local anaesthetic and a long hollow needle surmounted by a syringe is carefully inserted into the womb. Some women talk about a pinching feeling, others of cramping or pressure in the uterus as the half-ounce of yellow fluid is drawn out of the amniotic sac. It will then be spun in a centrifuge to separate the cells shed by the baby from the rest of the liquid, and the cells will be cultured for anything between two and five weeks.

The stress of waiting for the results at this stage in pregnancy is possibly the hardest part of the entire operation, and there is a 1 per cent chance the cells will not grow sufficiently for diagnosis to be given. (Laboratory technicians can also tell the sex of a baby from the cells.) Occasionally the amniotic sac itself punctures: bed rest will allow the fluid to replenish itself with no ill-effect to the baby.

In 2000, 16.5 per cent of women gave birth over the age of 35 and nearly all would have been offered an amniocentesis to test for Down's syndrome. Now that more reliable non-invasive tests are available the proportion of mothers opting for an amnio purely because of their age is likely to be lower.

With Martha the fear of having a baby with Down's syndrome obsessed me throughout the pregnancy. Greg's mother, Rosie, had taught mentally disabled children for many years, so we had both seen the reality of mental disability. In the very early days of the pregnancy I'd also heard of a local woman of 27 whose second child had been born with Down's, and this subconsciously affected my confidence. When Felix was conceived, I still felt that I would like some preliminary screening.

15 FEBRUARY 1992: I don't think – I hope – the thought of the baby having Down's syndrome is going to obsess me quite as much. It can't. I don't want to ruin this

pregnancy with the ache of worry. But I'm going to
have every test going, all the same: then, when they're
all negative, I'll have proved that I was right not to
worry.

The probability calculated by my Triple test was 1 in 30,000
as compared to the bald statistical likelihood (going by age
alone) of 1 in 800. Since 1 in 250 is the dividing line, I was
reassured!

## Why Me? Why Not Me?

Sharon, whose twins are now eight, feels that she would want
more tests if she was to become pregnant again.

> A friend of a friend of mine, who's younger than me,
> has just had a Down's syndrome baby completely out
> of the blue, which really brought it home to me.

Having nursed severely disabled children, Jane too decided
that she did not want to go through that herself as a
mother.

> I definitely wanted an amnio, because there has been
> some vague research that you can have a chromosomal
> defect if the father is a lot older too, and Matt is in his
> forties.

Jane's GP forgot to send her booking letter to the hospital
and she was already 18 weeks pregnant when she had her
first scan and an opportunity to ask for an amniocentesis.
Huge pressure was put on her – the Registrar himself was
even drafted in – not to go ahead. They said that, at 32, she
was too young and that she was in all probability putting

a healthy child at risk. Jane knew that the increased risk of miscarriage is greater than the statistical risk of having a child suffering from Down's. She also knew that the lowest age limit of women routinely offered an amniocentesis had only recently been dropped from 40 to 35. But at the same time she knew that she could not cope with a mentally disabled child. The hospital went into explicit detail about how awful a late abortion would be, stressing that by 20 weeks plus it is safer for the woman to be put into induced labour, using prostaglandins, artificial rupture of the membranes and a syntocinon drip. Jane felt that they were using the demon of this deeply distressing process to upset her rather than trying to help her come to an informed decision.

> I felt bullied, I felt that I really wanted to have an amnio and I was being prevented from having one by somebody else's cock-up. I also felt that they were all so sure that it was a mistake to have one, and I just hoped that they were right.

Debra too met a lot of opposition to her request. Unlike Jane, Debra wasn't sure that she would choose to have an abortion if the result was positive, but she would have liked the reassurance.

> I did quite want an amniocentesis, but they put me off it. I think I would have gone along with the risks, actually, and hoped that I didn't have a miscarriage.

She thought about the possibility of disability throughout the pregnancy, and was amazed that nothing other than amniocentesis was offered to detect abnormality.

> It must be the most devastatingly awful thing that can happen to a family and I think it would be a real test for me and Hugo. I think he would feel that it was something to do with him, but I didn't feel like that at all. I think it would be just terrible bad luck.

Sometimes it was the partner who was most worried about the possibility of having a child with a learning disability. Every woman I interviewed did feel that their partner's anxieties should be taken into account, although many also felt that it was their body and so the ultimate decision about whether or not to have tests should be theirs. As one woman said, 'I think it's different when you're the one carrying a baby that's not right inside your body.'

Surprisingly few couples actually discussed how they would react to a test result revealing abnormality. Often this was because men did not feel they had the right to burden their pregnant partner with their own fears. Even fewer couples had discussed what they would do if they had a disabled child. Given that there is minimal state support and care for the parents of disabled children, several women commented that they knew that they – rather than their partners – would shoulder most of the burden. One woman knew that her partner would be against either abortion or adoption at birth in the event of disability, but

> I'm afraid I thought his reaction was very much based on the premise that I would cope with it, so it was all right for him to make that sort of decision because he wasn't going to have to do anything about it.

Lisa wasn't particularly worried about the possibility of there being something wrong, so although she had a scan she decided against having even the Triple test. She only discovered how preoccupied Rob was with having a disabled child at a weekly antenatal class for couples. They each had to pair off with someone else and talk about their worst fears. In a post-mortem in the car afterwards, Rob admitted that his nightmare was the fear of having a mentally disabled child:

> He also saw this thing in a newspaper, this – what seemed to me – appalling insurance thing which you could take out against your child being handicapped. It's literally a new thing that's come out a month or so ago, and all the societies like Scope and spina bifida and things like that are really anti it.

Pam's partner, Gérard, was worried about disability. Despite being 41 Pam knew that she didn't want a routine amniocentesis, but was happy to have the non-intrusive Triple test. In the event, the Triple test came up with a probability of having an affected child of 1 in 800, compared with Pam's statistical odds based on age alone of 1 in 85. This helped reassure Gérard and gave Pam the confidence to turn down the offer of an amniocentesis.

> I didn't want to have any chance of there being an abortion, not one little chance. Because whether the child – and it took me a long time to decide – had anything wrong with it or not, I was determined to have this baby. And I also had this stupid idea that if I was going to have a Down's syndrome baby, or one with spina bifida, or whatever, then again that was for a reason: that I needed that sort of experience in life.

Some women, like Nicki, did feel that they would be able to cope with a child who had Down's syndrome. Jenny too did not consider asking for screening other than a routine blood test, for the same reason.

> I wouldn't want a Down's syndrome child, but I've looked after one before in Sweden and she was very sweet, so I wouldn't mind and I think I could cope.

Siân, like Joanne and Caroline, just couldn't see why they would have a mentally disabled child since there was no history in either family, so only really worried in the odd flash from time to time.

> You also realise that even if you did have a Down's syndrome child you'd love it as an individual just as much. You just have to keep your fingers crossed.

Lee felt confident that her body would be telling her if there was a problem in any case: 'I would have known if things had been desperately wrong.'

Many people's attitude to disability changes when they already have a child, when practical considerations rather than unspecified fears tend to take over. Tessa was not over-worried in Joe's pregnancy. In her second, however, the prospect of how her family as a whole would cope loomed larger in her mind and she decided to have the Triple test.

> I did it because it existed and to alleviate my worry, although had it been worrisome and had I been forced to have an amnio and that was positive, I honestly still don't know what I would have done. I did it more because I hoped it'd be negative. I look around me and all the children are well and healthy, and I just don't think we can all be that lucky. It's mostly that, really – it's like

thinking one of us will die of cancer and it will probably be me.

She also realised that when she was still a mother-in-waiting she'd had a slightly romantic view of how she and Mark would have coped with a mentally disabled child.

> When I look at any family I know who's had a disabled child of any measure, even a very unseriously damaged Down's syndrome child, still you're looking for schools for them all your life, still you're moving for the child; and then all your other children suffer because that child's life is so important. It's the amount of time and energy you spend on a handicapped child, the amount of money, and not being able to go to work.

Sue, who had had a 'magical pregnancy' with her son Nick, was haunted by the thought of disability through Hannah's nine months. But because she felt her worries were ungrounded, she didn't feel able to ask for any additional screening.

> My reaction was I wouldn't want to know, I'd almost rather it didn't survive. I know that sounds really harsh, but with one child already I kept thinking 'well, it's not just you it's going to affect, it's going to affect him too. He's going to have to live his life round a handicapped brother or sister.'

The only woman interviewed who did ask for – and was given – an amniocentesis was Sasha. Her history of miscarriage made it a traumatic procedure, but with her and Lou 38 and 43 years old respectively, they felt it was the most sensible course to take.

## Genetic Disorders

Not all fears about disability can scientifically be laid to rest. Screening still cannot detect genetic disorders if neither partner has previously been identified as high risk, and there are approximately 3500 different single-gene disorders.

Single-gene disorders fall into three basic categories: those produced by a dominant gene, those produced by a recessive gene and those which can be carried by girls but appear usually in boys, such as haemophilia: if a man has haemophilia none of his sons will inherit it, but all his daughters will be carriers. With each pregnancy the daughter will have a 50 per cent chance of a daughter who is a carrier and a 50 per cent chance of a son who has the condition. With dominant gene disorders anyone who inherits the defective gene from either parent is extremely likely to have the condition. Examples are Huntington's chorea and brittle bones (osteogenesis).

Disorders caused by a recessive gene are those which the child won't inherit unless both parents carry the faulty gene. In Britain the best known are cystic fibrosis and sickle-cell anaemia.

## Cystic Fibrosis

Cystic fibrosis affects the lungs and digestive system and is the most common genetic disability in the Western world, where it strikes one in 2000 babies. One in 25 people is a carrier of the cystic fibrosis gene, and when it is present in both parents there is a 25 per cent chance that the child will be affected. The relevant gene was first tracked down and identified in America in 1989, making accurate carrier testing possible. It also allowed researchers to explore the possibility of using gene therapy – where a faulty gene is replaced by a healthy one – and clinical trials are due to start in 2007.

## Sickle-Cell Anaemia

Sickle-cell anaemia is another recessive gene disorder, which mainly affects black people of African descent. The most recent estimate was that 1 in 10 black Americans is a carrier. Those affected have a lack of red blood cells and the remaining cells, when short of oxygen, form a sickle or S shape. It is painful and debilitating, though not always fatal, and rarely appears before the age of six.

The chances of a child being a sickle-cell anaemia carrier or sufferer are the same as for cystic fibrosis, as they are for two of the less generally known recessive gene disorders, Tay-Sachs disease and beta-thalassaemia (the latter is a rare condition affecting people of Mediterranean origin). Blood taken at the booking visit is tested for both sickle-cell and thalassaemia if either or both partners are considered potential carriers. Tay-Sachs disease usually affects children born to Jewish couples (and, more rarely, if only one partner is Jewish). Babies can be born seemingly normal, but progressive cerebral degeneration starts to begin at the age of about 6 months and few children live beyond their fourth year. The Tay-Sachs test is not routinely offered in Britain, but there has been an intensive and successful screening programme in North America since 1969 where, at one time, an estimated 1 in 30 Ashkenazi Jews was a carrier: the figure for non-Jews was one in 300.

Ironically, for most pregnant women these are calm, enjoyable weeks, despite the needles. Most women are not affected by – or manage to live with – their concern about chromosomal or genetic disorders, but it is rare that a woman never worries at all. I have given so much space to anxiety about disability and testing because it is one of the emotional areas of pregnancy most overlooked. Health and family history are often not what determines the level of worry, and many women are made to feel silly by a medical establishment which often does not take the emotional stresses of pregnancy seriously enough. In some cases dreams are the only outlet, and nightmares of giving birth to a disabled child are very common. If a woman feels that she is experiencing such dreams because her subconscious mind is preparing her for giving birth to a disabled child, then health professionals should find the time to be reassuring and supportive. This is why tests can be so important.

## The Baby

As the halfway mark approaches, for some women the baby is becoming an individual with a character. For many, the scan gives a visual representation of the baby they are getting to know through its movements. Lee had an early scan at 14 weeks which introduced her to her baby: it was some six weeks later that she first felt that bubbly feeling:

> It was at 11.40 p.m. on the 25 November 1989. I was alone in bed and was so overwhelmed that I ran downstairs to get my diary to record the event. It became quite a regular occurrence after that, lying on my back in bed.

Sue felt Nick 'bubbling around' at 20 weeks and her third child, Lottie, was a 'real wriggler' from 16 weeks. Jenny's first child James started at 20 weeks, her second at 18, and Joanne first felt Rowan – nicknamed Stephanie Gertrude – at about 20 weeks. Having felt stirrings at 9 weeks, Nicki did not feel her twins starting to move regularly until 20 weeks. She knew which was which and the fact that one – John – rarely moved did worry her. Her daughter Anna took advantage of the extra space, and 'rolled around like a football team'. With Matthew, who moved at 16 weeks, Fran said, 'it felt like someone was tickling me from inside.'

By 20 weeks I was still wrestling with swollen labia. Some days it felt as if a speculum – that corkscrew thing they insert into your vagina for internal examinations – was stuck inside me, and my navel was flattening itself every day. Felix's movements, however, were wonderful, not so much kicking or tickling as a gentle pushing, as if he was shifting position to get comfortable.

By 18 weeks the baby's arms and legs are well formed; it can now twist and frolic inside the uterine sac. By 20 weeks it is nearly 10in (25cm) long and about 12oz (340g) – the weight of a pack and a half of butter – so it is not surprising that many women emotionally feel that their child is making its presence felt as itself. Some babies spend as much as 90 per cent of their time tumbling about, although the average is nearer 20 per cent. It is at this point that speculation about the baby's sex can take on a different character, where instinct and physical reactions combine to build up a sense of the child as a person.

Tessa's first baby, Joe, moved at 20 weeks, softly at first then increasingly strongly:

> I joked that it was a boy; I said no girl would hurt me like this. It was very active and very gentle, and I knew straight away it was a nice person. You're always right, aren't you, because you always remember the things you were right about.

# Girl or Boy?

## Weeks 20–24

31 MAY 1992: Last night, snuggling on the sofa with Martha, the baby suddenly flipped over in one big, turning movement – like a cat settling down to sleep. Martha looked up at me with real joy on her face. 'The baby's talking to me?' She pulled up my T-shirt, placed her hands either side of my navel and shouted 'Hello', as if down one of those old calling trumpets used to summon staff in huge Victorian houses. She hasn't asked whether it's a girl or a boy, but she is very smug about the idea of being a big sister. I think she's a she . . .

Some of us have an unshakeable gut feeling by now as to whether we are having a girl or a boy. Others have extremely strong convictions but they change from week to week, day to day even. Many have no idea whatsoever. And most of us are influenced, often subconsciously, by the so-called old wives' tales – which of course we don't really take seriously

– as well as by local folklore and friends, who assure us that their predictions 'are never wrong'.

For reasons of filial inheritance, national interest, male primo-geniture, family preferences and economics, people of every period in history, in every country in the world, have tried to predict the sex of a baby. Most superstitions reflect the value society places on supposed female and male attributes: a lively baby is more likely to be considered a boy; a quiet baby, a girl.

## Divining the Sex

In many cultures, even today, it is considered preferable for one's first child to be a boy, and late abortions once a girl has been discovered are still not uncommon.[1] But in many Western societies the desire to know the sex of one's baby is more an emotional than a social issue. Wondering about gender is one way in which some women involve friends and family in their pregnancy. Others feel that knowing the sex of their child will help them adjust to the idea of parenthood. But most speculate for fun, and listen to predictions with a combination of interest and detachment.

In Egypt 4000 years ago physicians would recommend putting wheat and barley seeds into separate cloth purses for the woman to urinate on every day: if the wheat sprouted first, it was a boy. (Needless to say, wheat was a more valued grain than barley.) In Mesopotamia, it was considered that if the forehead of the mother-to-be was heavily freckled then she was carrying a boy. In nineteenth-century Denbighshire, a sheep's shoulderblade was scraped clean, scorched, pierced through the thinnest part, then suspended over the front door. The first non-family person to come through the door the next morning was supposed to be of the same sex as the child.

In Nepal a craving for spicy foods indicates a girl, as does the baby moving before the sixth month of pregnancy or the mother-to-be dreaming of necklaces (dreams of vegetables mean a boy); in Britain, however, the view is that women crave sweet things for a girl, spicy for a boy. Fran had to take three jars of cocktail gherkins with her to school every morning during Matthew's pregnancy, yet didn't develop a sweet tooth during her daughter's pregnancy.

In his wisdom the father of medicine, Hippocrates, pronounced that if a pregnant woman's left eye and left breast were bigger than those on her right, then she was carrying a girl. Serbian folklore has it that first being aware of the baby moving when you are at home means a boy, outside a girl. Nineteenth-century Americans thought dreams of apple pie indicated a boy, cherry pie a girl.

There are of course only two sexes to choose between in this game and superstitions of this type are just as likely to be wrong as right. After all, the odds are even. None of the women interviewed actually believed that they could divine sex, although many commented that the test they had done had been accurate.

The lore that came up most frequently among the women I interviewed was that girls were carried low, boys high. The Ancient Egyptians thought it was the other way round. Another common tale was that women having boys had lumps that stuck out in front and they gained little weight elsewhere, which was true for Debbie and Lisa; a wider lump and larger weight gain – particularly on the hips – signified a girl (presumably the genesis of many a mother/daughter conflict). Caroline, who has two girls and two boys, said that her pregnancy lumps were exactly the same shape every time. So were mine.

For fun, several people – married and not – had let friends do the wedding ring test, which has its origins in sixteenth-century Europe: the ring spins round and round for a girl and up and down for a boy. Alternatively, people used a penny instead of a ring: clockwise revealed a boy, anticlockwise a girl. A friend of Siân's did the Spanish napkin test for her. He draped a napkin over his hand and invited her to take it from him. She took it holding the edge, which indicated that she was carrying a girl; if she'd picked it up from the middle it would have meant a boy. Katherine was born the following October.

A widespread and quite false myth is that boys are more likely to be overdue than girls (Siân's Alexander and Fran's son Matthew were both nearly two weeks late; Tessa's son Joe was nearly three weeks early, her daughter Matilda was late). But some women had been influenced by a more scientific approach, for example that girls' heart rate averages 140 beats per minute and above, whereas boys' rate tends to be lower. Sarah, the trainee NCT teacher who had learnt about these things, was convinced that both her high heart-rate babies were girls, and she was right. But a baby's heartbeat will vary at different times of the day and there were just as many people whose diagnoses had been wrong. Eve's absolutely definite no-two-ways-about-it slow-beating boy turned out to be a daughter and my fast-beating girl was a son.

Among other medically based guestimates Nicki thought that Anna would be a girl because her breasts were much more sore than they'd been with the twins, Max and John. She put this down to an excess of female hormones. Sasha commented wryly that she'd heard that you got worse morning sickness with girls, but after nine months of daily vomiting Freddy was born . . .

In her first pregnancy, Jenny was wrongly convinced that she was having a girl.

I was crossing the road one day and it suddenly flashed into my mind – wrongly – that it was a girl, and I was quite positive from then onwards that it was a girl. We nicknamed her Jules, short for Julia.

Lee and Simon didn't really have a strong gut feeling.

But I'd had a couple of dreams and she looked quite similar to Hannah, although she was a lot plumper, in this grubby white dress with biscuit all over; and that was twice, the same dream, the same child, so then I thought it might be a girl.

## The Baby

Though we don't necessarily trust them, we are all more swayed by our own instincts than by the speculations of others, even our partners'. Between weeks 20 and 24 the baby, although still thin, is doing an awful lot of growing and changing and is becoming much more of a person. The teeth start to form in the jawbone, hair starts to sprout on its head, it can suck its thumb and even hiccup. Tiny creases are beginning to appear on its palms and fingertips. Every woman should have felt pushings and flutterings by 24 weeks, and many comment on how reassuring it is that the movements can be so definite, so firm.

By 24 weeks the fetus is over a foot long (33cm) and weighs around 1.25 lb (570g), a little less than half a bag of flour. It is now that the eyes first open, fluttering their delicate eyelashes. Rapid eye movements, the kind that signify dreaming in adults, might also begin. The baby is aware of light and dark, so if you are facing towards a bright light it will be bathed in a warm, rosy glow. Many women say that this is the time when they really start to have a sense of their baby's individuality, as it makes its character known. Fran had a strong relationship with her first child by this stage.

> With Matthew we were intensely close as a pregnancy. I did everything for him, all the rubbing and patting and talking to the bump, and cuddling; and Jim did massage. Sometimes we used to joke that he tapped back.

## Knowing Your Baby's Sex

They knew that Matthew was a boy, because he presented himself in a very immodest way on the scan and the radiographer commented on it.

> I always wanted a girl and when we saw Matthew was a boy I was so disappointed. But it gave me a couple of months to get over it and prepare myself. I think if I'd found out after I'd given birth, I would have been really upset in the delivery room.

In the second pregnancy both Fran and Jim wanted to have that adjustment time again, so they asked the radiographer if she could assess the sex of their second baby. A girl. Fran was delighted, but at the same time said that having a strong preference *in utero* made no difference at all once the babies arrived. Knowing was more a matter of being able to prepare, and most women who had a preference qualified it by saying that they knew that they would have loved their baby equally whatever its sex. Jane asked to know the sex of the baby at the scan for the same reason: 'Because I wanted a girl, and if it was a boy I would have had time to get used to the idea.'

The radiographer told Pam and Gérard that he would lay a bet on it being a girl, so from that point on they referred to it as Manon and didn't even choose a boy's name. For the next 27 weeks they lived with the idea of a daughter in their heads, until their son Jackson arrived nearly three weeks late.

## Maternal and Paternal Bonding

During this period Gérard formed a strong pre-natal bond with Manon, imagining them all walking out together in the park. Pam never felt that she developed any sort of relationship with the baby:

Not even secretly, in quiet moments on my own, did I feel a deep connection with it. The closest I could get to allowing myself to feel anything was when I let out an involuntary gasp of 'that's my baby' when we first saw it on the screen.

It is perfectly normal to feel ambivalent about a baby during pregnancy, as normal as it is to worry that the antipathy or lack of love will continue after the birth. Psychologists, such as the American Warren Miller, suggest that most women shift towards increasingly wanting the baby as the months pass, regardless of earlier ambivalence.[2] Equally, some women will not feel strong emotion towards their baby until they hold it in their arms.

Many of us fluctuate between loving the unborn baby passionately and resenting it fiercely, often at the same time, and Jenny was worried about being an inadequate mother for this reason: 'Because I did quite resent being pregnant and I didn't like it. I think I thought I'd resent James.'

The important thing to acknowledge is that the experience of pregnancy does not define the relationship a woman will have with her flesh-and-blood child. Women are under a great deal of pressure to love their babies throughout pregnancy for fear of being categorised as an unloving parent. Much of this pressure is caused by the images of maternal perfection that our society encourages women to measure themselves against.

In the 1950s another of the male childcare psychologists, D. W. Winnicott, described a gradual shifting of a mother's sense of self on to the growing baby throughout the pregnancy as an appropriate preparation for motherhood. Contemporary opinion considers that what Winnicott termed 'primary maternal preoccupation' could happen at any time during the pregnancy, but that even if it never happens there will be no ill-effect on the relationship between the woman and the child once it's been born.[3] Pregnancy and parenthood are two wholly different states.

But, like Jenny, most women who experienced little or no sense of connection with their growing babies did feel guilty about it, even if they knew that they were deliberately keeping their feelings at arm's length. On top of the burden of her repeated miscarriages Sasha had powerful fears about abnormality or about the baby dying – she had frequent dreams about giving birth to a monster – and she just couldn't allow herself to think of the baby as a person.

> I wondered why I wasn't able to make a relationship with this thing that was living in me – I was too used to being my own body. I welcomed any sign that he was there, but I think from a totally self-centred point of view; that I was doing it OK, again achievement, some sense of, well, I'm getting on all right with this job.

Eve also didn't bond pre-natally with Annie in any way, and resented the fact that her husband seemed so preoccupied by the baby's welfare:

I didn't have any of this talking to your tummy business, getting to know your baby, it was just this lump growing and I was totally detached from it. And I worried that Stephen would love the baby better than me, and how would he have enough love for both of us.

These worries about ambivalence, this lack of so-called maternal instinct, often surface consciously when fetal movements make the baby hard to ignore. Kicks and pushes testify to the fact that something is living inside your body, a truth which alarmed Jenny first time round.

It felt like a bubble bursting in the same place, over and over again. I felt it was revolting to start off with, like aliens. Second time round the idea wasn't so strange.

I was overwhelmed with a sense that it was ridiculous that my body now contained someone else's body, especially since Martha's movements were more akin to those of a bag of puppies scrambling over one another than those of a tiny baby. Sue also felt that the idea of some living thing in her stomach was bizarre: 'I felt that I'd been invaded, but I didn't feel terribly negative about it.'

Sue's pregnancies were psychologically very different and often it is around this stage (from 20 to 24 weeks, past halfway) that the variations become truly pronounced. For Sue ironically it was the planned pregnancy – Hannah's – that was the most worrying and the one she least enjoyed. She often didn't feel Hannah moving for 24 hours or so, so had little sense of her character. She was also extremely worried about not being able to love this second child. For Sue, the word that most summed up Hannah's pregnancy was guilt.

> I found it difficult to talk to people about it, because I wasn't sure if they'd react badly to me and I didn't need someone being critical – I needed reassurance.

Rachel was tyrannised by both the presence and the absence of fetal movements: she loathed them, but when they stopped she immediately assumed that the baby had died.

> I thought 'There's an alien inside me', and at times I thought it was taking over. I didn't refer to the baby very much: in the later stages I referred to it as she, though.

While not allowing herself to form any sort of bond with Rose, Rachel desperately wanted everything to be all right.

> My public face was I'm me, I can cope in the same way that I ever could cope with things, I'm not different at all. But I was secretly obsessed. All I did at home was lie on my bed and read pregnancy books. I was all on my own with this secret obsession.

## Choosing Names

In many European countries there are registers of acceptable (i.e. Christian) first names that parents can choose from. Any name not on the list is not legally acceptable and the child will be registered as unnamed. (During the first Gulf War a French Muslim tried to name her child Saddam Hussein and was prevented by law.)

There are no such restrictions in Britain, but a baby has to be legally registered by the time it is six weeks old in England and Wales, three weeks old in Scotland. If married, either parent can register the birth. If unmarried, both partners have to go to the Register Office together if both want to be named on the birth certificate. If a couple subsequently marries, they must go back to the registrar to get a new birth certificate for their child.

Of course this paperwork is all some way off. Most people choose names for reasons of taste, not practicality. Siân and Peter didn't feel sure of the sex of either of their children in advance. With Alexander they had a good selection of approved boy's names but had no instinct for a girl; with their second child Katherine the situation was reversed. It was as if subconsciously they knew which names they would need.

Some children have names-in-waiting, one for a girl, one for a boy. Other parents draw up a shortlist and feel that they will take a look at the baby before deciding. Others, for reasons of superstition or boredom with the whole matter, decide to wait until the day.

In 2005 the most popular girl's name in England and Wales was Jessica, followed by Emily and Sophie. Among boys there were more Jacks than any other name, then Joshuas and Thomases. In Scotland, Sophie and Lewis topped the lists.[4]

## Nicknames

With Martha I was too superstitious to choose names, although we mused endlessly and I even scoured the credits on television programmes looking for inspiration. There was also a part of me that felt that it was somehow rather presumptuous to choose both a girl's name and a boy's name, since the baby had a sex and it wasn't the baby's fault that we didn't yet know it. The nickname Bean had appeared at some early stage in the pregnancy – perhaps descriptive, perhaps sarcastic, we can't remember. It was universally used partly to avoid 'the baby' or 'it', and partly in response to my mounting irritation every time someone asked if 'he' was kicking yet.

When people referred to my baby as 'he', they were using the male pronoun to encompass both the masculine and the feminine. To me, this is a powerful and subversive way of ensuring that the norm is presented as male, as if everyone and everything is masculine unless stated otherwise. Our baby was certainly not going to be categorised in this way, even if it did turn out to be a he. So Bean it was and – until she started 'big school' – Martha, the name on her birth certificate, was plucked out of the highly charged air of the delivery room, never having been mentioned before.

Lynne and John nicknamed their baby Pandora: John had always wanted a daughter called Pandora but Lynne hated the name. 'So this was a compromise; he was allowed to have a fetus called Pandora.' Ironically, Lynne commented that several midwives had cautioned against referring to the baby as 'she', just in case it was a boy. She joked that she was only redressing the balance, since most pregnancy books and magazines use 'he' to represent both sexes. The confident rejoinder was, 'Ah, but that's different . . .'

Debbie was convinced that Jack was a boy, so before he was born he was nicknamed Billy Badger. She was only half-sure about David being a boy, so he stayed as 'the baby' or 'the bump'.

Ten years before, when teaching in China together, Joanne and Georgina had called the child that they would one day have Stephanie Gertrude. Despite choosing a unisex name, Rowan, for their real baby, the ever-faithful nickname Stephanie Gertrude was still used during the pregnancy, even though Joanne was sure they were having a boy.

Sarah was convinced that Kirsty was a girl, so although they referred to her as 'it' their shortlist of boys' names was really rather short. Then with Abigail, they both thought they would like another girl: 'I think Mike was quite bowled over by this charming little girl he'd got, so wanted another.' Again they kept their options open with a long list of girls' names: Kirsty was named on the third day, Abigail on the second.

In subsequent pregnancies, some women felt that they would be more comfortable having the same sex again since they knew what to do. There was a sense that as the mother of a daughter, another daughter would be easier. Others felt that it would be easier to have a child of the opposite sex, so that each child could be distinct and special in its own right.

After the twins Nicki was hoping for a daughter, but she was also worried that if she had a third boy then he would not feel different: the twins were special because they were twins, a daughter would be special for being the only girl. In fact throughout the twins' pregnancy both Nicki and Mike were convinced that they had a girl and a boy; so Max and Sally they were called, and Sally only became John – much to everyone's surprise – once he'd been born.

Sharon had no feelings about the sex of her twins and found it difficult to identify one set of thumps from the other. She was anxious about her lack of instinct, worried that it intimated that she wasn't going to be a loving mother. From time to time she wished she was only having one baby, which exacerbated her feelings of inadequacy: 'It was a very odd feeling: what if they're ugly, what if I don't like them, what if they cry all the time?'

The guilt was fuelled by the fact that she desperately didn't want two boys. She and her husband could only agree on the names Charlotte and James, good solid names, so when two daughters were born they were stumped. Gary asked the wonderful, supportive student doctor what she was called: when she replied 'Katie' the second twin was named.

Since we have no choice in the matter most of us try to want a boy and a girl by turns. And we can think of positive reasons for preferring either. Whilst wanting a girl, Tessa at the same time thought it would be special for her first child to be a son, partly for her parents' sake. This was not because the potential grandparents thought that boys were better than girls, but more because of the cultural and social significance of sons within the Jewish community.

> There's something public about a boy. Having a girl is like having yourself, and the thought of a girl inside me felt very normal. The thought of a boy inside me felt like something from outside was inside me.

But Tessa and Mark did want a name that could be as Jewish or non-Jewish as their child wanted it to be. They settled on Joseph, abbreviated to Joe.

As Catholics living in Northern Ireland, Debbie and Patrick were faced with another sort of choice. With Jack and David they chose names that would not, as they saw it, label their children as belonging to one community or another: there is a tendency for Catholics to choose traditional Irish names.

It is also true that however strong a woman's preference for one sex or the other, once the baby is out most of us cannot imagine it being anything other than it is. Your child is not a girl or a boy, it's simply and obviously your baby. I was convinced that Felix was Florence, right up to the point when he was born. I looked down at my new daughter after the birth and what went through my head was that she had a penis. Immediately I couldn't imagine why I had ever thought he was a girl. Since both Martha and Felix dislike the name Florence, they've often joked that he had a lucky escape!

## Family Pressures

Of course family prejudices are another matter, and many relations do unwittingly – sometimes deliberately – exert pressure both on names and on sex. If there are already four granddaughters then perhaps the birth of a boy will be hailed with greater enthusiasm. Many women and men find this pressure upsetting for emotional reasons, intolerable for political ones. It implies that the baby will be valued more for its sex than for its individuality. Caroline admitted that she partly wanted girls because she was worried that her two feminist sisters wouldn't show any interest in a boy.

If the parents show any hesitation about names, the 'why don't you call it . . . ?' question can soon become oppressive. Many women commented that their parents continually asked them if they had decided on names for the baby, then criticised every one and suggested alternatives. As one woman said,

> I went along with their questions at first, but my mother and father hated every name. They're real snobs, and all their ideas were snobbish, I thought. It was like they wanted to make the baby sound upper-class or something. I didn't think it was their business anyway.

Others don't mind the continual phone calls, and welcomed the involvement. Debra both comes from a close-knit, loving family and has married into one. She felt that discussion over names was one of the most natural ways in which to express interest.

> My sister said, 'I hope you don't choose a name that sounds as if it's nothing to do with us. It's just got to feel right for our family.' And I think she was right.

They called their son Edward.

### The Surname

In the end, choosing a baby's first name is usually less stressful and challenging than the problems that can arise over the surname. If the two parents are married and both use the same name, there isn't anything to discuss. For some, changing one's name is an important rite of passage, visibly marking the psychological shift from child into woman. Many women also feel that the honorific 'Mrs' gives them status in the adult world. But more and more married couples use separate surnames today, not just for professional purposes but in all spheres of their lives.

History is a pattern of male lines, of 'who giveth this woman to be married?' followed by the bride's name being subsumed into the male dynasty, a practice now rejected by many. And increasing numbers of women do not want their status defined by the title Mrs.

For countless people – married or not – the politics has been easy to accommodate until the decision is made to have a baby. Some women realise only at this point that their male partners expect the child to bear their name.

Greg and I were not married at the time – in fact we waited until 2001, when Martha and Felix were old enough to be the witnesses and make the speeches before we made a formal social commitment – but four months into the pregnancy Greg decided that he would like to change his surname to Mosse by deed poll: partly because he had no positive attachment to his surname; secondly, because he felt it would minimise the practical difficulties; and thirdly emotionally, because he wanted to have a visible and identifiable connection to his family. For others the problem was harder to resolve.

It had not occurred to Jeremy that his and Rachel's baby would not have his surname, despite the fact that Rachel had legally kept her name when they married.

It threw into sharp relief the whole reason I'd kept my own name; I always assumed it was a feminist statement, but it's not really. It's more to do with feeling a part of the Scottish heritage than anything and I quite wanted the baby to have my surname. But Jeremy absolutely wouldn't countenance it, even for one second.

Lisa and Rob decided to double-barrel their surnames for Harry: the issue was whether or not they should retain their own names, or double-barrel too so that the three of them had a common family name.

Nicki and Mike, although married, have different surnames and as they put it, 'didn't want to lumber their children with a double-barrelled moniker'. Instead they decided to use both names – without a hyphen – but as soon as the twins went to school only the second of the two names (Mike's) was used, a situation that doesn't entirely satisfy Nicki.

Eve and Stephen, whose daughter Annie is now four, faced a similar problem.

I was not going to lose my name, which Stephen quite understood, but didn't see why I should want him to lose his name on the same principle. And then you start getting into these grand philosophical and political debates about who's oppressing who . . .

Eve's name is the one used on forms. Stephen, like Nicki, feels unhappy.

There was never any question over Rowan's surname. The name of Joanne's sperm donor does not appear there or on the birth certificate itself. Georgina's surname, however, is one of his middle names.

Of course for many women it is just not an important issue. Jane, like Sasha, kept her own surname when she married, for professional purposes, but didn't care at all if Sophie had Matt's surname or hers. Pam was equally happy for Jackson to have Gérard's surname, even though they weren't married.

Names are often one of the things that people first ask about when you tell them that you are pregnant. It's an easy way to initiate conversation. The ways people react can be very disappointing, not least if they reveal their image of you as being qualitatively different from your self-image.

## Breaking the News

The question of when to tell people that you are pregnant will eventually be superseded by your expanding waist measurement. It may also be forced on you by the exhaustion of your supply of excuses for absences from work caused by morning sickness and antenatal check-ups. You will have to judge at what point reliably discreet friends and relations can be told if you want to guard against the all too probable 'leaks'. People can become competitive, anxious to show that they are the most important friend by boasting that they were the first to know.

If you are no longer on your first pregnancy you may find that your audience was much more excited first time round and your proud announcement is greeted with comments such as, 'Another baby, that's marvellous . . .' or a surprised 'Already?' So it can be a finely balanced decision as to when to break the news.

There is a tradition that you don't tell people in the first three months in case you miscarry; others who have decided on screening tests and know they would have an abortion for severe disability may feel that they would rather wait until – if – the baby is given a clean bill of health. But although some of the women interviewed did follow the three-month disclosure rule, women mostly felt that if they did miscarry or have to terminate they would rather that people knew and could share in their grief.

Lynne and John started telling people as soon as they knew

they had conceived. Obviously they hoped they wouldn't have to go back to people to tell them that something had gone wrong, but they still very much felt 'that at least this way they know the good bit before the bad bit'.

Caroline too broke the news immediately: 'Although I didn't get the phone book out and ring everybody. I told family, then friends, as and when I met them.' Caroline found that people's reactions varied enormously, particularly on her fourth pregnancy when people assumed it was a mistake and few responded with any level of enthusiasm. When pregnant with Anna, Nicki found that people assumed it was an accident since the twins were only 20 months old, and in fact looked no more than 16: 'People would come up to me and ask how I would manage when the next baby was born, or ask how old the twins would be when the baby was born.'

Some families subtly or explicitly pressurise their adult children, by hinting at how much they would like to be grandparents or implying that they expect their children to produce children of their own. One woman thinks that her mother actually needed her daughter to become a mother. 'By having children she thought that I was somehow endorsing her, by choosing to do the same as she had done.'

Others were surprised at how important an issue it seemed to be for their parents. Most women interviewed admitted that when they broke the news their thoughts were wholly – and rightly – for themselves as mothers and fathers-to-be: they did not consider how complex their own parents' emotions might be about being grandmothers and grandfathers-to-be. Some women admitted that they – and their partners – had unrealistic expectations of how their respective parents would react to the news, as if the knowledge itself would immediately make them closer. As one woman said of her partner:

My husband's not got much of a relationship with his
parents. But when we went to tell them I still think he
expected his father to be interested and pleased for us.
He wanted them to throw their arms around him, to be
parents in fact. But it would have been out-of-character
for them. They were as lukewarm as always. Afterwards
he said he was embarrassed at minding so much.

Eve was disappointed by her parents' inability to celebrate.
They had always hinted at how much they would like grand-
children, so she expected excitement, endorsement even. She
and Stephen tried to make it a special occasion, going over
on Mothering Sunday with a bottle of champagne to break
the news; their response was the same noncommittal 'oh
that's nice' they'd given to her A-level results, her degree,
her PhD . . . 'I wanted someone to hug me, someone to burst
into tears, someone to open the champagne.'

I was surprised and upset by my parents' reaction. Their
first comment when I told them about being pregnant with
Martha was, 'are you going to get married?' Second time
round, though, they were unreservedly delighted. And that
meant a lot to me.

Lynne was irritated, more than upset, by her parents' bland
response.

They were far worse than I thought they'd be. My
mother had always wanted me to have a baby, and she
used to do this awful thing like grab people's babies
and say 'oh Lynne, isn't this baby lovely?' and I'd say,
'yes, and it's not mine'.

Lee and Simon also told people straight away. But since they
had just married after nine years of living together they didn't
anticipate that anyone would be surprised. Debbie and Patrick

told their families immediately, but did wait until the so-called danger period was over before telling friends and colleagues. Debbie, like several women, rather liked having such a special, secret, piece of news. 'It's quite nice to keep the knowledge to yourself for a while.'

Jenny, on the other hand, would rather not have told anyone for as long as possible, but the decision was taken out of her hands.

> I found it quite difficult to tell people – in fact, I felt sort of quite difficult about the idea of me being pregnant – I just couldn't cope with the image of me being pregnant.

Because Jenny didn't find out about James until she was 12 weeks pregnant, and because of her worries about having had antibiotics and the mini-pill during that time, she and Bruce had decided not to tell anyone until after the 16-week scan. Since they were living in South Africa, with most of their family and friends based in England, there was little pressure to explain her persistent sickness. Then, at about 14 weeks, a colleague who was also pregnant decided to tell their boss. After the customary congratulations, the boss joked

> 'Pippa's just told me she's pregnant. I hope you're not!' And of course I went bright red. But I couldn't lie to her, then a couple of weeks later tell her I was.

Joanne wasn't superstitious about telling people, but she did want to keep it quiet for as long as possible at the primary school where she worked as a music teacher. Few people knew about her domestic situation and she didn't relish the sorts of questions she might be asked.

At her primary school Fran told her headmaster at 8 weeks. His only reaction, rather snidely given, was that she would have to change her title from Miss to Mrs so as not to offend parents . . .

Many women who do decide to keep the news to themselves find it slipping out because, as Tessa says, 'it's the nicest news to tell people'. Rob and Lisa had made a practical decision only to tell family and close friends; emotionally, though, they wanted to tell everyone straight away. Then when Lisa was 8 weeks pregnant they went on holiday.

> In Morocco we told everybody, every single Moroccan we met, the whole world, because it just didn't matter. I was incredibly ill at that point, but I used to think about this little thing growing inside me and I just used to skip for joy, over and over again, I just felt so happy.

## Keeping it Quiet at Work

For many women the worry about how and when to tell employers can be extremely stressful. In 1996 women's pay, hour for hour, was still only 70 per cent of men's. Only six High Court Judges were women, the House of Commons was still 91 per cent male and a mere 1.7 per cent of science professors in universities were women.[5] The unwritten subtext was that mothers were still a third-rate choice for employers, after men and childless women.

Some women felt that the discrimination against working mothers started as soon as they announced their pregnancy, and that the timing of the announcement could make a great deal of difference to their professional futures. As Jane said, 'people look on you as suddenly having less ambition, as being more staid and stable.'

In 2006, women's pay in comparison to men's has risen slightly to 74 per cent and there are just as many women working as men. Even so, women make up just 26 per cent of senior civil servants and 23 per cent of top management posts so we still have a way to go.[6]

## Maternity Rights

Women are allowed paid time off for antenatal care however long they've been in their jobs and however many hours a week they work. But the new rules and regulations governing who gets what from whom are extremely complicated and are being updated all the time, partly because of home-grown pressure and partly because of the influence of Brussels and the European Union.

Many professional women will have specific employment contracts that cover their maternity rights and provisions. Always – always – check the small print. For those without personalised contracts, there are two basic provisions – Statutory Maternity Pay and Maternity Allowance – as well as the unpleasantly-named Incapacity Benefit.

Leaflet NI17A covers all aspects of current maternity provision and is available from social security offices and antenatal clinics. What follows is just a digest, although wholly indigestible . . . I've also listed benefit helplines in the address section at the end of the book – altogether more human and easier to understand.

## Statutory Maternity Pay

If you have been working at the same place without a break for at least 26 weeks (including and ending with the fifteenth week before the week your baby is born) and you have been paying national insurance contributions, then you should qualify for Statutory Maternity Pay. If you have more than one employer, you might – only might – be able to get SMP from both of them.

For women due in or after April 2007, SMP can be paid for up to 39 weeks, starting at 11 weeks before the baby is due at the earliest. Usually, though, SMP starts from the week following the week you stop work. You will get 90 per cent of your average weekly earnings for the first 6 weeks, then a reduced flat rate after that.

You don't have to claim SMP as such, but you must tell your employer at least 28 days before you intend to leave work. In most cases, of course, they will have noticed . . .

## Maternity Allowance

If you are self-employed or have recently changed jobs, you might find that you don't qualify for SMP but instead can go for Maternity Allowance. This does involve form-filling (form MA1) and you must have earned an average of at least £30 per week in the 66 weeks before you give birth or, if you are self-employed, paid enough Class 2 national insurance contributions to be eligible. It can be paid for 39 weeks, starting from the eleventh week before your baby is due or later if you're still working. The money will be paid either directly into your bank or building society or can be cashed at your local post office. If you don't qualify for either SMP or Maternity Allowance you may be entitled to Incapacity Benefit around the time of your baby's birth.

Most of the women I talked to had done their maternity paperwork, but most admitted thinking less about their financial positions than about how their professional images might change once it was known that they were pregnant. As Eve said: 'Mothers are not taken seriously at work. There are a lot of unreconstructed men around who make it difficult and who disapprove.'

There is no more fundamental psychological and social shift than that of non-parent to parent, and the first time round you have as much mental adjusting to do as physical and practical. Until you are comfortable with your changing status it is difficult to convey the news to an employer, especially if you think they might be unsupportive. But once you have a child, your status as a parent in your own eyes and the eyes of the world is already established. Friends and colleagues will not be surprised if you announce that you are pregnant again and, since you have already successfully balanced career and parenthood, fewer assumptions will be made about how you will cope. On a second or subsequent pregnancy, the adjustments are predominantly, although not wholly, practical: the cost of childcare for two, the difficulties of getting two children out of the house in the mornings and still arriving at work on time, tiredness, having enough love for both of them . . .

## Telling the Boss

When I became pregnant with Martha I was working for a publisher and my rights on paper were extremely good, well above the state minimum. But I was involved in negotiating a deal on maternity leave on behalf of the workforce, and I didn't want the strength of the case undermined by the management feeling that I had a vested interest. I also knew that carrying on as usual when pregnant – before anyone knew I was pregnant – was the most effective way of signalling to my employers that my ambition and commitment were unchanged even if my figure wasn't. I made the announcement officially at 20 weeks, when the pallor, untucked shirts and avoidance of coffee were beginning to tell their own tale anyway.

Many women still feel guilty about being pregnant and taking leave, as if they are somehow letting their employer down. And if the company has an established pattern of women leaving when they become pregnant, or refusing to take anything more than limited maternity leave, then it is especially difficult to insist on one's full entitlement. On the other hand, if the company has had experience of women whose careers have continued to flourish despite having been pregnant and who have taken sensible maternity leave, the pressures about when to make the announcement are less pronounced. Siân, a senior television producer, was not worried about her boss's response for this reason.

> There were so many women who'd had kids over the past few years that I didn't feel that I was blazing a trail. I was certainly aware that I'd had a role model, a woman who had two children and who managed to carry on holding down her job and committing herself to it totally. So I knew it could be done.

Still, she was in no hurry to tell people at work while she was still coming to terms with it herself:

> You do feel different, you are aware that your body is sheltering something else, and even at the early stages there are times when your mind is elsewhere: and you can't really cover that up I don't think.

Siân finally broke the news officially at 13 weeks, when she was about to be sent on an assignment to Mozambique and would have had to have inoculations, such as that for yellow fever, which are contraindicated in pregnancy.

Rachel, who works in the City, wanted to keep the news secret from people at work for as long as possible, especially since she'd just started a new job. She was not worried about losing her job or not receiving maternity benefit; but she was more anxious about the long-term effects on her career.

I wanted to get something under my belt, I wanted to prove myself in some way before they knew I was pregnant. I didn't want to talk about it even, I didn't want anyone to make allowances for me – and I didn't even acknowledge it really. I just wanted to carry on, to prove myself. I just put it out of my mind.

Because Rachel put on weight so noticeably and so quickly, work colleagues had in fact guessed by the time she was about 13 weeks pregnant. Sasha, who stayed extremely small, managed to keep the secret until about 22 weeks.

It's a lot to do with this bloody working woman business, and having to keep up the front that you haven't gone woolly-edged, that your brain is still functioning, you aren't emotionally about to burst into tears all the time – which you are – that you can still concentrate. You have to be even more the things you're supposed to be because you're pregnant, and so I had to work harder, I had to be a better artist, I had to be a better teacher, to take on more challenges . . . and I had to not look pregnant.

Because of the fear that her pregnancy was ectopic, Tessa felt it only fair to tell her employers why she had to be away from work for so long.

Mistake. That was my first big mistake. To be alone and emotional in Glasgow and tell people at work. Ideally, the fact that you had a baby on your hip and a script under your arm would make you be seen as a better person. I don't think that generation has arrived yet, but perhaps we might be it.

Tessa paid the price for her honesty and good faith. When she came back from sick leave certain things she'd been promised – maternity leave for the future, a renewed long-term contract, relocation expenses for moving to Glasgow – had been withdrawn; or, rather, no one claimed to know that they had been offered in the first place.

> It's typical of large institutions not to care about women. Which means that even if I'd had seven consecutive contracts over seven years I still wouldn't have been entitled to maternity benefit.*

The best she could do was to try to negotiate as favourable a financial deal as possible, but there was no possibility of her job being kept open.

Many women, including Lynne, faced a similar sort of disapproval from their employers. Another woman found that although the company was legally bound to keep her job open, it was clear that her career there was considered over.

> The offer was there, however it came with all sorts of conditions attached such as returning in a changed role. My boss basically didn't like women with children. I was written off the moment I told her.

Professional women are too often expected to keep their personal and working lives separate. The visible evidence of a growing stomach defies this and challenges colleagues to

---

* Short-term contracts, whereby people are employed for only 11 months then their contracts renegotiated, are becoming more and more popular with employers. In this situation companies do not have to pay statutory maternity benefits or redundancy payments because an individual's employment is not deemed to have been continuous in the eyes of the law.

distinguish the mother-to-be from the pre-pregnant woman. As Tessa found.

> It's very hard to be taken seriously at work, big, so that was a big problem. The bigger you get, the more difficult it is to sit with authority in a meeting.

I now regret hiding, then ignoring, my pregnancy. As Rachel, who did the same, commented: 'Part of me felt I was denying my real self. Deep in my heart I wanted this baby and to be a mother more than anything.'

It might well be true that a particular company or department will suffer if a key woman is away on maternity leave, but our working practices are hardly exemplary, often not cost-effective and few workers have the sort of job satisfaction and quality of life they deserve. Working patterns in the so-called developed world need reforming. So why do we agree that our pregnancies are inconvenient, reassure that we will take the minimum leave, allow our bodies to be used as 'proof' of mental incapacity? It is actually an excuse for discrimination, on the principle of divide and rule. And those senior female executives who allow themselves to be manipulated into working until 24 hours before delivery and being back at their desks within two weeks of having given birth, are helping to ensure the longevity of this anachronistic system. The Ancient Egyptians, the Romans and the American Confederate South all made the same claims for the efficiency of their economic systems: that productivity would suffer, that society would crumble if they changed their working patterns. Of course they were talking about slavery . . .

Most working mothers have done a lot to challenge the prehistoric prejudices against women who have children. They have disproved the thesis that working mothers are unreliable, unambitious or that their commitment is questionable. If things are to improve further, it is the turn of fathers to put their careers on hold by refusing to work longer than their contractual hours in order to play an equal role in childcare. Since the introduction of paid paternity leave there have been great improvements, but men must also talk about being expectant fathers. It is only in this way that parenting will no longer be seen as women's business alone.

Every professional woman interviewed acknowledged that there were obstacles, even if their careers had continued to follow their chosen path without being impeded by pregnancy. Becoming a mother does not automatically make it harder to pursue a career, although being aware of potential difficulties can help a woman to circumvent them. Many women also felt that the sense of perspective that parenthood had given them had made them better at their jobs, and widened their expertise and ability to face challenges. Despite her experience Tessa was positive.

> My career has not been damaged yet, at all; I imagine it could be damaged now with a second child, except that I feel that I'm in a position of a fair amount of experience.

As a freelance stylist for pop videos, Pam felt that her position and experience were unassailable. She was able to stop working when it suited her and still hold on to clients. Nicki, a manager of a large college, said, 'I have achieved everything I could possibly have achieved by this stage in my career anyway, regardless of having children.'

Eve acknowledged that her attitude to her career had changed, but felt that the promotions she had been offered since having Annie were appropriate to her expertise.

So now in a sense although I'm more senior, have a much rosier future ahead of me, I have a feeling of why should the career always take priority, why should I sell my soul to a company that may or may not make me redundant? Whereas in a way now what I would like in an ideal world is to have enough money to be able just to quit for two years and not to have to worry. What I don't want is this awful juggling. So it's not my career for the sake of my career any more, it's more material concerns.

## The Macho Work Culture

The hours people spend at work in Britain are the highest in Europe. For many women, particularly those with high-powered careers, the atmosphere at work is often very competitive. It is not so much the job itself that is demanding, but the number of extra hours they are expected to put in as a sign of their commitment: staying late, going for a drink after work, going through things at home in the evenings, always being available at short notice, and so on. It is clearly impossible for most parents to work in this way, but the pressures exerted by this sort of macho work culture take their toll even before the baby has been born. As one woman put it:

I suddenly realised that I wasn't seen as a high-flier any more the minute I said I was pregnant. They were suspicious of anyone whose No. 1 priority wasn't getting on in the company. I got through all my work as usual, but I didn't want to spend half the evening in a smoky pub any more. I was just too exhausted by the end of the day to do all that boys' stuff, and it wore me out trying to keep up.

However well you feel, pregnancy is tiring. The temptation to try to carry on as usual is very strong, but it is hard to live by the 'work until you drop' philosophy as pregnancy progresses. For women who spend much of their working day on their feet, or have jobs with little flexibility, the physical demands can become too much.

> My direct boss was awful. I felt I had to make excuses for feeling tired – for being pregnant, in fact – because I'm out and about all the time in my job. I even tried to make all my antenatal appointments early in the morning or after work. Then I thought, I wouldn't be doing this if I had flu or something.

The most important thing at work is to try, in so far as it is within your power, to balance your needs as a pregnant woman with your ambitions as a professional one.

## You're Going to be a Big Sister/ Brother

If the timing of your announcement at work is a delicate issue, your older child's reaction can be an even greater challenge. Many parents have mixed feelings about having a second child. They may feel that their existing child will feel inadequate or abandoned. If you express your ambivalence to your child then she or he is likely to feel threatened rather than excited by the prospect of a sibling. But if you allow them to share in the pregnancy, then they are more likely to be welcoming and enthusiastic.

The age and maturity of your other child or children are obviously important factors. If they are old enough they might hear from other quarters, so need to be told as soon as possible: then you risk them becoming bored with waiting. If they're still babies themselves they're just not going to understand, so you can delay telling them: but they might resent you being more tired and having less emotional energy. Most young children like tiny babies and are quite possessive: if they feel you are still very interested in them, they are more likely to boast about becoming a big sister or brother than they are to feel jealous.

The best rule of thumb is to let your child decide when she or he is ready. I am pretty flat-chested normally, but blew up as soon as I became pregnant. Martha was delighted by these wonderful, cushion-like things that had suddenly appeared. I don't know whether or not this fascination was spurred by a subconscious memory of having been breastfed, or whether it was simple curiosity on her part. But it made it easy to explain that my body was changing shape because there was a baby in it.

Debbie and Patrick found it easy to tell Jack, not least because they live in a Northern Ireland community where babies and children are part of everyday life.

> The family's all-important still and if you go to a family there's even teenage boys cooing over babies. It's a really different society from Britain, and everyone's been in contact with babies really.

Fran and Jim talked to Matthew a lot about the new baby. He seemed to take the news with equanimity until about 24 weeks. When they started to get the cot out and prepare practically, he developed a bad stutter, especially on the letter 'm'. The stutter disappeared two days after his sister Rowan's birth.

Siân and Peter told their son Alexander just before his second birthday, when Siân was about four months pregnant. They introduced the subject gradually, and although he showed little interest the information did gradually sink in.

> A few weeks before the birth we were sitting on the couch. I was reading a story to him when he said 'baby sit there, Alexander here', as if I was in the middle. So he'd made a place for the baby on the couch apparently, although I've still no idea what that meant or what he'd thought to make him say that.

One woman was worried about how her daughter would react to another child, especially since as a full-time mother they spent most of their time in each other's company. 'She very much hated me touching another child, or picking up a baby, so it was a worry.'

A close friend had a baby when she was about three months pregnant, so it was at that point that they started to talk gently to her daughter about having a brother or a sister. 'She was too young for me to see if she understood: whether or not she did, I still don't know. But she was fine.'

Jenny also spent most of her time with James, so was worried about him feeling left out and displaced. She too used the occasion of having visited a friend's newborn baby to start explaining that she was pregnant and they were going to have a new baby too. James asked how it would get out, and when Jenny said that a doctor would help, his response was, 'what, take the lid off?'

Sue and Max had a difficult choice as to whether or not to go ahead with her third, unplanned pregnancy, so they decided to involve Nick and Hannah, who were by then six and four. Nick was very keen on having a brother, Hannah was equally keen on having a sister: the decision was made to go ahead, even though one of them was bound to be disappointed! Both children were extremely interested in the baby all the way through pregnancy, loving to watch Sue's stomach lurching from side to side.

## Physical Changes

While your mind and emotions are occupied with all these decisions, your body is changing, although perhaps not as dramatically as during other four-week periods. Often it's a matter of women catching up, when those whose bumps had not been very visible will start to look pregnant and those lucky souls who have escaped heartburn and indigestion up to this point – like Debbie – may suddenly become aware that the baby has displaced their stomach:

> There's an old wives' tale in Ireland that heartburn means a lot of hair on the baby, but in fact I had less heartburn with David and he had more hair.

Several women said that it was at this point that they started to be cursed by cramp, and Sarah developed painful sacroiliac joints in her second pregnancy at about 22 weeks: 'One week I just couldn't move. I don't know how I got through the week, I could hardly get up the stairs.'

I found that the skin round the side of the bump was starting to feel tight. Some skin obviously stretches more easily than others: the average woman has 17 square feet of skin on her body, which stretches to 18.5 square feet by the ninth month of pregnancy!

By and large most women felt that these weeks were physically enjoyable: they looked properly pregnant but didn't feel too heavy and uncomfortable. They had acclimatised themselves to the physical niggles of pregnancy, the inconvenience of twinges, trapped nerves and surprising jolts when leaping rather than rolling out of bed. As Jenny put it,

What I learnt from pregnancy was nothing stays the same for very long. So when you've got this pain in your side, you think it's going to be there for the next six months, but it isn't.

## Colostrum

The one distinctive physical change that can happen between 20 and 24 weeks – although it is usually noticeable much later in first pregnancies – is for the nipples to start to secrete colostrum. Colostrum is the form of milk which will feed your baby in its first few days before your proper milk comes in. I didn't notice it until I was 30 weeks pregnant with Martha. Lying in a bath one night, this pale, white liquid seeped out of my breasts without invitation, like wreaths of cigarette smoke floating on the hot water. I had no idea what it was, and at once hauled myself out of the bath and over to my nearest pregnancy book to see if it was normal. If this was supposed to happen, then surely someone would have mentioned it at my antenatal visit. With Felix I could express colostrum two months earlier, from about 22 weeks.

> 5 JUNE 1992: it's really hot and close. I'm feeling pretty heavy and breathless, and the stairs are crippling me. Breasts very sore and heavy, then when I squeezed my nipples yesterday I discovered to my horror that my colostrum has already come in. Why so early, it's not as if it's of any use ...

# Anyone for Sex and Love?

## Weeks 24–28

> My mother, heavy with me, cried for apples. She did
> not mind if they were Coxes, Granny Smiths, or even
> Bramleys, just so long as they were crisp, sharp, and
> there in front of her. While she does not openly boast
> of her cravings, she was clearly pleased that she did
> have them, as though they helped to confirm her role
> as a mother. Personally, I suspect they were also a way
> of involving my father, by making him drive through
> suburban London before dawn in search of an all-night
> greengrocer.
>
> Jeremy MacClancy, *Consuming Culture*[1]

For most women these are tranquil weeks. You are over
halfway there. You are large, but you're not yet too big to
be comfortable. (Every other person you meet will pronounce
– undeterred by science or experience – that you are small
or big 'for your dates'.) Most of the physical discomforts
have been assimilated into your daily routine: the odd twinge

here, heartburn after a rich meal, stairs torturing your calves, the frequent visits to the loo. Most of the inconveniences specific to later pregnancy have not made their presence felt. Jenny even climbed Table Mountain when she was six months pregnant!

## Physical Changes

By 25 weeks into pregnancy your heart and lungs are doing 50 per cent more work, which means that not only do many women feel hotter and sweatier than usual, but foot ache, leg ache and backache might begin. These problems – breathlessness too – were much, much more severe for those women whose babies were born in the summer and early autumn.

Caroline and Tessa, who had September and August babies, started to suffer from cramp. Salt and a high calcium intake, in the form of a calcium and magnesium supplement, can help avoid cramp in the long term, as can adding wheatgerm to your food. Herbalists might suggest a decoction of cramp bark, but the only immediate remedy is to flex your foot or calf backwards, as Tessa found.

It was only because I read in a book not to point your toe but to move your foot backwards that I was able to deal with it, because it was really sudden and painful.

Eve, returning from a holiday in Italy at 26 weeks, noticed that her lower limbs were swelling into special effects for a horror film:

I remember sitting in the car then suddenly looking down at my feet, and I couldn't see my ankles. It was the most frightening thing I'd ever seen, mutant feet, little blobs of jelly!

### Backache

Backache affects the majority of pregnant women at some stage during their pregnancies. After the sixteenth week the weight of the growing baby pushing down in the pelvis can tip the pelvic brim forward. Together with the ever-growing weight as the pregnancy marches on, this puts a strain on the muscles and ligaments surrounding the lower spine. The hormone relaxin, which is present in high levels during pregnancy, has softened the muscles and ligaments around the back in preparation for labour, and this general elasticity means that they are all more liable to be stretched and to ache. It takes until three to five months after the birth for the relaxin levels to go back to normal, so backache can continue to be a problem even when you are no longer pregnant.

If you do suffer from backache try putting your feet up on cushions when you can and avoid sitting cross-legged. Don't stand still or sit in the same position for too long. Let your legs not your back take the strain when picking up heavy, awkward-shaped objects (such as other children) and take regular exercise. I felt crippled by backache in Martha's pregnancy but with Felix, when I had the time to go swimming most days, I had backache on no more than about five occasions towards the very end.

Women with multiple pregnancies often find that most symptoms are exaggerated. Nicki, who is only 4ft 9in, had a lot of backache with the twins, partly because of the additional weight. 'Have you ever worn an X-Ray apron? It was like that with the twins, like sleeping under concrete.'

At 24 weeks with Felix my bump was beginning to feel uncomfortable when I lay on my side, so I started to wedge a small cushion under it in bed at night. Because my abdominal muscles had already been stretched by my first pregnancy I needed the cushion six weeks earlier with Felix. I also started to be aware of strong and regular Braxton Hicks contractions at this stage. I liked them. They boosted my confidence that my body was preparing itself for labour. I did not like the two painful attacks of indigestion which – psychologically – had the opposite effect.

## Indigestion Attacks

The attacks started off as straightforward abdominal pain, as if I had an unfrozen lump of ice-cream sitting at the bottom of my stomach. But within ten minutes they had built up into circular waves, working their way inwards from the outer limits of my uterus to a central point about an inch above my navel. This was accompanied by clean back pain, as if someone had pressed a plank horizontally across my lower spine, and sharp, neat, regular stabbing pains slicing down through my cervix.

Sitting propped up on pillows, stoically chewing a couple of chalky indigestion tablets, I found that the attacks passed within an hour. Luckily I knew what was happening, so I wasn't frightened. In the first pregnancy I'd had one, far less painful, bout of indigestion which had terrified me. The worst thing then was the conviction that I was going into premature labour. Although I knew that indigestion is common in pregnancy, I underestimated the level of pain I might experience. Several women commented that they had called out their doctors, terrified that they were miscarrying.

## The Baby

Since 1992 any baby born dead after 24 weeks' gestation is considered a stillbirth, not a miscarriage. The limit was dropped because the extraordinary advances in medical technology had made life possible at this point, although most women admit that they still see the end of the second trimester (28 weeks) as the watershed.

According to the premature baby charity BLISS 50 per cent of babies born at 25 weeks have a chance of survival, and at 30 weeks the vast majority will live provided they are given special care immediately after birth. Of course physical survival is not the same as healthy survival, and in June 1993 the largest study of premature births carried out in Britain, at the National Perinatal Epidemiology Unit, revealed that two thirds of babies born before 29 weeks' gestation suffered some mental or physical disability. The risk rose with declining gestational age.[2]

By week 28 the baby inside your womb is 14.5in long (37cm) and weighs about 2 lb (900g). Its head is no longer so out of proportion and seems smaller in comparison with its body. It can hear and recognise its mother's voice, and perhaps other people's. With the gushing of liquid and food, the regular pumping of your heart, the gentle throbbing of blood circulating, it is surrounded by noise. It also responds to loud sounds in the world outside: cars backfiring, fireworks. The baby's translucent skin is damp and shiny, tiny veins are visible, and patterned downy hair covers the body. Fists may punch the side of the uterus, as if it's trying to attract your attention. Dr Thomas Verny and Dr John Kelly suggest that it can even kick in time to music and respond to its mother's changes in emotion.[3]

## Mood Affecting the Baby

That a woman's emotional well-being has an effect on her physical well-being and that of her baby has been acknowledged throughout history. The Hittites had to pay 10 shekels of silver for inflicting actual or emotional harm on a woman in the later stages of pregnancy, only 5 shekels if she had not passed her 'sixth moon month'. In 1818, the Physician-Accoucher, Augustus Bozzi Granville, carried out his own survey of miscarriage amongst the women he treated at the Westminster General Dispensary in London: 28 per cent of women attributed losing their babies to emotional factors such as shock or worry.

There are a great number of superstitions surrounding the effects of maternal shock or emotional distress on the growing baby. In sixteenth- and seventeenth-century England it was a commonly held belief that birthmarks were caused by the mother being frightened by a particular animal or occurrence during her pregnancy. In Hertfordshire as recently as the 1960s, a woman claimed that her child's throat ailment was caused by her being frightened by a snake during her pregnancy.

The International Society for Prenatal and Perinatal Psychology and Medicine (ISPPM), founded in 1971, has been conducting an intensive field study into how the mother's mood affects fetal consciousness, and many women today are convinced that their distress transmits itself to their baby. For this reason Siân felt protective during her two pregnancies.

> I did worry about reading things and watching things that could affect the babies. With Alexander, Pete was reading a book on the Holocaust and I desperately wanted to read it too. But I didn't because I thought I just couldn't subject the child to the emotions of the horrors of what people do to each other.

It is one of the paradoxes of pregnancy that outward physical development and psychological development often do not happen in tandem. It is the first three months that are often the hardest emotionally, yet the woman has nothing to show for her changed state: everything feels different, nothing looks different. It is often all too easy to blame hormones for emotional change during pregnancy. Feminist thinkers and writers have rightly challenged historical and contemporary schools of thought which have portrayed women as fickle creatures entirely at the mercy of their untrustworthy bodies.

## Always in Tears . . .

Although the link between pregnancy harmones and mood is only just beginning to be understood, every woman I interviewed did say that she was much more sensitive when pregnant. For some, it was the only time in their adult life that they had ever cried, and most said that the behaviour of their friends and even of people with whom they only came into sporadic contact took on greater significance. As Fran put it, 'anything set me off, from cats with wounded paws to mass murder I found upsetting – I was emotional over everything.'

Many women commented that they responded to world events on a personal, intimate level. During Sasha's pregnancy the Berlin Wall came down, Nelson Mandela was released and the so-called Velvet Revolution was liberating Czechoslovakia: on each occasion she cried and cried. Many women could not watch the television news – I had to leave the room when reports on the famine in Somalia were being broadcast during my pregnancy with Felix – and others, like Sue, had a sixth sense for anything on the television involving pregnant women or children, however mundane. 'I would dissolve into tears over anything slushy – I even cried in *Crossroads* once . . .'

Most women need a compass for their changing emotional map. There is still a tendency to treat pregnancy and all issues to do with becoming a parent as 'natural', a matter of course: the implication is that so long as you are physically

comfortable there is nothing else to worry about. This attitude is reinforced in medical circles and books which focus
predominantly on the physical condition of pregnancy rather
than the mental one. This concentration on the visible as
opposed to the invisible challenges of pregnancy has been
questioned by many sociologists, and was one of the recurrent issues of a ten-year study undertaken by American
psychologists Carolyn and Philip Cowan. They followed
96 couples becoming parents from 1979 to 1989, after a
successful three-year pilot scheme. The study analysed the
main emotional and practical changes in the relationships of
couples making the transition from partners to parents.

> Expectant parents talk primarily about the psycho-
> logical and emotional changes they are experiencing and
> what is happening to their relationships with the people
> who are important to them. Doctors and childbirth
> educators focus primarily on the physical, physiological
> and medical aspects of pregnancy and delivery, paying
> attention to women's emotional reactions only when
> they are unpredictable or disruptive.[4]

Pregnant women do have the right to expect those around
them to be solicitous and responsive to their emotional
needs. Pregnancy is not an illness, but any extreme physical
change is challenging to the person experiencing it. It is just as
manipulative to demand that women appear totally unaltered
by the experience as it is to behave as if the pregnancy is now
the woman's sole defining characteristic. As Sharon commented,

> When you're pregnant lots of people, especially men,
> tend to think your brains have disappeared and that
> you're no longer Sharon, a woman, you are just a carrier
> of a baby.

## Relationship with Your Partner

Some women, through choice or necessity, decide to have a child alone, but the majority still embark on pregnancy with a partner. If you are in a couple, your partner's responses to the changes pregnancy is wreaking during these emotional times can be crucial and their every throwaway comment can take on huge significance.

What a woman can – and should – expect from her partner obviously is governed by a web of interconnected issues: the nature of their relationship in the first place, the financial and social pressures on them as individuals and as a couple, whether or not the baby was planned and the feelings that each has about being a parent.

A pregnant woman, whether or not she is happy about the pregnancy, whether she is acknowledging or denying the baby, is emotionally and physically pregnant every second of every day: it is an internal experience. But a partner can only think about the pregnancy, he or she cannot live it: it can only be an external experience. Adjustment cannot help but happen at a different pace. And the schism is immediate, even if on the surface both partners appear to be responding identically. Many couples will not expect to share the emotional experience, and will be comfortable responding as individuals. If partners are emotionally separate already, even estranged, there will be few expectations.

Even while accepting difference, most women and men hope that they will have a common preoccupation, that they will share the experience of moving towards becoming parents. If they feel divided by the experience – even temporarily – destructive resentment can quickly build up. The more symbiotic and dependent the pre-pregnant relationship, the greater the sense of loss is likely to be.

The pregnant woman may assume that her partner's

responses to the baby are identical to hers; he or she, on the other hand, may be unable to empathise with the invisible physical and psychological changes taking place. To the partner, the pregnant woman looks physically the same as the pre-pregnant one, yet she is making demands that are out of character. Simultaneously the expectant mother may feel let down, disappointed, if her needs are not instinctively understood; she might even feel undermined by the fact that she craves continual emotional support and reinforcement.

When she was nearly 10 weeks pregnant with Nick, her first baby, Sue wrote in her diary:

> I'm feeling in need of lots of love at the moment – it's a frightening time . . . I'm glad Max is working but I do feel as if we lead totally different lives that are poles apart. Maybe he finds me boring – what have I got to talk about other than trivia and everyday stuff? God help me if I turn into a cabbage and a prize bore.

I was surprised that Greg and I were so out of kilter with one another during the first few months. Having decided that we might want a baby, we had been stunned with Martha when my body outstripped our minds and I conceived almost straight away. Neither of us was emotionally prepared. And because Greg's reaction to the positive test result was less enthusiastic than mine I felt abandoned, as if the decision to have a child had been mine alone. Expectation did not concur with reality: I expected emotional parity – that we would experience the same emotions at the same time, react as a couple – whereas of course we responded to the situation in character, as individuals.

In the early days of my pregnancy with Felix it was even

harder. I felt starved of love, care and attention, as if Martha and Greg were ganging up on one side, leaving me on the other with the baby.

> 25 FEBRUARY 1992: Martha's birthday. Felt dreadful – dizzy, sick, weak, tightness in my stomach and in my throat – and passed out at her party at nursery. Very weepy. Wanted Greg to make everything all right. He's not well, not to mention doing all the day-to-day practical parenting things so that I can rest and look after myself, so I feel mean being pissed off. But I want to be looked after too.

Yet it is crucially important that the individuals retain their sense of self, as Sasha acknowledged:

> In the same way that having a child and being pregnant alters the balance of your entire life, it alters the dynamics between the two people who love each other and the way they love each other and what that loving is based on. And it can tip into something where you're into role playing that isn't either of you.

The challenge is that while most couples are prepared for their relationship to change once the baby has been born, few expect this shifting to start before the morning sickness does, as Debra found:

> At first it was very distant for Hugo as it was not physically evident, and he was irritated by my seriousness and worries. Later, he was interested and shy. My feelings went from psychological to purely physical as the baby started to move more.

Because they were so near the beginning of their relationship, Jane and Matt knew that it was important not to make assumptions about each other.

> We just decided to make a concerted effort to maintain as much of our life as we could individually and as a couple without a child. I didn't have the right to step into his head; his head's his own. I was interested in what he had to say, but I didn't want to invade.

And Eve too felt that she and Stephen reacted in character to the pregnancy rather than suddenly starting to think as one homogeneous parent-to-be figure: 'We slipped into extremes of our roles anyway, which is always me as the neurotic one and him as the very calm one.'

For some, the extension and exaggeration of their ordinary roles was not positive. Several women commented that they resented their partners assuming that they would take pregnancy in their stride, that nothing would change until the baby was born. They were extremely excited about the idea of becoming a father, yet simply carried on their lives as normal. For one woman, whose husband works long hours, normal meant him being physically and emotionally absent for much of the pregnancy. 'I had to push him – no, nudge him rather than push him – to be supportive.'

Another felt that her husband made no allowances for how drastically her life had changed already.

> He never took on board that not only was I a full-time working pregnant woman, but I was someone who was bearing the financial responsibility for our future too. He would never accept that that made a difference to my pregnancy. Yet I knew it right from the start.

Sharon's husband Gary was excited about the twins in a rather macho way, as if it was a reflection on his virility to have fathered more than one child. Once the initial euphoria had died down, though, resentment started to set in. 'He actually said that I was getting the attention and he wasn't.'

They were living in a small maisonette and the prospect of having twins brought forward distant ideas of moving to more spacious accommodation. But somehow all their future plans were put on hold by Gary. He became increasingly unreliable, started not to come home some nights and Sharon had to face the fact that he was having an affair. But by six months into the pregnancy, feeling vulnerable and intensely protective of her babies, she no longer had the strength to confront him.

> I was extremely suspicious, but I felt completely power-less. I had no job, I had no financial means of supporting myself really other than the small amount of maternity benefit and what have you.

The situation worsened, right up to the evening at 34 weeks when the girls were born.

> I didn't know then that he was cancelling a date. But I did know that he was put out because he was going off to do something and I was most inconsiderate to go into labour on Friday night . . .

It was only after the twins came out of the special care unit that Sharon started to regain her self-confidence. When they were seven weeks old she left him.

> I felt I was supposed to be playing this role of the help-less little female, barefoot and pregnant almost. But I

finally thought well, I can bring up two children on my own better than I can with you.

Most women hope that emotional estrangement during the pregnancy will disappear once the baby has been born, so are prepared to put up with a feeling of being let down. As one woman said, 'I thought the baby might bring us together again, and I wanted that.'

Caroline was disappointed by Malcolm's lack of excitement on each of the four occasions when she gave birth. Others took steps to ensure that the second time wouldn't be a repeat of the first. Not only had one woman's husband been drunk during her first labour, he took only one day off work despite having agreed to take leave.

I was very, very angry. Upset as well. I made it clear through my second pregnancy, quite clear, that the same thing couldn't happen again.

There is cause for hope though. A recent report by the Equal Opportunities Commission showed that, following the introduction of paid paternity leave in April 2003, 70 per cent of new fathers now take some or all of their paternity leave entitlement.[5] Also, with the increase of men working part- or flexi-time, it means that many can be around in the early weeks.

But for most women the situation is fluid. As before the pregnancy, the relationship continually changes as both partners adopt and assimilate new roles. A pattern of separateness during the first few months is not necessarily the pattern that will continue for the rest of the pregnancy. Confidence in asking for what you want, and security in accepting what is offered, are the most positive ways to help the pregnancy develop emotionally. Many women uncharacteristically allow themselves to be mothered.* In common with many women, Debra was surprised that she enjoyed it.

> Pregnancy made Hugo softer and more attentive – he treated me like a baby. He said he couldn't relate to the bump, but I said it's me he has to cope with anyway as it is not a whole person until it's born, it's just the changed me. You feel like a child in your wants – food, sleep and love. You even look like a child in your clothes.

When she was pregnant with Lottie Sue told Max that she wanted to be spoiled rotten since this would be her last opportunity. Jane also liked Matt's increased awareness of her needs.

> Throughout the pregnancy he was more concerned about me than the baby, and I was pleased about that because I was doing enough worrying for both of us and it was nice to have somebody whose sole apparent concern was myself.

Lynne loved being looked after by John, although she was disappointed that she couldn't send him out to find her weird and wonderful food fancies. 'We were remarkably in tune; I was amazed.'

With a successful freelance career behind her, for the first six months of her pregnancy Pam was extremely confident and did not need Gérard for practical support any more than she had in the past. The only practical change was that they decided that they would live together in Pam's flat while his was being renovated, then move into his and sell hers.

---

* I hope our children will truthfully be able to use the word 'parented' to put across the idea of unconditional care and support; that mother and father will come to denote gender rather than role.

I knew as long as I didn't rely on him, or depend on him – which I wasn't used to doing anyway – I could rely on myself.

Pam then had the shock of discovering the fibroid in her womb and, later, the discovery that it had grown. Pam slid into an emotional decline and a period of agonising self-doubt began.

I was all over the place, very unstable. I was very emotional in that I would cry all the time about feeling a failure about the possibility of not being able to have a vaginal delivery. And again it was only in retrospect that I thought that I'd been using the process of labour as a mega-therapy session for me – you have to open up to give birth. Gérard was the only one who saw everything. He was extremely supportive.

Other women, like Jenny, remained opposed to being looked after throughout:

I felt that women perhaps used pregnancy as an excuse to sit and get their husbands to run around and to eat chocolate, whereas I just didn't want that for me.

### Sharing the Housework

Many women felt that practical support – going to antenatal appointments, cooking meals with minimum nausea value, fielding telephone calls, making sure that they could rest if they needed to – was the most positive contribution their partners could make. And although many surveys sadly suggest that a pattern of more equal distribution of household chores during pregnancy does not tend to continue after the birth (particularly if the woman has elected to be a full-time parent),[6] several women commented that their confidence about the division of labour after labour was hugely affected by the level of practical responsibility their partner took on during the pregnancy.

It is depressing that at the start of the twenty-first century, so many pregnancy books still talk about asking your 'husband' to 'help' with the housework. But it seems this picture of British home life is accurate. Figures released in 1996 revealed that over two-thirds of women with full-time jobs were mainly responsible for general domestic duties: 59 per cent usually made the meal every evening, and 79 per cent usually did all the washing and ironing.[7] More recently, research has shown that it is predominantly women who take time off to look after sick children and that working mothers do twice as much housework as working fathers.[8]

In retrospect many women wished that they'd looked beyond the birth during their pregnancies to visions of how the nitty-gritty of their lives as parents would work. Both parties often make inaccurate or incomplete assumptions about the other person's expectations of life with a baby. As Cowan and Cowan comment: 'Many women and men neglect to share with each other their notions of the ideal family.'[9]

## Co-Parenting

Occasionally both partners choose to be full-time parents. Lee and Simon made the decision that there was more to life than making money, and that so long as they could survive on odd jobs here and there they did not want to be part of the system. More often, however, it is a question of adapting individual circumstances as efficiently as possible.

Finance permitting, the decision whether or not the woman would return to work after the birth was often seen as hers alone, rather than a parenting decision to be made jointly. The majority of partners expected to continue their professional lives unchanged. Many men had a laissez-faire attitude to the practicalities of childcare and its costs. In some cases this sprang from an unconscious conviction that it was the woman's task to deal with it, to provide a replacement for mothering should she decide to return to paid employment – a childminder, nanny, neighbour, whatever – even if during the pregnancy the couple had talked about a 50/50 parenting arrangement.

Women who felt they were given little practical and emotional support during the pregnancy tended to have less confidence in the idea of joint parenting. As one woman put it:

> If he couldn't shape up as far as the pregnancy, then I didn't think he was going to shape up as far as being a father was concerned.

Others were surprised and disappointed when reality failed to fulfil their expectations:

> It was supposed to be both of us, we'd agreed. But I was at home with the baby, he made no effort whatsoever to do much when he was home. He did things to 'help' me, like it was my job and made out he was being really great just changing a nappy or something. It really depressed me, especially when he thought it was my job to find someone to look after the baby when I wanted to go back to work. It was clear that he thought I would pay for it out of my salary.
>
> It wasn't that he thought that I should be a full-time mother, it's like he didn't see it was anything to do with him. And that was almost worse. For the first six months

> I was really bitter. I didn't think we would be the types
> to make rules beforehand, but I wish we had.

Many women reluctantly had to accept that their partners couldn't take much time off, for fear of losing out in promotion stakes or getting a reputation for being unreliable. As another woman put it: 'I'm as happy as circumstances dictate. It makes sense for him to be out doing the job, because he can earn more than I can.'

In many ways it is a question of priorities. This woman's husband set up his own business, supposedly so that he would have greater flexibility:

> The whole point about him going solo was so that he
> could be involved. The truth is he chose to use it as an
> excuse, that he had to work long hours otherwise he
> wouldn't be offered any more work. This New Man
> stuff is really a myth, isn't it? They're all for change just
> so long as they're not the one to have to make it . . . The
> idea of whole days with no one but a baby for company
> bored him rigid. But it's boring for me too. He didn't
> even realise that he was behaving just like my father
> did with us.

Even in 2007 – and with the many shifts there have been in social attitudes to parenting and parental responsibilities – with two professional parents (as opposed to those who are self-employed or who have some measure of control over their own working day) it is still more often than not the mother, rather than the father, who leaves the meeting early to pick up the sick child. Back in 1992, Greg and I knew that if he wanted to play an equal role, then it would be easier for him to give up his job and set up on his own, than try to fight against the prejudices of employers. Many men and their partners have come to the same sort of conclusions, helped enormously by the advent of flexible working, technology and email! It was surprising how many friends, male and female, asked Greg if I paid 'his' part of the mortgage and although things have moved on in this area, the idea that women shouldn't earn more than their partners still persists.

## Talking About Childcare

While you are still pregnant it is difficult to know what arrangements will or will not suit. Rachel had intended to work up until the last possible moment, then take six months' maternity leave on full pay, gradually easing back into her work as an editor in the fifth and sixth months at home. She didn't think she would need six months off, but she thought it more responsible to be generous to herself.

> I'd met people before who'd said they were going to be back in two weeks and hadn't, and I knew that the repercussions of that from a work point of view are much worse than someone saying I'm going to take the proper amount of time off then the office getting cover.

Neither she nor Jeremy considered childrearing exclusively a woman's job but Rachel did worry that practical responsibility for Rose was going to fall squarely on her shoulders. She wanted to allow herself enough time to make arrangements without feeling pressurised.

Eve fell into the trap of assuming that nothing would change, so refused to plan for a different sort of lifestyle.

> I thought I'd be back very quickly, six weeks after, all part of the not being changed; then afterwards I very

quickly knew that I never wanted to work again, I never wanted to leave the house again, I wanted to stay with this baby forever. I kept saying 'oh, I'll be back next month, I'll be back next month.' I wasn't brave enough to say I want six months off . . .

Jane and Matt did discuss how to organise childcare. They agreed that Jane would go back to work full time after three months and that Matt, who is a freelance journalist, would look after Sophie one day a week.

The only problem was that Matt found it quite difficult to come to terms with the fact that while he was looking after her he couldn't do any work, so as soon as the childminder had another day available, she went there instead.

Chatting with her boss at an office party a few weeks before she was due back, Jane remarked that she'd arranged for Sophie to be left with a childminder for four days a week. In the general hubbub and boozy atmosphere, wires got crossed and the assumption was made that Jane was not coming back full time. Unknown to Jane, alternative arrangements were set in motion at the office and, actually, she was thrilled.

There was – and still is – a part of me that wants to be a full-time parent in a way, although it would drive me barmy. Ideally, I'd like to do 2 or 3 days a week.

Because there was no question of going back to the BBC, Tessa was in the invidious position of attending job interviews when she was visibly pregnant. Mark was away filming in Italy from about six months into the pregnancy until ten days before Joe was born. They both knew that the sorts of unsocial hours Mark was expected to work would ensure that his contribution would remain small in the foreseeable future. So although there was no question of Tessa not pursuing her career in the long term, she didn't put herself under any time pressure to get back to work immediately.

> We needed the money, and I needed it for me. It was almost as if I recreated my professional self in the time that I had off.

Debbie and Patrick were both teachers. They tried to arrange both pregnancies around school terms to allow them both maximum time off, but Debbie still only had six weeks' leave for her first child Jack. Although in retrospect she thinks she was probably suffering from mild postnatal depression during the first 18 months after his birth, Debbie was surprised not to enjoy her maternity leave. Seen from the outside and with hindsight it is not surprising: she was on her own during the day, in a new community, a different country, away from her family and friends, isolated and unsupported.

> I always thought it would be natural to love Jack, but I found it very difficult to love him to start with. I really resented the fact that he totally took over my life and I never seemed to have any time for myself. I have lots of hobbies and I never seemed to have time to do anything, and Jack just used to cry the whole time. And I thought, is there ever going to be a moment when he doesn't cry? I thought I'd be able to cope better than I did.

Sue also enjoyed the early months less than she expected. Max was a company director and they both assumed that he would continue as usual and that Sue would look for a job some time after the baby's birth when she was ready. Initially, she'd thought she would be ready after staying with Nick until he was 12 months old. Not only did Nick scream and cry a lot, however, but Sue was also driven out of her mind with boredom. So when he was 16 weeks old she arranged for a neighbour to mind him part time and found a job with a local newspaper.

Fran took statutory three months' maternity leave from her teaching post. Her husband Jim, who as a postman worked shifts, rearranged his working life so that between them and a childminder they could care for the children.

> I wouldn't have minded going part-time, but there wasn't any choice because of the mortgage. But I don't think I would have wanted to stay at home. By the end of my three months at home with Matthew I was more or less going up the walls with boredom because I didn't have a network of friends who were doing the same thing.*

Joanne, also a teacher, knew that she would be away from work for three months (having cleverly already been off for the summer holiday). Georgina, despite choosing not to claim any rights as a co-parent from her employer, reduced her days to a four-day week.

Nicki and Mike wanted to have flexible roles, and planned ahead. Mike worked as a carpenter when they returned from travelling in South America so that he wouldn't be restricted by office hours once the twins were born. Pam and Gérard,

---

* There is no doubt that for many new mothers the experience of the first few months is defined by the presence or absence of similarly occupied friends and acquaintances. Often the value of antenatal classes only becomes apparent after labour when the people you shared the pelvic floor exercises with become your support network once you have had your child.

who already had flexibility, discussed in detail how the workload would be divided up once Jackson had been born. Pam acknowledges that their plans were hopelessly idealistic.

> Again due to these fantasies we both had, which had nothing to do with the reality. That the baby would sleep when you put it down after it had been fed, that we would walk out together with the baby in the pram, and it would be laughing and gurgling and adoring us and we'd be adoring it.

John, who worked for himself, and Lynne intended to share childcare, even though she didn't mean to go back to work until Michelle was at least 18 months old. To her surprise, she found that she wanted to be a full-time mother: 'I felt, I haven't produced this baby just to see it in the evenings.'

## Whose Word Goes?

But joint parenting obviously throws up its own challenges. Traditional attributes of mothering and fathering are deeply ingrained in our subconscious, however confident we are that we have rejected the stereotypes. Men who passionately believe that they should play an equal role might feel guilty if they feel unfulfilled by it; women who want to share the responsibility might feel undermined at realising that in fact they want to be the prime carer. Siân admitted that the reality of shared parental responsibility was harder than she'd expected. She and Peter had discussed how they were going to divide up their responsibilities once Alexander was born. Siân was taking statutory maternity leave, with holiday on top, before returning full-time to her television job. Peter was a writer working from home.

He was very insistent that he got as involved with the kid as possible during my maternity leave, which actually led to a lot of clashes. I sometimes resented him telling me to go away and that he'd deal with it. So although I wanted him to, it was hard to allow him to have a role.

The psychologists Cowan and Cowan acknowledge that many couples are reluctant to intrude upon each other's decisions. Once there is a child, however, someone's view has to take priority.

Becoming parents not so much raises new problems as brings old unconscious or unresolved issues to the surface. Before children come along it is possible for a couple to deal with differences or disagreements by avoiding them or by simply accepting the fact that each partner has a different view. But once children are part of a family, most of us discover certain disagreements have to be resolved on the spot.[10]

Much of the conflict is caused by the malevolent expectations of others. Many women are frightened at relinquishing their traditional mothering roles, just as many men are reluctant to abandon the path society has indicated for them and embrace what they see as femaleness. Society still fashions itself on a gender-defined division of labour and those who step outside their roles are considered exceptional and eccentric. Couples who do attempt to co-parent are often critically observed, not least because many people genuinely believe that parenting roles are not acquired but instinctive. A supermarket checkout assistant said to one husband who regularly shopped there with his three-month-old daughter: 'But can you really look after her, you know, like her mother could . . . ?'

Again at the supermarket, another father was told, in doom-laden tones: 'She'll know you better than her mother.'

He explained that the child was with her mother at home, it was just that he – the father – did all the shopping!

At this stage in your pregnancy the logistics of juggling washing up, shopping, a baby, a relationship and a career are a long way off. Some couples can't even believe that they are going to have a real child to deal with in sixteen or so weeks, let alone contemplate how their lives will change. But there are practical arrangements that do have to be made now: if you qualify for maternity benefit you can claim at 27 weeks and, by 24 weeks, you must write to your employer stating when the baby is expected, when you intend to stop working and if you are intending to go back. For many women this is the time when conflict or difficulties over their physical relationship with their partner came to the fore.

## Sex

Polygamous societies tend to regard sex during pregnancy as contraindicated. In China in the first century BC, when the prudish Confucian philosophy started to triumph over the mild and indulgent Taoism, pregnant women were forbidden to have sexual intercourse. The same goes for twelfth-century Muslim societies, the Aztecs in fifteenth-century Mexico, the Incas in sixteenth-century Peru and Mormon communities in America in the nineteenth and twentieth centuries. Male, not female, sexual needs were the issue: all these societies clearly felt that so long as a man had more than one wife to satisfy him there could be no reason for a pregnant woman to make love. Even today, some men use their wives' pregnancies to justify extra-marital affairs.

From Athens in the fourth century BC to the *yoshiwara* – pleasure quarter – of seventeenth- and eighteenth-century

Tokyo (then known as Edo), most cultures in which courtesans were accepted or where female – sometimes even male – prostitution was tolerated have tended to see sex during pregnancy as unnecessary, if not abhorrent. Of course attitudes to sexual intercourse in general have a direct correlation with attitudes to lovemaking during pregnancy. A ruling of the Christian church in the first century AD declared that 'religious women' should be chaste for three months before birth. But by the fifth century, St Augustine's view that sexual intercourse was fundamentally disgusting had taken hold in much of Europe: Arnobius called it 'filthy and degrading', Methodius 'unseemly', Jerome 'unclean', Tertullian 'shameful', Ambrose 'a defilement'. Of course when sex is acceptable only for the purposes of procreation, such as in middle-class Victorian England, a ban on the 'ungodly' practice of making love when pregnant was readily enforced.

Today attitudes still vary wildly. One book *Mamatoto* quotes a woman of the Santhal tribe in India:

> Of course we make love when we're pregnant! Without love, how can you get through life?[11]

On the other hand, it quotes Nyinban women in Nepal saying they don't make love during pregnancy for fear of breaking the child.

The West is becoming better at talking about sex in pregnancy, although it is still a subject that many authors and researchers seem to find embarrassing. A major history of sex in Britain in the twentieth century, published in 1993, did not even have an index reference for sex in pregnancy[12] and a national survey of 20,000 British men and women did not even ask what they thought about making love during pregnancy[13]. Since then, though, women's glossies – not just mother and baby magazines – have included the odd article.

Taboos are often based on invalid physical considerations. In a healthy pregnancy there is minimal risk of penetrative sexual intercourse triggering either a miscarriage or premature labour, despite the fact that semen contains prostaglandins similar to those used in Prostin pessaries designed to ripen the cervix and induce labour. Orgasm stimulates and exercises the muscles of the uterus, keeping them supple, and several women commented how surprised they were when they first noticed that their uterus became hard as a rock for the first five minutes or so after a climax: this is due to the release of oxytocin at orgasm. In *A Woman's Experience of Sex*, Sheila Kitzinger comments that men often have an exaggerated sense of their own size.

> They worry that their large penis might somehow dislodge the fetus. But it doesn't happen like that – although rough sex is potentially dangerous as well as painful.[14]

Many books caution that libido might fade during the first and third trimesters, when nausea, tiredness and bulk can diminish sexual desire. Others suggest that because of the added spontaneity that comes with contraception-free sex or because of the high level of circulating hormones, pregnant women are more easily aroused, so sex will be fun. As Caroline put it, 'there's a lot more blood flowing around . . .'

Juliet Rix interviewed a wide range of women for her book *Is There Sex After Childbirth?*

> There are two main patterns of sexual activity during pregnancy. There's either a steady decline in interest from start to finish, or it dips during the first trimester, goes up in the middle period and then dips again in the last trimester.[15]

No one can predict what they will want sexually during pregnancy. It is no more nor less normal to have a sexual appetite that rockets through the roof than it is to find even the slightest sexual touch intrusive. All that matters is that you feel emotionally comfortable and adjusted to your body's needs, that you don't feel pressurised or abnormal. If both partners' needs dovetail rather than conflict, sex or lack of it will not be an issue. If they don't, the only answer is to try to talk the issue through.

In Martha's pregnancy, once the nausea had stopped at 12 weeks, I really enjoyed sex: no spermicidal jelly to think about, no diaphragm pinging out of your hands and getting covered with fluff from the carpet. Then, unfortunately, I was hospitalised for unexplained vaginal bleeding at 30 weeks and was advised to cut out sex. I expected to feel the same second time round. But in common with many parents who find it hard to have a spontaneous sex life, although I physically wanted to make love I often didn't have the energy to enjoy anything more than gentle massage. I was just too tired.

Lynne and John liked her changing shape, but lovingly rather than sexually, with more kissing and cuddling. On the other hand, both Caroline and Malcolm enjoyed sex during all four pregnancies: 'In fact I think that's the only reason that I've been allowed to have four children . . .'

Mark was away for a lot of Tessa's first pregnancy, so when they did get to meet up they tended to leap into bed at the first opportunity. In both pregnancies, Tessa always felt attractive and Mark made her feel wonderful.

Even at 11 weeks he'd look at my tummy, which I thought was a fat, ugly one, and say 'see, it looks like a baby already' with complete excitement.

Fran and Jim both went off sex: they were a little disappointed since friends had said that they had had fantastic sex lives when pregnant and, like most heterosexual couples, they'd been looking forward to contraception not being part of the equation.

> My sexual appetite totally disappeared, immediately, both times. I couldn't bear to be touched in a sexual way at all. Anyway, to Jim, the idea that the baby was coming down the way he was going up was too much.

Both partners may be surprised at their reaction to the woman's ever-changing shape. In the same way that emotional needs do not necessarily synchronise, partners may require different levels of physical involvement. Some women find their bodies attractive, others do not. Sue was undermined by her lack of sexuality, as she wrote in her diary.

> I look totally different now – my belly is getting rounder and my boobs are enormous. The one main change is in my view of myself. I feel totally asexual, and that's awful. I can't understand how anyone can find me attractive.

Feeling aroused during pregnancy, intimidated or not bothered are all equally valid responses. How one feels about the baby's movements can be a crucial factor. Some women and men find the idea of a third party utterly off-putting:

> I felt disgusting, like the baby was there watching me. I just couldn't enjoy it, although it didn't seem to bother him much.

Others rather like the sensation of the baby reacting when they're making love. For the rest it's just too funny to be able to take seriously.

## Sexually Explicit Dreams

Interestingly, many women said that regardless of whether or not they were making love regularly, they had a significantly higher number of sexually explicit dreams and fantasies, very often involving other women. As one woman, who felt that her partner was unable to meet her sexual or emotional needs for much of the pregnancy, put it:

> I found that I was much, much more sensitive when pregnant. Things that I might enjoy when I'm not pregnant, I didn't like. What I wanted was to be licked, sucked; even being touched with fingers could be too intrusive and painful. I used to think I wish I was with a woman. I had this feeling all the way through my pregnancy, and this was for two reasons: one, all my women acquaintances, friends, were so appreciative of my changing shape. I had so many compliments about my bump, I can't tell you, but they genuinely mean it, they genuinely think it's beautiful. And two, because I just thought a woman would know how to make love in such a way.

It can obviously be frustrating, at worst deeply wounding, if only one partner feels sexual. Eve and Stephen were emotionally and physically close through Annie's pregnancy, but deep-seated worry about penetrative sex damaging the baby inhibited Stephen: 'Right from the beginning I was randy as hell, but Stephen was scared stiff of intercourse. He treated me like Venetian glass.'

A few women felt, rightly or wrongly, that their partners actually found them physically repulsive. So not only
did they feel frustrated, they also felt hurt and physically
undermined.

> Sex was dreadful, which didn't help. I felt quite sexual,
> but he just wasn't attracted to me at all. Sex had always
> brought us together, sex had been very positive before.

When I asked women about their sex lives during pregnancy,
as a postscript a few added how they worried that the baby
would perhaps spoil the relationship, dilute it, that lack of
spontaneity would stifle intimacy with one another. They did
want the baby, but they were aware that things were never
going to be the same again. Joanne and Georgina found themselves going out to cinemas and restaurants a great deal just
before Rowan was born. And by 28 weeks pregnant, many
women have a sense of time running out. Nicki, who had to
go into hospital twice in false labour with the twins, felt that
on each occasion they'd somehow been reprieved: 'Part of
me didn't want to share our flat with anybody.'

# Who Am I?

## Weeks 28–32

I am a woman
of thirty years
proud with flesh
breasts and glistening belly distended
and from them my nipples and the navel-knot
just startling out
for these months the three targets
of my bloodstream

Lesley Saunders, from 'Voices'[1]

The beginning of the third – and last – trimester brings with it a sense of relief for some. No one wants their baby to be born prematurely, but at the back of one's mind is the knowledge that statistically from now on it would have a fair chance of survival if it did decide to come out.

These last three months also bring mild panic. They are the countdown to labour and birth, the finishing line is in sight. Even though most mental and ceremonial preparations for birth happen only in the last month – from the bizarrely named American baby showers to the Zulus who hang coloured beads and engravings around the birth room – some women feel a kind of crescendo building throughout these 12 weeks.

However confident a woman is about her pregnancy and labour, most experience some sense of apprehension. You may swing between wanting to precipitate events and wishing that D-Day would never arrive. Some of the most impatient expectant mothers I spoke to had to endure the cruel irony of overdue babies, extending their final trimester into as many as 14 or even 15 weeks of pregnancy yet to be negotiated. One said she felt like a runner finishing a gruelling 10,000-metre race only to be told she had to go round again.

Sudanese women make no allowances for late deliveries. Their ritual preparations are carried out in the seventh month of pregnancy. They henna, scent and braid their hair and take to wearing a special bracelet on their wrists for protection. They also knot a leather thong around their waist.[2] Their wise example could be usefully followed by many in the West whose attention is focused on the baby at the expense of the mother. The ritual physical pampering carried out in Sudan must be a tremendous fillip for the woman enduring the soreness, aches and breathlessness of the final weeks.

## Physical Changes

For many women physical discomforts increase with the passing days. A sense of having been pregnant for ever coalesces with absolute disbelief that your bump can possibly inflate any further. At 28 weeks – not least because it was an extremely hot and humid July – I started to feel that someone was kneeling on my chest when I lay down flat on my back, as if Felix had his map upside-down and was planning on exiting through my throat. He became a presence it was impossible to ignore. Whenever I sat down at my computer to write it felt like I was squashing a bag of chicken bones and beaks under my breasts, a hotchpotch of spiky twigs. It was as if he was complaining at being condensed into such a small space.

At this late stage my breathlessness made me feel like a 40-a-day smoker and the puffiness around my legs and feet reached grotesque proportions. Each night, several times a night, I was obliged to undertake a stumbling obstacle race in the dark to the loo. I suffered pins and needles when I leant on an arm or a leg for too long. Trapped nerves irritated my crotch and a series of domestic disasters – a flood, a chain of power cuts and our third car in a row being written off when parked innocently outside our house – should have put the lid on a miserable four weeks. But I didn't feel miserable, not in the least.

I felt amazingly energetic and fit. I was enjoying work, and revelling in Martha's company. She was extremely loving of my daily changing shape and very solicitous, stroking my head if I was at the bottom of one of my emotional roller-coaster rides. Spurred on by observing a couple of our friends feeding their new babies, and a wonderful *Sesame Street* sketch on introducing a new sister or brother into the family, Martha also took to breastfeeding her dolls and Duplo figures. Looking back, my body was fast disintegrating, but I hardly noticed.

In one survey about the sorts of physical symptoms women experience in the seventh month of their pregnancies: 68 per cent reported lack of energy; 43 per cent indigestion; 46 per cent breathlessness (with late summer pregnancies being more affected than winter births); 68 per cent reported leg cramps; 48 per cent backache; 55 per cent tired legs; and 66 per cent urgent urination.[3] Most of the women I interviewed had some – if not all – of these symptoms, but mostly they weren't depressed by their bodies' rebellion at this stage unless specific, new problems showed themselves. Sharon, whose twins were in fact born at 34 weeks, felt everything earlier than women with singleton pregnancies.

> I remember I sat reading a book the hospital gave me, which listed some of the things you may or may not get when you're pregnant. It was hilarious. It included breathlessness – yes, I've definitely got that I thought – backache, headaches – I used to get terrible headaches. I used to get so tired, bleeding gums, haemorrhoids and I was getting tearful like you do towards the end of pregnancy. I thought, well the only one I haven't got is nosebleeds; and I wiped my hand across my face and my nose was bleeding . . .

Jane, whose blood pressure had been low throughout her pregnancy, started to faint at about 30 weeks whenever she went out anywhere: she joked that she saw more loo floors and tiled ceilings in restaurants in the last 10 weeks of her pregnancy than at any time before or since. The problem was so severe that she had to stop working a couple of weeks earlier than she'd anticipated.

I had very low blood pressure too, making me susceptible to fainting and dizzy spells even early on (in the heat and humidity of Singapore I passed out three times in an hour at only 9 weeks). Lying on my side rather than my back with my feet in the air helped, as did making my bath water a little less scalding, wearing loose clothes and avoiding airless spaces. There is also a Bach flower remedy, which I never tried. Appropriately called Dr Bach's Rescue Remedy, it contains ingredients from five flowers – Star of Bethlehem, rock rose, impatiens, cherry plum and clematis – and may help persistent keelers-over.

## Threatened Premature Labour

In both her pregnancies Fran found herself having to stop work early due to the threat of premature labour. One night, having felt a little under the weather for a couple of days, she developed what she thought was indigestion alongside a sense that something was not quite right. Since we all analyse our physical symptoms on a regular basis and diagnose ourselves as suffering from the most life-threatening problems our handbooks have to offer, she thought she'd sit it out. But then contractions started, not the usual Braxton Hicks tightening, but painful, labour contractions. Dispatched urgently to hospital by her GP, she was given an internal examination and told that her cervix was softening – that if they didn't do something she would deliver the baby.

Perhaps the most worrying aspect of delivering a seven-month baby is whether it will be able to breathe unaided. In hospital the doctors gave Fran a shot of steroids to help try to mature Matthew's tiny lungs, just in case they couldn't halt things. Inside the uterus a baby's lungs have a pink waterproof lining. Just before the birth, agents are produced which naturally scour away the lining so that when the baby is born the surface of the lungs is exposed and air can pass through them. It is possible to mature the lungs within a 12-hour period if a baby is born before 32 weeks – the critical time for lung development – by administering drugs intravenously.

> They kept saying to me, look if he does come out now,
> he's old enough, he will live. They kept trying to re-
> assure us, but I was terrified and crying.

By now the contractions were coming every five minutes and
getting progressively stronger. An intravenous drip was put
in to slow labour down and for the next eight hours they just
watched and monitored.

Some of the most commonly used drugs to slow down
or halt labour are ritodrine and salbutamol, both of which
relax the muscles of the uterus. However, these drugs can
also have unpleasant, and occasionally dangerous, side-
effects and doctors are increasingly using drugs like
nifedipine and atosiban, which have fewer side-effects and
according to some studies are more effective. A stiff drink
(although this is not likely to be prescribed by obstetricians)
might also help, since alcohol has an inhibiting effect on
uterine contractions. Nobody could tell Fran why it was
happening.

> They said to me, because it happened again with Rowan,
> that either I've got a hormonal defect which short-
> changes me by 10 weeks, or I've got a basic womb shape
> problem so that the pressure of the baby by 30 weeks
> is too much.

Matthew was active throughout the crisis, which reassured
Fran and Jim. But after a brief stay of execution, the contractions started up again. The key observation was, however,
that her cervix was not dilating. This was the first indication
that her body didn't really want to go into full-blown labour
yet and, like many women who experience the signs of premature labour, she began to believe she would in the end go to
full term. She was encouraged by the knowledge that the

cervix is able to close up again after dilating and that ruptured membranes can heal themselves.

> One doctor said to me 'it's like a team of rowers, with one person rowing the wrong way and three people trying to row the other way. So you are actually contracting, you are doing the work, but you're not going to get anywhere.'

Fran's cervix did harden up again and she was discharged to bed rest at home. For the next 10 weeks she had proper, painful contractions twice a day until Matthew was born at 39 weeks.

There are several herbal remedies which are recommended for coping with painful contractions during the latter stages of pregnancy, such as an infusion of black horehound and ladies' slipper or a decoction of half an ounce of false unicorn root to a pint of water, simmered for about 15 minutes then strained and sipped.

## Fear of Something Being Wrong

This sense of things happening before they should, before one is ready, is one of the most unnerving things that can happen in late pregnancy. Many women in these situations talked about resenting the medical profession for not being able to explain exactly what was going on. I was briefly hospitalised in Martha's pregnancy at 30 weeks, for bleeding. I was given a scan, told that my cervix was tightly closed and that the blood wasn't coming from the placenta.

On first noticing the blood I had self-diagnosed antepartum haemorrhage due to placenta praevia, on the basis of the books I had read. So initially this was a relief. But as I lay in the postnatal ward – the only available bed – listening to the cries of other women's newborn babies, I became angry that the doctors, with all their science, couldn't tell me why it was happening. After all, if they couldn't say why I was bleeding then how could they know that it wasn't going to happen again? How could they tell me that it was 'nothing to worry about'? And what was the point of interminable queuing in depressing waiting rooms for antenatal appointments if this could happen out of the blue? It was all very well for books and doctors to talk about babies having a good chance of survival by this point, but Martha wasn't ready to be born: she was my baby and I was just sure it was too early.

As well as being haunted by that dangerous thing, a little knowledge, I was also half aware of my mother's distressing gynaecological history: she suffered three miscarriages (one at 20 weeks). I had been born six weeks premature, my mother unconscious and not allowed to see me for five days because of her physical condition: my father's strongest memory was of the consultant in his white wellington boots tipping a teaspoon of brandy down my scrawny throat to shock me into breathing.

Many women, as they make the transition from daughter to mother, talk about their need to connect their experiences of pregnancy and birth with those of their mothers and grand-mothers.[4] Although I had not consciously been aware of how my mother's experiences had been colouring my pregnancy, lying in the hospital bed I realised that I thought history would repeat itself: like mother like daughter. I hadn't been frightened of labour, but now there was a chance that it might happen before I was mentally prepared for it. I was terrified, of everything and nothing.

But the bleeding stopped. I went home the following day and was back to work 24 hours later. Only the fact of having been admitted to and discharged from hospital was recorded in my notes, but I'd learnt a valuable lesson: that pregnancy, and by extension labour and birth, is unpredictable. The best one can do is to allow oneself to respond, partly instinctively and partly based on appropriate advice.

Pam, who had been so confident for the first six months of her pregnancy, feels that her physical problems had subconscious, emotional roots. The fear of losing control was preventing her from adapting to the physical truths of her situation:

> I wasn't aware of being frightened of labour and pain, but I must have been worried because I set this fibroid up to prevent me from having any labour, I'm convinced of that. But I wasn't aware of there being any fears around the pregnancy, the birth, until I had this fibroid: and then I just panicked.

## Superstitions

Some women are convinced that things are going to go terribly wrong, whether by embarrassing oneself in the delivery room, having to have a caesarean, or paralysing fears of the baby being disabled or dying before or during birth. By the end of her pregnancy Lynne was overwhelmed with panic: 'The fears were really, really awful. They just grew and grew.'

In Lynne's case her irrational fears, the sense of the odds being against her, were exacerbated by having had two friends who'd had normal pregnancies but had given birth to severely disabled babies: one was born brain damaged and the other had a growth on his brain stem. She became superstitious about actually having things ready for Michelle: so although they had bought a cot, they didn't make it up until Michelle was brought safely home from the hospital; Lynne sewed curtains, but didn't decorate Michelle's room in any other way. Rationally she knew that she couldn't influence events by these sorts of appeasements, yet she couldn't take things for granted.

> I don't know why I was that superstitious though, because I did all that for my friend and it didn't make any difference.

Other women find that their worries come and go, yet they are still surprised at how instinctive and fundamental their responses become. Most ancient myths and rituals governing behaviour in pregnancy and childbirth encourage women to cheat fate by taking actions diametrically opposed to those they want to do. Given that as recently as 150 years ago a child only had an even chance of reaching the age of five, it is not surprising that so many superstitions linger in our unconscious minds only to bob to the surface when we are emotionally at our most vulnerable. As Lisa put it:

> A sense of physical vulnerability started almost instantly. I became nervous crossing roads before I even had anything to show for it. At the end, with reason, because if I tried to cross a busy road I wouldn't be able to scarper across in the usual way. But I'm normally really brave.

The desire for other people's goodwill, for universal approval, to appease gods that you don't believe in, afflicts many pregnant women and grows with the maturing baby. You are more reliant, less independent, less yourself. In sixteenth-century England it was believed that a woman who drank from a jug or a cracked cup was risking her child being born with a cleft lip. In Yorkshire in the nineteenth century the cradle had to be paid for before it came into the house, otherwise the child that slept in it would be a pauper and too poor to pay for its own coffin. Prams were always left outside for fear that the baby would be stillborn. Sue remembers that in her first pregnancy the pram did sit outside the house until Nick had been safely born. In subsequent pregnancies a more pragmatic approach took over.

> You start thinking 'I've got to buy these things now because if I don't I'm going to be left with a hell of a big shopping list afterwards and three children in the way of getting it done.'

I was so superstitious that we bought nothing at all for Martha, and even clothes that were given to us remained unwashed in sealed black bin-liners. With Felix I felt no need to store borrowed baby clothes and the Moses basket outside the house; I just didn't have such a strong sense of fatalism. Eve too couldn't let herself take anything for granted: 'My waters broke at 7.30 in the morning, and I had to spend that day going round Mothercare and Boots buying nappies and sheets, everything really.'

Lisa had many friends who showered her with nappies, sanitary towels, romper suits. But although she and Rob did make some practical preparations, she felt that all animate and inanimate objects around her were potential harbingers of doom:

> I was incredibly superstitious. I saw this dead fetus of a little baby bird, I saw the egg which had been broken. And I just thought this is a really bad omen. Then I was down in Shropshire and a friend found this lucky horse-shoe. I put it by my bed to be really near me when I was in labour. I'm not a superstitious person, but I became one.

## Nightmares and Premonitions

Some women do not allow their waking hours to be haunted, but have vivid dreams of giving birth to monsters, headless babies, children they are incapable of looking after. Most women expected to have these sorts of nightmare as a means of unconsciously coping with the odds on something going wrong, a way of being realistic, not naive. In my first pregnancy I thought every day about Martha dying or being disabled, and sleep was filled with processions of grotesquely deformed, sad children. With Felix, when I was happier and more confident at being pregnant, I had only two nightmares:

> 7 AUGUST 1992: Had a dream about giving birth to a handicapped child last night, my first one, not bad for 31 weeks. I was actually there giving birth, but my sister came down afterwards to say that I'd had a boy which I was pleased about, and not surprised. When I got upstairs to the birthing tank, he had a mop of jet black hair, piercing blue eyes and clearly had cerebral palsy: the upper part of his body was huge, the lower part was withered. He was at least 30 years old, a wise face, and almost as tall as me. Greg and I had to convince everybody that there was something wrong, but we were very loving and happy. Oddly, I didn't find this dream particularly disturbing. In Martha's pregnancy I would have thought it a premonition.

Some women, like Joanne, commented that they couldn't remember having unpleasant dreams – 'like you're supposed to' – and others, such as Caroline and Lee, talked about never really feeling anything other than calm and peaceful in themselves. As with everything in pregnancy, it is no more normal to feel at peace and have complete confidence than it is to feel anxious, constantly teetering on a knife-edge. Fear defies logic, and no amount of stern rationality can banish the sinister chimeras. After all, everyone knows that flying is statistically safer than road travel, but for some of us statistics cannot make natural an essentially unnatural mode of transport.

## The Baby

But if your baby was born now, what would it be like? Of course most newborn babies at term look more like wrinkled, red slugs than children to everyone other than their parents. The floppy thing that emerges even at 40 weeks bears little resemblance to the mental picture most of us had of our strong, determined baby who's been shifting, kicking and grouchily jabbing us for the past few weeks.

By the thirty-second week the placenta has reached maturity and the baby's lungs are – or are nearly – developed, an important personal landmark. Even by week 34 the baby, who is responding to a great number of external stimuli, is still covered in vernix, the creamy-white substance which acts as a moisturiser and prevents the baby's skin getting soggy with amniotic fluid. Its fingernails are like tiny shells, and it weighs about 3.5lb (1.6kg), about as much as a large bag of potatoes. On average an amazing 16in (40.5cm) long, it is mostly curled up with its head on its knees and is very thin. It opens its eyes, plays with its fingers and thumbs, and some babies start to get hiccups from gulping too much amniotic fluid. A gentle, rhythmic tapping, both Martha and Felix had hiccups pretty much every night from about 30 weeks.

## Breech Babies

A definite disadvantage to giving birth at this stage is the increased likelihood of your baby being the wrong way up.

About 15 per cent of babies are breech at 30 weeks, where the bottom not the head is over the pelvis, although only 3 to 4 per cent remain so at term. It is not unusual for one of two twins to be breech at birth.

The commonest type of breech position is known as a frank breech, where the baby is bent shut like a penknife, its legs sticking straight up with its feet sometimes touching its ears. In a flexed breech the baby's knees are over its tummy, sometimes with the legs crossed. Most obstetricians will not be concerned by this position until about 32 weeks, since at the beginning of the third trimester there is still a lot of amniotic fluid relative to the baby's size, so it can swim and walk itself over in the uterus like a somersaulting acrobat.

A breech presentation used to be hazardous, and even independent midwives are loath to deliver known breech babies at home. The biggest danger is to the head which, in the normal head-down position, is the baby's most efficient tool for helping the cervix to dilate fully and open the exit. If the baby is coming down bottom first there is a danger that the head may become stuck in the birth canal. If the head is expelled very rapidly through the pelvis the sudden cranial pressure can be damaging to the membranes of the brain, which has not gone through the usual, slow moulding process. Some doctors will automatically suggest delivery by elective caesarean section, particularly for first babies or if the baby is in the rare footling presentation (feet first, rather than bottom first). There is also an increased risk of cord prolapse.

The Royal College of Obstetricians and Gynaecologists (RCOG) now recommends that all women with an uncomplicated breech pregnancy be given the chance to have their baby turned manually. This is known as an external cephalic version. With her hands on the mother's stomach, the midwife will gently place one hand on the baby's head, the other on the baby's buttocks, and try to encourage it to turn by softly flexing and juggling. It feels like an extraordinary churning, as if your whole uterus is being revolved inside out and upside down. You can take things into your own hands and kneel on the floor, bottom up and head on your arms for ten minutes twice a day, which can encourage a stubborn baby to turn. Homoeopaths might recommend Pulsatilla 200 in two doses two days apart in the thirty-fifth week.

## The Importance of Fetal Movements

Not so long ago mothers who were worried whether or not their baby was moving enough would be given a kick chart, where you plot your baby's movements on a chart so the pattern is visible. These have largely been abandoned since they aren't reliable and can breed rather than soothe panic. These days midwives are more likely to recommend that you acquaint yourself with your baby's pattern during the day and sound the alarm if it changes significantly.

Some babies clearly appreciate order and routine more than others and their movements follow a regular pattern: 5am, 8am, 11am, whenever you lie down after doing something especially strenuous. Siân's second baby, Katherine, always woke up when she went to the loo at three in the morning, although obligingly settled easily as soon as Siân had groped her way back to bed. Other babies have a sense of humour, only wanting to play when you want to sleep or make love. Conversely, Sue's second baby, Hannah, did not move much, nor did Annie: both babies were fine, and are extremely active children.

## Clothes Bespeak the Woman

By 28 weeks most women look obviously pregnant. You are not quite big enough for passers-by to assume that the baby is due next week but your clothes – those you can still get into – hang strangely about your distended form. Some women felt that their status in society was enhanced as a pregnant woman, but for those who felt reduced to a stereotype one of the most irritating weakeners of self-esteem at this time was the problem of what to wear without either bankrupting themselves or losing their identity. As Fran put it:

> You either get tacky designs with flowers all over them and daisies on your chest, or nothing. I could never wear leggings because they were just too tight. I ended up walking around with the elastic under my bump, which gives a very baggy bottom, and they tend to drop down too.

For working women the issue is about authority and confidence, not just vanity, since in offices in particular the clothes bespeak the status. In 1977 a male fashion consultant, John T. Molloy, published a book called *The Woman's Dress for Success Book*. An instant bestseller, it remained on the *New York Times* bestseller list for over five months and outlined what women already knew: that if you want to be taken seriously professionally then you must look like a professional. Nothing has changed.

The problem for pregnant women is that these sorts of power-dressing clothes (if, indeed, you want to wear them at all) are not designed in maternity sizes – unless you have an unlimited budget and spend a good deal of time in Italy and France, where designer maternity boutiques are more common. All women who were working found it difficult to look smart enough, even if they were happily making do with baggy sweatshirts and loose-waisted tracksuit bottoms at home. Most women tried to adapt and borrow as much as possible, but lots of people commented on how not being able to dress like themselves gave them a sense of somehow being in disguise.

Eve felt that not being able to wear her sort of clothes greatly affected her self-image in the later stages of her pregnancy, aggravated by the fact that her mother continually talked about how petite *she* had been when carrying Eve.

> She had built up this glamorous image, so I had this awful beacon of my mother's beauty and I would have loved to have been like that.

Eve found it difficult to dress for work, and several women who continued working up until the last moment commented that there was a sense that men punished women for being pregnant and working. If you play the game – slipping into the role of the gentle mother-figure who needs to be protected in her fresh, pretty maternity dresses – then fine; but if you want to be yourself, to continue to work 'like a man', then you should be prepared to fend for yourself.

Eve commuted daily between London and Brighton throughout this seventh month, but rarely was offered a seat: you don't look like a mother, so don't expect to be treated like a mother was the hidden message.

> First of all I'd do the eye contact and poke my stomach up a lot further; then if they just put up their *Financial Times* a bit higher or ignored me, I'd say I'm pregnant, I want a seat. But the only people who volunteered to get up were women, women of all ages. Not one man offered me a seat, not once.

Rachel invested in special maternity suits in order not to look unprofessional, but she too experienced the prejudice against her as a woman continuing to work.

I hated being huge, loathed it. My experience was that
people would actually push you out of the way because
they thought, well, she's not going to be able to rush. I
was never, not once, offered a seat.

## I'm Still Me . . .

I was treated very differently in my two pregnancies.
Although my power suits no longer counted for much in the
office, to some degree they kept me safe from certain sorts
of stereotyping when expecting Martha. When I was writing
during my second pregnancy, slopping around at home in
grotty casual clothes, it was automatically assumed that I did
not work, that I had all the time in the world to stand in
queues, that I was 'just a mother'. And on the days when
two-year-old Martha was with me, I sometimes felt that I had
really, utterly opted out.

Sue, who in her third pregnancy was working from home,
was irritated by the assumptions that people make about you
when you're pregnant.

> Society has this rather romantic view of what a mother
> should be, which doesn't allow for the fact that there's
> an awful lot of guilt and inner conflict that goes on in
> most women when they actually become mothers and
> before: and that's part of the reason we all feel so terrible
> about it, because it's all shoved under the carpet. You're
> supposed to be this wonderful, placid, kind patient crea-
> ture. Well, if you've not been that before how is nine
> months of pregnancy going to change your personality
> like that?

Nicki, who was working for the now-defunct Inner London
Education Authority, was enraged – especially by market

researchers asking, 'what does the head of the household do?'
– that when pregnant with Anna and pushing Max and John
in the buggy people assumed she didn't work. Sharon, too,
couldn't believe how people thought her stomach was a reflection of her character.

> People expect mothers always to be calm, unflappable,
> perfect women who never swear or shout or feel angry,
> unhappy or want sex or whatever. You change phys-
> ically, you change emotionally, but you don't become a
> different person, you don't suddenly become Miss
> Advert on the TV.

How women saw themselves tended to influence how they
were treated. Those women who were emotionally at war,
who were denying that they had changed in any way whatsoever, were unhappier with how the world saw them and
were very harsh on themselves. In retrospect Eve is critical
about the pressures she put herself under, although honest
enough to admit that she would probably behave similarly
next time round.

> All the time I was at work I was behaving as if I wasn't
> pregnant; it was all this macho pregnancy thing, it was
> that this will not change my life, I'm still going to be
> this promising career person, I'm not going to be some
> dowdy mother. That was what it was all about.

## Feeling Fat

In our society girls are brought up to subscribe to fickle defin-
itions of beauty. For white women in particular the ideal is
still tall, thin and elegant with sophistication and sexual allure
thrown in. This is of course completely at odds with how any

pregnant woman looks, and the furore that accompanied the appearance of the heavily pregnant actress Demi Moore naked on the front cover of *Vanity Fair* highlighted the tyranny of society's views of female beauty.[5] The message was clear: we will allow certain sorts of women to pose naked, but not our mothers, not even mothers-to-be. Pregnancy as a public affirmation of sexuality is immediately submerged under the ideal of pure, chaste motherhood. Maternity clothes are designed to infantilise. That women still talk about succumbing to or managing to avoid the floral smocks and tabards illustrates the daily struggle many pregnant women feel they are engaged in to keep their character and individuality intact.

By around 30 weeks pregnancy has shifted women from the private to the public arena. Everyone has an opinion about how pregnant women should behave; everyone wants pregnant women to look well and to enjoy being flattered; everyone expects them to be available for and endlessly fascinated by discussions of dates and names and – where applicable – ages of other children. The double-bind is that, while we may resent conversation becoming limited solely to the sphere of our bodies and our babies, most of us do wish to be thought to look healthy, not least because it constitutes an endorsement of how well we are coping.

I looked dreadful all through my pregnancy with Martha, but with Felix everyone from the regulars at my local swimming pool through to friends and family remarked on how I was blooming. Although I would be intensely irritated in my non-pregnant state to have my appearance remarked upon, while carrying Felix I liked to be complimented, especially on those days when I felt like an extra from *The Wizard of Oz*.

Waiting in the dark for the curtain to go up in the theatre, Nicki can remember hearing herself described as Humpty Dumpty by a man talking to his companion. She knew it didn't matter, but felt crushed nonetheless. Tessa thought she looked brilliant when pregnant, yet became increasingly sensitive of her size as the months went on:

> I was carrying around a lump that was up to my chin and down to my knees, or at least it felt like that because I'm very short.

The hardest emotion to cope with is perhaps a sense of letting yourself down, that you are allowing your appearance to undermine your confidence when you'd convinced yourself that those teenage eating disorders had been banished for ever, the bathroom scales thrown away. But seven months is a watershed at which some women start to feel fat and unwieldy. The presence of amniotic fluid can't really be blamed for the fact that the tops of your thighs have started to rub together: that inconvenience has to be set firmly at the door of those Double Deckers, Mars bars and Kit-Kats you've been snacking on ...

Many women fight against the received wisdom of society and pride themselves on not caring about the opinions of others. But then pregnancy exposes vulnerability, a need to be approved of and endorsed. As Greg said of me, 'you don't give a damn what people think or say, as long as it's positive.' Contradiction is one of the strongest emotions of pregnancy. Although there were some women who felt wholly unattractive or wholly voluptuous, or found their sense of themselves completely unchanged, most women veered between all three attitudes.

**Join the Club ...**

Caroline liked her changed status. She felt fulfilled when pregnant, that she had a clearly defined place in society. Her assertiveness, general self-confidence and sense of self-worth completely changed once she became a mother: 'Until I'd had Emma I don't think I would have said anything to anybody. It made me more confident having had a child.' Lynne, Fran and Lee, amongst others, felt part of an élite, a special club where women smiled at them knowingly on the street. As Debra put it: 'Pregnancy is a great leveller amongst women.'

Lisa had mixed feelings about being seen as representative of a group: she enjoyed the way she was treated whilst being suspicious of the underlying politics.

> People on the whole are much friendlier to you. I went into a chemist's one day to get some eye drops, and there was the great breeze of smiles. 'When's it due?', and when I said 'any day now' they looked pleased. Men and women take liberties with you, but for the first time you don't feel 'how dare you?', because it's so unsexual, it's so unthreatening. Having said that, I felt like a pregnant woman, lumbering along . . .

Sue, although uncomfortable with her size, also felt special and part of a gang. 'On a human level, I think your status is slightly enhanced, because everyone is fascinated by a pregnant woman.'

Debbie worried about her weight, but liked the special attention she got, the consideration other teachers showed her at school, and was pleased to be complimented on how well she looked. She took as much trouble over her appearance as always. 'I still put my make-up on every day, and had my hair done.'

By 32 weeks, though, whatever emotions are in the ascendancy, practical considerations will probably start to take higher priority – finishing off all those last-minute work things; checking the address and time of your antenatal classes;

arranging a series of stand-by lifts to the hospital; inviting your older children to other people's houses for tea for when you go into labour. And all through this are the two-weekly blood pressure checks, the urine tests, the questions about the level of your baby's daily activity and the knowledge that, in Ziman-Tobin's words,

> Nothing any adult can do – male or female – compares physiologically to a woman's ability to become pregnant, carry and deliver a baby.[6]

# Visualise Your Bottom

## Weeks 32–36

When she was young and dancing,
Pregnant women sometimes took
The floor, shamelessly bouncing,
Treating it as a good joke.
Patricia Beer, from 'Jane Austen at the Window'[1]

Antenatal exercise sessions, waterobics, yoga, Active Birth classes, NCT couples' sessions, modules at the local hospital . . . There are many different types of pre-parenthood preparation available nowadays, even though outside the major cities the choices tend to be limited.

Women – and their partners – want a range of things from antenatal classes, most notably hard information, help with breathing and relaxation techniques and the chance to meet and listen to the experiences of other local pregnant women and first-time parents. It's not just a question of forewarned being forearmed, but also of emotionally preparing yourself for your imminently changing role and of committing time to your pregnancy. As Sue put it, 'it gave me a chance to sit and think about that baby [Hannah], just for one hour a week.'

Many women commented that they and their partners enjoyed sharing a set period of time in which to sit and concentrate on the baby together as a couple. Classes can be a constructive way for a partner to assimilate information and to be involved. Several men found it liberating to be allowed to talk about their feelings: their dread that something would go wrong, their fear that they would not be able to cope with their partner's pain, their apprehension about becoming a father. As one woman commented:

> He never seemed to have the time to read any of my books, although I did keep leaving them lying around the house with the pages turned down. But because of the classes at least I knew that we both had the same information about epidurals, what hospital policy was for certain things, what have you. He felt he was making a proper contribution and that he'd have some sort of idea of what I wanted when the time came. On Wednesday nights it was our baby, not just mine.

So far as facts are concerned, it is all very well having read about pain relief, elective caesareans and birth plans, but unless you know something about the procedures at the hospital where you will be having your baby the information could be useless. It was a common complaint that no one ever had time to answer questions about delivery and birth at routine antenatal appointments.

> I kept saying 'I've got a few questions to ask and when can I ask them? Can I ask you now? Should I wait or is there somebody else? And I've got a couple written

down.' And the midwife said, 'well, tell me a couple,'
so I told her and one of them was I'd like to have the
choice of forceps and the vacuum thing, that I wanted
the vacuum thing because I didn't fancy the forceps
and she went straight down my throat. She was really
against me wanting to know anything, and she said
'don't worry about it, forget it all, leave it, you don't
want to know.'[2]

## Hospital Antenatal Classes

Most hospitals run their own antenatal classes, lurching from
the unimaginative but helpful to the surreal. Expecting
Martha, Greg and I attended a couple of sessions at our local
hospital where the senior midwife, Miss Brown, tried to
explain in 1950s BBC euphemisms what pelvic floor muscles
were and how to exercise them. Then, careering into some
peculiar antenatal vernacular, she explained that the increasing weight of the baby and accoutrements was roughly equal
to carrying a shopping basket of five grapefruits, two bottles
of stout, a bunch of bananas (and a partridge in a pear tree,
we muttered under our breath). Imagining that selection of
groceries bearing down on my cervix and bladder exceeded
my powers of visualisation.

The prim assumptions Miss Brown made about the class's
personal circumstances were painfully inappropriate. The
women were collectively referred to as 'girls', and the single
parents were no doubt gratified to learn every now and then
that 'your husband can help you with this one.' Greg was
the only man present, skulking uneasily by the door. Miss
Brown offered him her chair and – though she clearly thought
him odd – referred to him deferentially as Mr Mosse.

The reward for having survived the comic introductory
session was a guided tour of the delivery rooms (sometimes

referred to as delivery suites or birthing suites) and postnatal wards. When we turned up for my actual labour it was extremely comforting to have been in the rooms before. On the day of Martha's birth my waters broke and I was transported from out-patient registration to the labour room in a wheelchair, seated on top of a pile of sodden towels. Having already undertaken the journey under my own steam I felt much less vulnerable in the wheelchair than I might otherwise have done.

In the hope of more practical information we returned – not without trepidation – for a second instalment. Miss Brown had promised us the presence of an anaesthetist, and the prospect of interrogating the person responsible for pain relief kept us sane through more imaginative euphemisms designed to avoid saying vagina and anus. Before the next session, Martha decided enough was enough and got herself born rather than go through any more.

Sue and Max had a similar experience at St Bartholomew's Hospital in London. There the room was so stuffy that several women actually passed out: they scarpered, never to return, after only one session. Jenny attended hospital antenatal classes from six months in Cape Town, where she had her first son. She found the class on pain relief – which is covered in detail in the next chapter – most helpful, although given the technological bias in South Africa it was heavily tilted against drug-free labour.

> They showed two videos, one with a woman having natural childbirth who got into awful trouble and one where the woman had an epidural. There's no doubt which you'd choose after that!

All women who were having hospital births were critical of the social and emotional aspects of the antenatal classes, and this was one of the reasons that so many women, like television producer Siân, didn't attend.

> It was probably very snobby, but from what people said I had this idea that if you went to the hospital ones you'd be stuck there with all the sixteen-year-olds, that there'd be loads of people and you'd just sit around for a long time waiting for things to happen. And you don't have much time.

Most women and their partners did enjoy being shown round the delivery rooms and postnatal ward, commenting that it made it all less intimidating when the day of reckoning arrived. They also thought it important that they had the opportunity to gauge the staff's attitude to everything from caesareans to enemas.

## Birth Plans

In the struggle to release women from a conveyor-belt attitude to birth, an acceptance that different women want different levels of involvement from health care professionals has been slow in coming. But it is one of the reasons that so many hospitals have now introduced birth plans, written by the parents-to-be.

Some women – and their doctors and midwives – have been uneasy about the increasing domination of medical technology, feeling that it has been allowed to triumph over the instincts of the women actually experiencing labour. A birth plan gives the woman a chance to weigh up, before being in the thrall of the heightened emotions of the delivery room itself, what sort of birth she would ideally like. Some hospitals even try to assign midwives on the basis of the tone of a woman's birth plan, a midwife with a very hands-on approach probably not being the best choice for someone who wants no drugs unless absolutely necessary.

The questions included in birth plans vary from choices about pain relief and forceps to whether you would like to see the placenta or not. Obviously it is no more than a list of preferences and no one can predict what will actually happen, but women who encouraged pre-labour planning did say that it gave them confidence, a sense that they would be in control. If medical circumstances dictate alternative action or the woman decides she does want an epidural after all, then there is nothing binding. Birth plans also give partners an opportunity to discover what is expected of them, what sort of role they will be playing.

Lynne attended classes at her local clinic, rather than at the hospital where she was going to deliver. She found the breathing exercises rather silly, and didn't really like the fact that they were only for women: 'I think it would have been more fun if the men had been there.'

Tessa also attended informative and helpful classes from 32 weeks, run at the private clinic attached to the hospital.

> The women were all exactly like me, spoilt middle-class educated girls, not at all the people I'd have as friends but very nice to talk to about babies. There were breathing exercises, but it was clear that virtually all of us were not intending to breathe and wanted epidurals anyway.

Many women, however, are just as interested in helping their bodies feel less cumbersome and pain-bound throughout pregnancy and labour as they are in gathering and absorbing facts. Having fled the airless confines of her hospital classes, Sue felt so shocked and unprepared when she finally went

into labour first time round that she decided to go to Active
Birth classes from 12 to 35 weeks in Hannah's pregnancy.

## Active Birth

Founded by Janet Balaskas in 1981, the Active Birth Movement
runs private classes for small groups of women at different
stages in pregnancy from its London-based Active Birth centre.

> An Active Birth is nothing new, it is simply a conveni-
> ent way of describing normal labour and birth and the
> way that a woman behaves when she is following her
> own instincts and physiological logic of her body. It is
> a way of saying that she herself is in control, rather than
> the passive recipient of an 'actively managed' birth on
> the part of her attendants.[3]

The groups concentrate almost wholly on physical preparation – yoga, massage, breathing awareness – and the possi-
bilities of having a drug-free labour. They also run postnatal
seminars and a breastfeeding and parenting telephone
helpline. Although Sue found it all 'a bit brown rice and
sandals', she thought the relaxation and breathing techniques
were fantastic and that they wholly transformed her second
and third experiences of labour: 'I still use the pain relief
techniques now. I never need an injection at the dentist, for
example.'

As well as doing yoga for pregnant women, both Pam and
Lisa attended Active Birth couples classes, which they
enjoyed. And Sarah, having attended NCT classes in Kirsty's
pregnancy, also decided to try Active Birth for Abigail's pregnancy from three months onwards to complement what she
already knew.

I wanted to do something and I felt that a yoga-based approach would be good for my back. Also, it was a way of giving some time to this baby as well.

A huge number of women who attend antenatal classes of all sorts want to meet other local women who are going to become parents at the same time. A majority want to hear the experiences of women who have gone through pregnancy and birth, to learn and be reassured. As Lisa said:

The best thing was when one woman came back and told her birthing story. That was when it all became a bit more real in a way. I loved the personal stories; some women told them better than others, but I thought they were fantastic.

## National Childbirth Trust

Founded more than thirty years ago, the National Childbirth Trust (NCT) is an important charity which offers support, information and practical help. As the introduction to their own pregnancy handbook says:

The Trust aims to help parents experience greater confidence in, and enjoyment of, pregnancy, childbirth, and the early days of parenthood.[4]

Almost all major cities now have NCT antenatal groups, as well as counselling and postnatal support networks. They also produce leaflets and books, initiate research and campaign on specific maternity issues. Over the past five years, their influence and scale of operation have grown.

The physical emphasis is based on psychoprophylaxis, breathing techniques pioneered in Russia and introduced in the West by Dr Fernand Lamaze. The philosophy of NCT is to encourage women to take responsibility for themselves, to prepare their bodies during pregnancy to respond automatically to each type of contraction they will feel in labour, and to be confident about their ability to give birth. Partners are expected to act as coaches and emotional supports during pregnancy and labour, and there is strong emphasis on introducing parents-to-be to other couples. Aspects of pain relief, problems that could come up during labour and listening to women who have just given birth are all integral parts of the course. The NCT also runs a postnatal counselling service.

Most NCT antenatal classes start at around 32 weeks and are held in the evening so that working partners can attend too. Women have the legal right to take time off work to go to any form of bona fide antenatal activity, but most said that they found it too distracting to be relaxing on the floor practising breathing when they were due at a key meeting 45 minutes later.

The majority of NCT teachers are women who have enjoyed the classes themselves, rather than health care professionals. The training takes a couple of years, and teachers are paid for the classes they take. Sarah was so impressed by the level of information she and Mike got at their local group, and the friends she made, that when Kirsty was a year old she decided to train as an NCT teacher herself. 'Once I'd given up my job I wanted to do something, and it seemed an ideal way to keep my brain going.'

Lee and Simon enrolled for the eight-week NCT course in Nottingham at 32 weeks. They didn't feel that they learnt anything they didn't already know, but did enjoy meeting other local parents.

Having abandoned yoga because of problems about not being able to follow instructions to 'visualise her bottom' without laughing, Eve and Stephen then tried NCT from six months in Brighton. Although they haven't stayed in touch with anyone from the class Eve did enjoy hearing about other women's experiences – not least about how badly most of the male partners were coping! She was interested in the attitude towards pain relief, which she agreed with and found to be in sharp contrast to the advice she was getting at the hospital:

> Some people obviously feel they're in control if they're not in pain, and other people feel that they're in control if they're not on drugs. And that's definitely how I feel, the second one.

But here Eve touches upon one of the biggest criticisms levelled at NCT classes. Some women had a sense that having pain relief was seen as in some way opting out. Jane got a great deal out of NCT classes socially, and went from 30 weeks onwards. She has stayed in touch with women from her group, but did comment on the lack of unbiased information she felt they were given about pain relief.

> I was definitely frightened about the pain in labour – I'd decided I was going to have an epidural from the minute I found out I was pregnant – so I went to NCT and sat there throughout all the classes saying, yes, very interesting, but I'm having an epidural.

Although Nicki went to NCT because she was interested in drug-free birth, she too thought that too little information was given about pain relief, and what there was was delivered in a negative way. Several women commented on friends who attended NCT classes and who, having given birth, felt disappointed and believed that they'd failed just because they'd had an epidural. And despite the fact that there had been sessions on stillbirth and other problems during labour they felt that they'd been presented with a rather idealised image. Debra elected not to go to local classes for this reason.

> I really feel from reading about active birth and all your natural chemicals and hormones balancing, that drugs and over-hospitalisation is a mistake. But you cannot predict it. Hospitals do a good physical job and you may need it. You must be more fulfilled as a woman to get the choice to do it naturally, but friends in London doing NCT seemed to be pressurised into doing it at home and not having any drugs whatever. I wasn't brave enough to demand too much and I was relieved not to have to choose.

Siân enjoyed the information on the pelvic floor exercises, thinking about a birth plan, meeting similar sorts of people. But at the same time she thought that there was far too much concentration on the birth itself and not enough attention paid to what it would be like once the baby was born. This feeling was borne out five weeks after the birth when, at her wits' end, she phoned the local NCT breastfeeding counsellor for help.

> She couldn't make it over to our house because she had her own children and things, and I didn't feel any resentment about that because it obviously was difficult. But suddenly I realised that, despite NCT being a great institution, at the end of the day the statutory bodies were much easier to deal with, the health visitors and other professionals who are actually paid to come and help, rather than a woman who has so many other demands on her time. For me, in the end, the whole idea of a voluntary network of women helping each other just didn't hold up.

The point is that different philosophies are appropriate for different women. No organisation, whether independent or part of the National Health Service, can possibly cater for every woman's needs and that is why it is sometimes sensible to attend more than one range of classes if you have the time. There is no doubt that helping new parents integrate into their local community is invaluable for many women, who are frightened about feeling isolated at home once their baby is born.

Sasha went to special breathing classes, her local NCT group and a series of eight classes at her local hospital: she feels she got something out of all of them. As Dr Miriam Stoppard says:

> Shop around for the classes in your area that empha-
> sise the aspects of pregnancy and childcare you feel
> most unsure about. Ask your doctor or midwife or at
> your local health centre.[5]

But despite an increasing emphasis on antenatal education, fewer than half of all pregnant women actually attend ante-natal classes, according to Mary Nolan, an NCT teacher and author of *Antenatal Education: A Dynamic Approach*, partly because they are increasingly hard to find:

> Money has never been so scarce in the NHS, and the
> first things to go in maternity services are always ante-
> natal education and postnatal care. Four years ago,
> we were running three courses a year. This year, we
> ran ten and could have run three times as many very
> easily.

Women from ethnic minorities, those with disabilities and young women find it particularly hard to find classes to suit their specific needs, as can single mothers and those with multiple pregnancies.

Expecting twins, Sharon did attend classes, but was given no information on how her experience might be different from the generally discussed norm:

> Only one person actually said anything to me that made any sense, which was at my last visit to the breathing classes. She was a health visitor, I think, and she said, 'everything we've talked about for women, it's going to be different for you. But one thing I know is you're not actually going to go full-term, you're not big enough, you're not actually tall enough to carry two babies.'

Debbie said that antenatal classes didn't really exist in her part of Northern Ireland – although she thought there were better facilities in Belfast – partly because there was an assumption that pregnant women would have been in the company of other pregnant friends and neighbours and would know what to expect. Caroline, who lives in West Sussex, felt the same. Many of her friends locally had been pregnant and had children, so she couldn't imagine what the hospital antenatal classes could have to offer. 'It worries you that you're doing it wrong. I'd just much rather get on with it than have all that fuss.'

I briefly thought that I would sign up for some other classes after the abortive hospital foray, but nothing really appealed. In retrospect, I realise that I actually wanted to cope with the experience of pregnancy and childbirth in my own way, and that subconsciously I somehow thought that any sort of group session would interfere with that. Already quite emotional, I didn't want to be pressurised or annoyed by assumptions about what would suit me.

4 AUGUST 1992: Every Tuesday afternoon I look at my watch at about 1.30 and make up some excuse why I can't amble up to the antenatal class – I've got too much work to do, it's too hot, I don't feel in the mood . . .

Why this reluctance, I wonder, to accept that I simply don't want to sit listening to a room of pregnant women? I'm warmed by the feeling of being a member of a special club, all bumps together, as if we're all in on some wonderful secret. But swapping smiles with a pregnant woman as you pass at the checkout till is somehow still private. That's it, really. Being in a contained group within four walls would be uncomfortably un-private. Intrusive. Yes, it would somehow intrude on us, me and the baby.

Instead I concentrated on my own daily exercise programme, feeling that the best I could offer myself was a body that I felt comfortable with going into labour.

## Two Laps Around the Park and Back

One of the advantages of exercise is that it regulates one's appestat, the brain centre that controls appetite, and I found that the periods when I didn't use up energy were those where doughnuts and chocolate featured more prominently. I swam regularly carrying Felix, greatly helped by the warm summer weather. Freezing changing-rooms that have your nipples and uterus rigid before you've even got into the pool rather spoil the sense of relaxation and pampering yourself, not to mention adding to the likelihood of cramp. I concentrated on the baby as I swam up and down, as if I was ferrying him across the water, and it made me think about breathing.

Worried about putting on too much weight, I hoped that I'd feel able to do more vigorous – aerobic – exercise in the early months of Felix's pregnancy. I remembered huddling under a horse chestnut tree in Greenwich Park when I was a few weeks pregnant with Martha, feeling the rain dribbling through the leaves and down my neck. Being British summer-time, it was settling in for the afternoon so there was no point in waiting. Yet my illogical self was convinced that if I ran the baby would drop out. Even as a novice to pregnancy I knew this was stupid, of course, but false instinct was more powerful than knowledge. With Felix, I was embarrassed to admit – even to myself – that I still didn't believe that it was safe to jump up and down. I missed a lot of buses . . .

Those women who didn't get very big, and therefore didn't find themselves with a new centre of gravity, were obviously able to continue doing their normal exercises: Lee was out riding on her mountain bike two days before Hannah was born. I don't think I could have reached the handlebars.

Physical preparation for childbirth has always played an important role in most cultures. Women of the Stone Age hunter-gatherer tribes were not expected to sit idle, as women in parts of the developing world cannot afford to today. Two thousand years ago Plutarch advised that women should 'harden their bodies with exercise of running, wrestling, throwing the bar and casting the dart' so that they would be fit for childbirth. The Ainu women of Japan still exercise strenuously when pregnant in the belief that it will encourage swift labour. The belly dance (otherwise known as the *danse du ventre*, *ventre* being the French word for stomach or womb) is believed to have been practised not only as a rite through which the Mother Goddess was worshipped with pelvic rocking and rippling of abdominal birthing muscles, but also as a form of childbirth preparation.

For the women I spoke to, as often as not it was time that stood in the way of fit, lithe bodies. For working women it is hard to find the energy to shoot up to the local sports centre for a lunchtime swim, and for those looking after older children it is often impossible to remain unencumbered for long enough to take regular exercise. Many women put great strains on their bodies during pregnancy, but not of a constructive kind. Standing on a commuter train or lugging a wounded three-year-old up from the playground floor is exhausting and does little to improve fitness. Several women commented that they'd always intended to be fit during their pregnancy, but when they did stop working they found that the sofa and a blanket were more inviting than bracing fresh air.

## Physical Changes

Exercise can mitigate the increasing numbers of aches and pains that women experience in the last few weeks of their pregnancies. Most of these are caused by the increased weight of the baby and the strain on your whole system (cramp, restless legs, backache). Some women, though, did have one-off problems, as when Lynne suddenly had a burst blood vessel in one of her eyes.

Lisa was hospitalised at 32 weeks for a suspected urinary infection. She had severe abdominal pains, but there were no indications that she would go into premature labour; although the pain went on for two weeks and Lisa stopped working, her pregnancy continued quite comfortably until she gave birth to Harry, at home, at 39 weeks. She thought that the worst thing about the illness was that no one could tell her exactly what was happening, so it sapped away her confidence in her body's ability to cope.

Some of the women who had previously remained in tune with their inflating stomachs, at this stage suddenly felt enormous and uncomfortable. This was often exacerbated by the anxious look in the eyes of passers-by who plainly believed that labour was imminent, not still a month away.

Breathlessness takes a few new victims, leading to increased fatigue. Some were afflicted by bouts of weepiness – for some women the first of the pregnancy – and a feeling that the whole of their pelvis was about to drop out on to the pavement.

In the eighth month Sasha and Joanne were still vomiting regularly and with Felix I still felt nauseous. Joanne was also diagnosed as having carpal tunnel syndrome, caused by the increased supply of fluid to the extremities during pregnancy. Pressure is exerted on the nerves and blood vessels which pass through the wrist canal (known as the carpal tunnel), resulting in numbness, tingling or sometimes pain in the hands, fingers and arms. Massage can help, especially in the neck and shoulders, to reduce tension, and for severe symptoms homoeopaths might recommend taking aconite 6X three times daily for five days.

Alongside the niggles, there are several serious problems that could develop now, which is why standard antenatal care at this point in pregnancy allows for two-weekly instead of monthly checks.

## Pre-Eclampsia

Any variation in blood pressure is closely monitored and signs of protein in the urine are analysed. A careful watch is kept for oedema, the slight puffiness or swelling that is normal in pregnancy and can be exacerbated by hot weather, prolonged standing and fatigue. Herbal remedies include dandelion leaves, golden rod, corn silk and couch grass. If you have generalised oedema, and if when you apply finger pressure to the puffy areas white indentation marks appear (known as pitting), and if you have protein in your urine, this may be a sign of the potentially very dangerous pre-eclampsia. A sudden rise in blood pressure of more than about 20 points after resting is also one of the warning signs. The normal systolic/diastolic pressure for pregnancy is between 110/70 and 140/90 depending on the trimester: blood pressure remains the same or drops slightly during the first, reaches its lowest point in the second, then works its way back up during the third. Many women with high blood pressure are consistently slightly higher and those of us with low blood pressure can be as low as 90/50. The systolic figure is a measure of the pressure generated by the heart as it pumps blood around the body; the diastolic figure denotes the pressure in the arteries when the heart is at rest.

Eclampsia is a potentially life-threatening condition peculiar to pregnancy which leads to convulsions in the mother. In the misogynist scientific journals of Victorian England eclampsia was often called the 'epilepsy' of pregnancy. The convulsions may be preceded by severe migraine which won't respond to analgesics; visual disturbances such as flashing lights; abdominal pain and swelling; and protein in the urine. It used to be extremely serious and, up until the mid-twentieth century when antenatal care improved in most industrialised countries, was responsible for many neonatal and maternal deaths.

In 1914 one of the leaders of the Women's Co-operative Guild, Margaret Llewellyn Davies, made a public appeal for direct experiences of childbirth and childrearing as a means of proving to the Liberal government of the time that maternal and infant care was virtually non-existent for poorer women. She had a particularly good response from the wives of manual workers, many of whom had suffered from – or known women who had died from – eclampsia.

... falling out of one fit into another, and at last, after her baby was born, she lay two days quite unconscious

– in fact they never expected she would recover. She had two doctors, and they gave her every attention, and then when she was getting better her own particular doctor told her that if she had only consulted him beforehand he could have saved her a lot of pain . . . He said it was some kidney trouble which had been the reason of all she had suffered. In both her case and mine we could have had advice, as far the expense was concerned, but it was sheer ignorance and the idea that we must put up with it till the nine months were over.[6]

These days, between 5 and 10 per cent of pregnant women are affected although it only develops into full-blown eclampsia in about 1 in every 2000 cases. About one third of cases are identified during pregnancy, another third are diagnosed during labour itself, while one third of cases come on after the birth.

In hot, humid Cape Town Jenny's blood pressure suddenly rocketed at about 35 weeks: when she went back a few days later for a follow-up check, they discovered protein in her urine and that her kidneys were leaking protein as well. Jenny had felt well throughout the pregnancy until this point, although she had experienced three or four debilitating migraine attacks. She was confined to bed immediately, and James was born on time at 40 weeks.

In her second pregnancy Jenny was given contradictory advice about whether or not she was likely to suffer from the same problem.

The consultant told me I was twice as likely to have it. My GP told me I was no more likely to have high blood pressure this time. In fact I was less likely having had it last time.

She actually had several migraine attacks, but her blood pressure remained at an acceptable level.

It is a more common condition in first pregnancies, and only 4 per cent of women develop the disease in second or subsequent pregnancies. No one really knows what causes pre-eclampsia, although there seems to be a genetic factor, as you are more likely to get it if your mother or sister has had it. The only thing Jenny could do was follow her instincts and wait and see. Although her blood pressure did rise a little towards the end, it was never a problem and Douglas was born on his due date weighing a healthy 7lb 15oz.

## Essential Hypertension

In a third of cases the cause of high blood pressure is never found, and it tends to be noted as 'essential hypertension', indicating the same treatment as for non-pregnant patients using anti-hypertensive drugs. You may be confined to bed either at home or, in severe cases, in hospital. Hypertension may interfere with the functioning of the placenta and prevent it from efficiently transporting glucose (food) and oxygen to the baby. Herbal remedies may help to reduce blood pressure, in particular those made with hawthorn leaves, flowers or berries, but should be taken only after consultation with your doctor or midwife. Horsetail tea, extra vitamin B6 and magnesium, and reduction in salt intake are also thought to help.

## Placenta Praevia

At this stage in pregnancy any vaginal bleeding should be reported immediately to your doctor or midwife. Repeated small haemorrhages of bright blood could indicate placenta praevia, bright red in colour because it is coming from so low in the uterus. Eve had a repeat scan at 34 weeks to check that she wasn't suffering from placenta praevia: as she suspected, the placenta had moved away from the cervical os [the opening of the cervix] and was now safely above the baby.

In fact, in most cases the placenta moves. A Finnish study of 8000 women scanned half the group between 16 and 20 weeks: 250 women were diagnosed as being at risk of placenta praevia. At delivery, only four mothers actually had the complication. In the non-scanned group, there were also four cases of placenta praevia. All eight women gave birth to healthy babies by caesarean.[7]

## Placental Abruption

Dark blood accompanied by abdominal pains can indicate placental abruption. The blood comes from a normally situated placenta which separates prematurely from the uterine wall. Sometimes the bleeding is concealed, but the woman has abdominal pain and is shocked. Very hard to diagnose, this is potentially an extremely serious condition for the baby, since depending on the degree of separation it can be cut off from its blood supply. Severe haemorrhage may also cause blood clotting difficulties for the woman, putting her at risk too. There is pain over the site of the placenta and the woman often goes into shock as the blood loss is internal as well as external. The baby will probably have to be delivered by caesarean section, although if the baby is mature, in good condition and there has been only mild separation, some doctors may induce labour for an attempt at vaginal delivery. Birth is often sudden, after a short labour.

## Early Deliveries

At about 14 weeks Rachel suffered from swollen ankles and prolonged tingling in her hands and feet. Since she was abroad working extremely hard in hot conditions she felt confident that things would calm down once she was home. For the next four months she felt well, although she was aware that she was putting on rather a lot of weight (she went from 9st 7lb at conception to 12st 3lb by 32 weeks). At 33 weeks she suddenly developed bad pins and needles in her hands and feet, her legs swelled up like balloons and her back became completely numb. Her GP confined her to bed for a week, took her blood pressure – which was high – and did a urine test, which was negative. Having read many pregnancy hand-books, Rachel diagnosed herself: 'I thought I was in the first stages of pre-eclampsia.'

She was sent to the hospital after the week's bed rest and was 'passed as fit', although she still felt that there was some-thing wrong: 'I felt like death.' She set plans in motion for finishing work at the end of her thirty-fourth week, rather than carrying on until 37 weeks as planned. She'd been smoking and drinking – both alcohol and caffeine – and paying no attention to her physical condition. Now she cleaned out completely and tried to take as much rest as possible. She went into the office from 10am until 3pm only on days when her husband Jeremy could give her a lift there and back. On Wednesday 15 August, her last but one day in the office, she went to the loo at about three o'clock to find that she was bleeding and passing large clots. Someone called an ambulance, laid Rachel down on the office floor with her feet in the air, then called a friend in another department who'd just had a baby.

I was absolutely in a state of shock, it was like being hit by a tree. I found myself saying – and feeling – things like 'This is the only thing that matters' and 'I don't give a fuck about work' and 'It's my fault'. Suddenly it was real, and the whole of work which had been a huge part of my life wasn't anywhere near as important as this baby.

Rachel cannot remember much of what happened next as her fear obliterated the flashing blue siren, the race through the hospital corridors. She does recall her friend holding her hand, and that it was reassuring.

On arrival at the nearest hospital they put in a drip then tried – unsuccessfully – to find a fetal heartbeat. Rachel knew the implications, but just couldn't take anything in until she asked to go to the loo and passed blood not urine into the bedpan.

It was too bad to be involved with, there was this distance. It was as if I was looking on at it and not really involved. But then when I passed all that blood, that was when it really hit me, in a real way, that this was happening to me.

At this point the Registrar arrived. Rachel was reassured because she felt that she would tell her the truth. The young doctor who'd failed to find the baby's heartbeat had made such a song and dance about there being something wrong with the machine that it pushed Rachel in the opposite direction and convinced her that Rose was dead. Violent, stabbing pains suddenly attacked Rachel, 'as if my insides were being ripped out'. Even then she clung to the hope that medical intervention would simply stop the bleeding and let her pregnancy continue. She couldn't accept that Rose had to be born.

I said to someone 'it's too soon, it's too soon, you can't do it', and I had this overwhelming sense of responsibility that it had been my fault because I'd been smoking

and working. I wanted to know if I was going to die,
if the baby was going to die.

With sensitive bluntness the Registrar firmly told Rachel that
both her and Rose's lives were at risk. Preparations began
for the emergency caesarean and finally Rachel realised that
she no longer had a choice. It was almost a relief.

The events of the next few hours she subsequently pieced
together from other people's reports. Her best friend had
joined the colleague who had accompanied her from the office
and both women were invited to stand outside the operating
theatre. The Registrar explained that women who had emergency operations and became mothers without the benefit of
preparation and labour often didn't believe the hospital staff
were telling them the truth when they said the baby was
doing fine. My mother, for example, wasn't allowed to see
me for five days after my birth and was convinced that I was
dead, that the doctors and my father were all trying to protect
her by lying.

The operation was incredibly quick. Rose was whipped
out weighing a creditable 4lb 5oz and taken to the special
care baby unit. Throughout, the Registrar treated Rachel's
friends as if they had a right to know what was going on.
She brought them a cup of tea and with the same unselfcon-
scious directness told them that both Rachel and Rose would
have died if the operation had been carried out five minutes
later. Her hands were shaking.

Rachel remembers coming round, clutching her friends'
hands, convinced that the baby was either dead or suffering
from Down's syndrome. By this time her husband Jeremy
had been tracked down and, after the difficulties of the pregnancy, she realised as he rushed into the room that all he
cared about was that she was alive. It made her feel curiously peaceful. Later, from her bed overlooking the river

Thames, she watched a beautiful sunset over the Palace of Westminster. Six weeks ahead of time she had become a mother, Rose had been born. Three years later, Rose was bigger than many children her age, a distinctive, intelligent and energetic little girl.

Sharon also became a mother earlier than she'd expected. Warned by the health visitor that she was too small to carry twins to 40 weeks, she had read that twins are considered full term at 37 weeks anyway. So although 34 weeks was still a bit of a shock, it was not too frightening.

Sharon had stopped working at 18 weeks and so when the moment came she was emotionally and practically prepared, with her bag packed for the hospital. 'It was quite exciting; I both wanted to get it over and done with, and I didn't want to get it over with after all.'

Two days earlier she'd had a show, where the blood-tinged gelatinous plug of mucus that blocks the cervical canal during pregnancy dislodged itself. In panic she rang the hospital, but they convinced her that she could still be a couple of weeks off going into labour so she carried on as usual. Her husband Gary had resentfully stayed at home that day, but by the Friday was so bored that he'd disappeared off to the pub.

Sharon was hoovering, having just had lunch, when her waters broke, a sort of whooshing noise then amniotic fluid all over the spotless carpet. She had no labour pains, but started to develop backache so she rang Gary at the pub. He begrudgingly came home to take her to the hospital. They arrived at about 3pm on a cold, grey November afternoon – an inauspicious start.

> You keep on thinking 'it's a false alarm, it's a false alarm',
> then suddenly you realise 'oh God, this is it!'

In many cases hospitals would try to halt labour by the use of drugs, and of course the earlier the babies are born the more likely it is they will have to be checked into the special care baby unit. In the past few years obstetricians have become more likely to let women go into vaginal labour, and several books, such as Elizabeth Noble's *Having Twins*, advocate the benefits of natural delivery for multiple births if at all possible.[8]

## Twin Labours

Twin labour is not necessarily longer than for one child, and there is only one first stage. The most common position is for both babies to be head down, with the second twin usually following within 15 to 20 minutes. So long as the second baby's heartbeat remains normal then – within reason – the amount of time separating the two deliveries is not important. But there is an increased risk to the second twin. It may, for example, be in an awkward position, or have shifted after the birth of its sibling; the woman's body may have less energy to push another baby out; there is a greater risk of cord prolapse and of premature separation of the placenta. Women delivering multiples are often offered an epidural just in case a caesarean becomes necessary.

In 1984, although caesareans for multiple births were not automatic, the latest improvements in the way many women in labour were treated had not really got very far and Sharon was put through an appalling labour. The midwife at first challenged Sharon, insisting that her waters hadn't gone at all. It was only after an internal examination revealed that her cervix was 2cm dilated that everyone went into immediate overdrive. Sharon was then assailed by a stroppy anaesthetist who arrived, without consultation, to administer the epidural.

I certainly wasn't a believer in natural childbirth. It might be OK, but not for me: I wanted pain relief, but I didn't know anything about epidurals. When I said this she said, 'Well, I'm not taking responsibility for you or the babies if you don't have an epidural.'

An epidural numbs the whole abdomen, giving the emotional advantage that the woman remains fully conscious and aware of what is going on as her baby or babies are delivered.

At 24 years old, intimidated by the very people who were supposed to be helping her, Sharon was terrified and desperate not to be told off any more. The epidural was set up, two drips and two monitors, but only one fetal scalp monitor because Katie, the second twin, was breech and they couldn't get the electrode on to her head safely.* By one o'clock the following morning, Sharon had dilated to 8cm, still 2cm to go.

The midwife then made a unilateral decision not to top up the epidural again, since she felt that somehow Sharon wasn't 'trying hard' enough. The pain, as it slowly seeped through her body, was unbelievable. Sharon knew she was going to be sick but the midwife took no notice: 'It was very much "We know what we're doing, you just shut up dear and do as you're told."'

Sharon's moment of triumph was managing to throw up all over the supercilious woman.

Shaking with cold and fatigue, Sharon desperately tried to push out the first of her babies. At 4am the medical personnel present suddenly noticed that both twins were distressed. Sharon was peremptorily told to stop pushing,

---

* A fetal scalp monitor provides midwives and doctors with a permanent digital readout of the baby's heartbeat and makes the traditional method of external checks with a stethoscope unnecessary.

which was incredibly difficult after three hours of being told the opposite. The anaesthetist – who had been so convinced that Sharon would need a caesarean that she had gone to bed fully clothed – was summoned to top up the now non-existent epidural. As the operating team assembled it was clear that several of the staff there thought the whole labour had been mismanaged. The student doctor helping was so upset that she whispered to Sharon, 'I promise you that I'll never let anyone else go through that. You shouldn't have been made to go through all that.'

There was a pause while someone plucked up the courage to ring the consultant for permission to operate. Next thing Sharon remembers is seeing her two babies being lifted out, Charlotte then Katie. She realised they were big (4lb 12oz and 4lb 15oz respectively) for 34 weeks, and quickly stole a kiss from Katie. Although the doctor told her that both babies were fine, they were immediately taken to special care: she could hear their cries getting more and more faint as they were wheeled away down the corridor. Sharon was amazed, delighted, that they were two girls. She remembers being surprised at how low the caesarean cut was, and that the sensation of being sewn up was like someone brushing their fingers across her skin.

Left alone in the delivery room Sharon felt shattered, relieved that the longest 14 hours of her life were over. She then realised that everything was different, that she was now a mother. Taken to the recovery room and wrapped in a silver insulating blanket, she was desperate to know why her babies were in special care: she'd been given photos – standard practice in many hospitals where mothers are separated from their children at birth – but it made her worry that they were going to die. The midwives and doctors said that both girls were fine, just premature, and she should get some sleep. The doctor had failed to sign the form allowing anything stronger than paracetamol to be administered, so it was only when a substitute doctor had been tracked down and he administered a shot of pethidine that the pain subsided enough for rest to be possible. The day passed in a haze.

## The Baby

Of course, the vast majority of babies are still kicking their mothers to pieces at this stage, and experiences like Rachel's and Sharon's are rare. By 36 weeks your baby will weigh about 5.5lb (2.5kg), will be getting plumper by the day and may have stretched to 18in (46cm). Its fingernails, like tiny shells, reach to the ends of its fingers, its toenails to the end of its toes. Its head may have engaged, which means that it has dropped down into the pelvis ready to be born, although many babies – especially in second and subsequent pregnancies – don't engage until labour is under way. It's clear when it happens, though, since breathlessness improves once the baby has sunk down a little.

Your baby's position will have been recorded in your notes from about 26 weeks onwards using an arcane shorthand. The most common terms – and the most common positions – are denoted by ceph, short for cephalic, meaning that the head is down, and anterior, which means that the baby's back is lying against the wall of your bump. The precise position of the head is described by the whereabouts of the occipital bone at the back of the baby's head (occiput). Positions to the left, right or front of your pelvis are known as left occiput anterior, right occiput anterior and occipital anterior. If the head is sideways across your pelvis so that the occiput is at one hip bone or the other, the positions are right occipito lateral (ROL) or left occipito lateral (LOL). Seventy-five per cent of babies go into labour as either ROL or LOL.

A less common cephalic (head down) position, when the

baby's back is towards your spine, is referred to as posterior. Three posterior positions are available, known as right occipito posterior (ROP), left occipito posterior (LOP) and occipital posterior (OP). Only 10 per cent of babies are in a posterior position at the start of labour, most commonly first babies. Although they usually rotate it can lead to a longer, more painful labour, with your back taking the strain. Indications of a posterior lie are a saucer-like dip around the navel and the kicks being obviously in the front rather than at the sides or back.

There has been a reported increase in the proportion of posterior babies since the 1950s. Some people put this down to the fact that women these days tend to spend less time on all fours scrubbing and polishing. This is undoubtedly good news for womankind in general, but tough on some in labour. You can adopt this position early on or, if you are suspicious about the lie of your baby in later months, try to rest on your hands and knees for ten minutes a day during the last four weeks: this might, by force of gravity, encourage the baby to spin round.

Alternatively, a stubborn baby refusing to budge could be a sign of things to come. After all, the next four weeks will take you – finally – to full term.

# Build Up, Count Down

## Weeks 36–40

Part of the paradox for a male doctor is one's knowledge that one will never experience the most important biological act that humans are capable of . . . Such
joy and physical creativity after the vomiting, piles and
stretching pains of pregnancy, the dreadful force of
labour and the blood and shit and waters of birth. To
the final shock and delight of suckling the immaculate,
slippery, vernix-coated living being: the proof that
bodies aren't just wonderful ideas but they *work*. Desire,
sexuality, fertility. Intercourse, conception, procreation.
The random sequence made circular and closed.

David Widgery, *Some Lives!*[1]

The emotions that build up in the countdown to birth are
anything but simple: desperation for it all to be over, desperation for it not to start. Perhaps being pregnant for ever
wouldn't be so bad . . .

There is excitement that you will soon be a parent, coupled

with paralysing fear that you simply won't be able to cope. Sometimes you are confident that your body will meet the challenge, but for many self-assurance is undercut by terror of pain. And from 36 weeks onwards, particularly with first babies, there is a sense of imminence, of the clock ticking away.

For me this incontrovertible timetable was one of the most satisfying things about pregnancy. Much in our daily lives, at home or at work, is artificially programmed to a degree. We can be late at work, we can fail to meet a deadline, we can decide when or if to visit friends, even when to keep going when a stinking cold makes bed the most sensible option. But pregnancy has its own timetable and seasons. Although science can delay – sometimes even halt – the rule of the physical, your body's instincts will ultimately hold sway.

Only 2 per cent of babies arrive on their estimated date of delivery (EDD), but most women expect their babies to put in an appearance around the 40-week mark. It is dispiriting to have to wait even longer, but equally disarming to find yourself in labour well before you'd expected. This inability to control the course of events is good preparation for parenthood, though, since there is always only so much planning you can ever do!

## Premature Babies

There is a certain amount of confusion surrounding the term premature baby. Rachel's and Sharon's daughters were classified as premature babies, not just because of the length of gestation but also because they weighed less than 5lb 5oz at birth. A real premature baby lacks subcutaneous fat, is still covered with a downy hair called lanugo and often has a thin, gelatinous skin. It is likely to need monitoring in a special care unit at a current cost to the NHS of approximately £1000 per day. Multiple births account for 25 per cent

of all premature births – 37 weeks is considered full-term by
many doctors and midwives – and the evidence now is that
babies born to mothers who smoke are twice as likely to be
born prematurely.[2]

In Britain 42,500 babies are born prematurely every year,
one of the highest rates in Europe. Tommy's (based at
St Thomas's Hospital in London) funds research in to why
Britain's figures are so bad. Leaving aside specific medical
problems such as pre-eclampsia or antepartum haemorrhage,
one third of premature deliveries occur for no known reason.

Sometimes doctors can tell if a woman is about to go into
premature labour by testing for something called fetal
fibronectin. This is a protein found in amniotic fluid and, if
detected on a swab from the cervix, can indicate that your
waters have broken early. An ultrasound scan to check the
length of your cervix is another method that's sometimes
used to predict early labour. Sadly, neither test is terribly
accurate and doctors tend to use them to identify women
who aren't at risk of premature labour rather than those who
are. In other words, if you don't have any fetal fibronectin
in your vagina and your cervix is of a normal length, you
are unlikely to be in labour.

By 36 weeks, though, the majority of babies born would
not be classified as premature. They might be small, but they
are as likely to be fully developed as a baby that has gone
to term, and they will look just like any other newborn child.
Martha was born at 36 weeks, weighing 6lb 10oz and was
clearly as ready to be born as she was ever going to be. Well
above the 5lb 5oz mark, she was not considered premature.

## The Nesting Instinct

One of the difficulties of having an early baby is that you
never get the time to plan and organise. In these last weeks

parents-to-be prepare in three ways: practically, emotionally and physically. Many people have decided that they will only start to buy things for the new baby, rearrange the furniture and so forth once they have stopped work and have time to enjoy it. Some, like me, never get the chance.

Jane admitted to developing an out-of-character obsession with cleaning and dusting: 'I was very much nesting. It used to be a joke in the household, what corner would I be cleaning next.'

Sarah was desperate to finish decorating the bathroom before Abigail was born and Debbie was sewing cushion covers for the new baby's room. But most women refuted the idea that their sudden interest in housework could be blamed on their hormones, as if being a mother was a pre-programmed instinctual, natural role.

Most of us, women and men, want to exercise control over our environment. Entering the uncharted territory of labour, birth and parenthood, it is natural for us to want our physical surroundings to be in order and comfortable. And if normally you work away from home the sudden impact of becoming more or less housebound with a heavily-pregnant stomach, then a baby, makes you more sensitive to piles of unironed washing or that infuriating chip out of the paint just by the kitchen door, right there, always in your line of sight . . .

Except for the most superstitious, who take nothing for granted, most women did want to have the basics ready for the labour and for after the birth, although the definition of basic varied greatly from person to person. Women all over the world prepare their physical environment, from the Mansi women of Siberia who decorate the birthing hut with their most beautiful handkerchiefs to women in America and Britain lighting candles, preparing cushions or setting up favourite pieces of music in the room in which they intend to deliver. Pregnancy handbooks often assume unlimited budgets and unlimited interest in pristine, perfect provisions to complement the experience of labour and birth. Take appropriate advice and decide for yourself. Also check with your hospital as to whether or not they have rocking chairs, a birthing stool, anything you think might help you through the labour. Many hospitals will be happy if you bring in your own beanbags and tape recorders; others are uncooperative.

If you are having a home birth, your midwives will have discussed what specific things you need – for example a sieve and a bucket for water births, plastic sheeting to protect the carpet – and you will need to ensure that you have sanitary towels, breastpads, nappies and a babygro or two, since there will be no one to borrow things from on the spur of the moment as there is in a friendly hospital labour ward. Most midwives will be grateful for the odd chocolate biscuit or piece of toast as well ... They will run through the sort of equipment they carry in case of emergencies, from plasma for maternal bleeding to oxygen in case the baby has breathing difficulties. For many imminent parents-to-be, knowing exactly what will be available is reassuring.

## Water Birth

When I was having Felix, water birth was just starting to become popular in Britain. There were an estimated 2000 water births in 1992, as opposed to a couple of hundred in 1987. Now, most hospitals have their own birthing pool and organisations hiring out pools – such as the Active Birth Centre, Splashdown and Birthworks – are doing a roaring trade.

Recent surveys show that 64 per cent of maternity units have at least one birth pool, although it's not known exactly how many women actually use them.[3] In one midwife-led birth centre – the Edgware Birth Centre in London – 80 per cent of women spend at least part of their labour in water.

Women have used water as a form of pain relief for centuries, but there are no historical records of women giving birth under water until the pioneering work in the Soviet Union of Igor Tcharkovksy in the 1960s. There are rumours, however, that South Pacific Islanders sometimes give birth in shallow salt water, and that the Maoris, American Indians in Panama and the Ancient Greeks may have practised water birth.

In Moscow, giving birth and suckling under water has been common for nearly thirty years. Michel Odent at his clinic in Pithiviers in France encourages women to use a uniquely designed birthing pool to help them during labour. The warmth helps the muscles relax between contractions and, because the water supports the body, some proponents claim that fewer women suffer perineal tearing when giving birth in water. It is less strenuous to give birth on all fours or in a supported squat aided by gravity in water. Many women talk of the privacy a bath or a pool gives them, with their terri-tory being clearly defined.

The temperature of the water in a birthing pool is like that of a warm bath, and it can be constantly topped up. The advantage of a specially designed pool over a bath is a matter of space: it is difficult to deliver a baby in a bath, even at home, as most are too small. And few women feel comfort-able in austere hospital bathrooms, even if the staff are prepared to deliver the baby there. In a pool, the midwife can either lean over the edge or get into the pool with the woman to help guide out the baby. Many women prefer to get out and deliver on dry land, especially if they have had a long first stage and have been in the water for ten hours or more; others couldn't contemplate moving into a different environment, and in fact stay put not only for the birth but for hours afterwards.

So long as the water is warm enough, there is little likelihood of the baby experiencing breathing difficulties because it is still receiving oxygen from the placenta via the umbilical cord unless it is kept under the water beyond the point when the cord has stopped pulsating. But, the midwife will guide the baby to the surface of the water within a matter of seconds and she or he will breathe as soon as air hits its face. To many, the advantages to the baby of being born into an environment similar to the one it has just left are obvious. And although obstetricians and midwives do need to feel comfortable assisting at a water birth no specific additional medical knowledge is required.

## Worries About Underwater Delivery

Shortly after Felix had been born, one of my midwives asked me to talk to her couples' NCT antenatal group about my experience of giving birth in water. Amongst the many questions were a few from partners voicing worries about hygiene or the possibility of a baby drowning.

Three years later a survey of water birth revealed that 12 babies died after their mothers laboured and/or gave birth in water, but none of these cases was thought to be directly related to the water birth itself. A further 51 babies either had some infection or breathing difficulties, but again exact causes were unclear owing to the retrospective nature of the research.[4] The same year at the First Annual Water Birth Conference, a makeshift sign pinned to the wall read:

Water birth is dangerous . . . for obstetricians.

Then Dr Geoffrey Ridgway, infection control specialist at University College Hospital, London, hit the news in April

1996 by insisting that all pregnant women wishing to give birth in water had to undergo tests for HIV and hepatitis B and C. He justified his decision in the press:

> We don't know what the risk of infection would be, but you can't just wait for evidence to appear ... My concern is that there would be a combination of faeces, blood and a baby in a body of water.[5]

Water birth enthusiasts were heartened when a review of eight clinical trials carried out by the Cochrane Library in 2000 concluded that there was no evidence that water birth jeopardised the health of mothers or their babies. And, finally, a joint statement issued by the Royal College of Midwives and the Royal College of Obstetricians and Gynaecologists in April 2006 gave water birth a cautious seal of approval:

> There is no evidence of higher perinatal mortality or admission to special care baby units (SCBUs) for birth in water. Women who make an informed choice to give birth in water should be given every opportunity and assistance to do so by attendants who have appropriate experience.[6]

I had known virtually nothing about water birth until I took the plunge myself, but until that moment in the NCT class the one thing that just hadn't crossed my mind was that it might be dangerous. Based on little other than instinct, I'd thought being in warm water would be a natural, almost enjoyable, way to work through labour.

My instincts were borne out by the statistics: in one study of first-time mothers, only 24 per cent of those using water in labour asked for pain-killers as opposed to 50 per cent of those on dry land.[7] Another study revealed that none of the water-birthers had episiotomies, whereas 27 per cent of the first-time mothers in beds and 8 per cent of the second-time round or more were cut.[8]

## Packing the Bag

Most hospitals provide clothes lists, which usually include night-dresses, maternity bras, pants and toilet bag. Because Martha was so early I went into hospital with nothing but a toothbrush and a big purple T-shirt that I intended to wear during labour. This meant that Greg had to charge round the shops six hours after becoming a father, buying feeding bras, nappies and a few baby suits. None of this really mattered, although it was stressful at the time. My trainers rather than slippers, raised a few eyebrows. But having personal things around you can make a big difference to how comfortable the hospital seems. After being in labour for 12 hours it would have been nice to have had a bath with my own soap and shampoo rather than indus-trial rent-a-block hospital soap. I would have liked cream to help prevent my nipples cracking and soft breastpads when my milk started to jet out, rather than a strange wadge of what looked like greaseproof paper shoved in an eminently unsuit-able and desperately tight sports bra. I would have liked my own salt to put in the bath to help my stitches heal.

Some handbooks suggest taking books, jigsaws or tapes into hospital to ward off boredom, but the women I met were too exhilarated or tired to focus on anything other than the baby itself and their aching bodies. Coins or cards for the pay tele-phone are useful – find out which – to maintain contact with your pre-parent life. Favourite snacks (Marmite sandwiches, in my case) can be smuggled in just in case the canteen food is awful. The husband of the Indian woman in the hospital bed opposite me brought her in a curry at about 6.45 every evening.

Practical preparation – or the lack of it – is an important part of emotional preparation. It can help instil a sense of order, of the time being right. With Martha I left my office on the Friday night with a breezy 'see you on Monday'. Everything was winding down, and I was now happily anticipating my final week at work. But by midnight on Sunday I had my child in my arms. The following Thursday my work colleagues went out for my good luck, pre-maternity-leave lunch – but without me.

It seemed rather lucky at the time; after all I'd avoided that awful, nerve-racking waiting. But the suddenness of Martha's birth made the first few months of her life extremely difficult for me. Emotionally I hadn't had the opportunity to draw the line, to tidy things up, to say goodbye to friends for the time being. In a way, it was my work persona which went into labour: as the monitor was strapped to my stomach, necessity was forcing me to write down a list of people for Greg to call so that meetings could be cancelled, tasks delegated. It stopped me being able to concentrate fully on Martha or myself. As Siân put it,

> You need to calm down, you realise that more second
> time round. You need to feel relaxed, turn your head off,
> so that you can cope with the sleepless nights that follow.

Eve stopped working at 37 weeks and Annie was born three days later. She still feels rather proud about her timing, even though she was not really mentally prepared either. But she is glad to have missed the growing fear of the pain and of something going wrong that assails so many women as the 40-week mark gets closer and closer.

## Pain

Tessa had complete confidence in the obstetricians who would be assisting her. In her first pregnancy she enjoyed her last few weeks, emotionally and sexually because her husband returned from Italy at 36 weeks, having been away for several months. But she was terrified of the pain and played games with herself, trying to imagine the very worst sort of pain she could have so that the actual pain of labour wouldn't be such a shock:

> I used to think what could be worse than being run over by a roller-coaster. Then my doctor said, 'Look, if you want to enjoy your labour have an epidural.' And he was right. You know there are so many books, so many articles, so many women who make you feel guilty for having drugs, and I think that's terrible.

Debbie tried to adopt a realistic attitude to the pain.

> Millions of women have had babies. You just have to think 'I can do it', and you just have to be positive and think he or she will come out somehow. But I think the books are unrealistic sometimes. They say this is going to happen and that's going to happen, but it's not really like that because every birth's different.

Sarah was also apprehensive about the pain. She didn't want a pethidine injection to dull the agony, because she had read that it crossed the placenta and therefore directly affected the baby. 'So that left me with either entonox, which might not be enough, or a full-blown epidural.'

There are many, many different ways of relieving pain in labour, and most women think about what they would or would not like before they actually reach the delivery room. The Bible enjoins women 'to bring forth children in sorrow', and although different cultures have had methods of minimising labour pain, historically women have expected to suffer. Then in 1853 Queen Victoria gave birth to her eighth child with the help of chloroform: to a certain degree, this helped legitimise pain relief in Britain.

Most good pregnancy handbooks have thorough explanations of the pros and cons of the three most commonly used chemical means of minimising pain, although for every woman who swears that her epidural was the best decision she ever made there is another whose experience was exactly the opposite. Labour is painful, and even though some women experience the pain positively most would say that there were moments when they would happily have swapped places with anyone else in the entire world rather than have another contraction. Only you can gauge the level of pain you wish to experience, how much is acceptable; only you know what form of pain relief will best suit you for that particular labour. Make no assumptions. Many women comment that a form of pain relief that was perfect for their first child proved wholly inadequate subsequently.

## Gas and Air

Entonox, a mixture of nitrous oxide (laughing gas) and oxygen, is generally known as gas and air. This is usually the first sort of pain relief that women are offered in hospital, and is also carried by most midwives for helping women giving birth at home. You inhale through a mask or mouthpiece, and it works best if you take several deep breaths as a contraction starts so that the gas is having an effect at the peak of the pain. It is effective for women who are happy for their heads to be slightly out of action, thereby dulling the messages of pain that their body is sending. I took one whiff with Martha, felt hideously drunk and nauseous, and that was the end of that. Caroline really enjoyed it in her second labour and felt she was controlling the pain by being able to choose when to use the entonox.

## Pethidine

Pethidine is a narcotic anti-spasmodic drug given by injection, usually into your bottom, which takes about ten minutes to work. It can be an effective block to the pain, and many women are happy with the pain relief it gives. But it is becoming less popular because of the possible side-effects on both woman and baby. It too makes some people nauseous and drowsy. Sharon, who had a pethidine injection post-caesarean, said that she was still aware of the pain but at a distance. Again, for women who do not want their heads to feel detached from their bodies it is probably not the best choice. If given between two and four hours before delivery it is also likely to affect the baby, possibly making it floppy at birth and depressing its respiratory centre. In this case, an injection would be administered to reverse the effect of the opiate.

## The Epidural

So what about the much-talked-about epidural? It takes about 10 to 20 minutes for a skilled anaesthetist to set up, and is an anaesthetic injection into the epidural space around the spinal cord inside the vertebrae. A fine catheter is threaded through the hollow needle and into the epidural space, then the catheter is fixed to your back, leaving a small badge-like object into which the drug itself is administered. The effect is usually felt within a few minutes, and the epidural can be topped up every few hours as necessary.

Many women are extremely nervous about something being inserted into their spine. At the hospital antenatal class I attended this fear was expressed and the anaesthetist told us we were free to sue him if we became paralysed. He did warn us, though, that in about 1 in 150 cases the catheter accidentally pierces the dura, a membrane around the spinal cord, leading to headaches over the following couple of weeks.

Some women found the sensation of being taped and wired up very unpleasant. With Martha the drug going down my back felt like someone tracing a straight line with an ice-cube: it was an enjoyable, sensual experience. Although my first dose was not 100 per cent effective – I had one patch below my left breast that was not numbed – they tipped me over on to my side and let the fluid swish around when they topped me up. Then I sat looking at the monitor, seeing that I was in agony, but feeling nothing.

The biggest drawback with an epidural is that it makes for a completely managed birth. You can't move about, as your legs are as numb as your abdomen, so you and your baby get no help from gravity. Your blood pressure may drop, and you will have a drip set up to feed you fluids to counteract hypotension. Your bladder will have to be catheterised and your baby will be electronically monitored to check for any signs of distress. Since I had also been induced with Martha, I actually looked like something out of an intensive care movie, with wires and tubes protruding from most parts of my body. A fetal scalp monitor looking rather like a blue and red striped bellringer's rope hung out of my vagina.

Epidurals do not always work, particularly if badly administered, and their effects can linger. Research done in the early 1990s suggested that women who had epidurals were more likely to suffer backache after labour although further research has since cast doubt on this.[9] Some women develop blinding headaches following an epidural – not what one needs when caring for a newborn.

Another survey suggested a further, alarming side-effect. Research showed that 30 per cent of babies whose mothers had epidurals registered a skin temperature higher than 38 degrees C; 10 per cent had temperatures of over 39 degrees C. Severe overheating (hyperthermia) is always potentially dangerous for a fetus.[10]

I did have a numb and tingling left leg for about three weeks after giving giving birth to Martha. Limp notwithstanding, I still thought my epidural wonderful in that particular set of circumstances . . .

## Forceps

When epidural anaesthetics are used it is extremely likely that forceps will be needed and an episiotomy performed. Forceps were invented at the end of the sixteenth century by an English obstetrician, Peter Chamberlen. Until the development of anaesthesia and caesarean sections, forceps were the only way of helping a woman in labour who could not push out her baby unaided. There are several different grades of forceps designed to correspond to how high up the birth canal the baby's head is located. Although there are the usual horror stories about obstetricians breaking babies' necks or causing brain damage, it is a safe procedure in skilled hands. Figures for 2004/5 show that 11 per cent of women have instrumental deliveries, which includes both forceps and ventouse.

Forceps resemble enlarged sugar tongs with the two blades held a fixed distance apart so that no compression is put on the baby's head. Some sort of local anaesthetic must be administered to the perineum, and maternal bruising is inevitable. Babies are often born with unsettling purple-red bruise marks on their faces, but these disappear within a few days of birth. Since midwives are not allowed to use forceps, only doctors, consultants and so forth, they have been seen by some as an example of male tools taking over from women's hands.

## Ventouse

An alternative to forceps used by more and more hospitals is the ventouse or vacuum extractor, invented in the 1950s. Many women feel that it must be less distressing for their baby than cold forceps blades, but its main advantage is that it can be used when there is still a rim of cervix left for the head to pass. As its name suggests, the ventouse looks and works like a mini-vacuum-cleaner. A vacuum suction cap is fixed to the top of the baby's head, and traction applied. The only likely after-effect is cosmetic: a small blister-like bump on the top of the baby's head which goes down within three or four days.

## Episiotomy

A common bedfellow to the forceps is the episiotomy, a small surgical cut made between the vaginal opening and the anus designed to help the baby out and to minimise the risk of tearing. Thankfully fewer hospitals now use it routinely: only about 13 per cent of women giving birth in England have an episiotomy these days compared with 52 per cent in 1980. About 80 per cent of women who have an episiotomy have one prior to a forceps delivery.[11]

Experts disagree as to whether cuts or tears are the most painful, and which heal more effectively. One's point of view will, of course, depend on the size of the tear and the competence of the obstetrician performing the episiotomy. Sheila Kitzinger's survey of 2000 women who'd had episiotomies came to the conclusion that they were more painful to suture and heal than tears. Caroline, who had an episiotomy for her first child, certainly felt that being cut was more painful, whereas Tessa was delighted with her obstetrician who decided not to risk a tear.

It was such a brilliant episiotomy that I was making love within three weeks. Now I do think that is brilliant. Mind you, I don't know anyone else who had such a good experience.

Her partner Mark, who was watching, was also impressed:

He said it was time. It was definitely a good idea. He just made this little cut and the baby shot out.

## Transcutaneous Electrical Nerve Stimulation (TENS)

Other methods of pain relief include TENS, transcutaneous electrical nerve stimulation. This reduces pain levels by interrupting pain transmission and by stimulating production of the body's natural painkillers, endorphins, by a small electric current transmitted to strategically placed electrodes on the woman's back. The sensation is like butterfly wings or pins and needles. Many hospitals now hire out TENS machines, and there are various firms like MamaTENS and Tens-Hire.co.uk, which do them too.

TENS has been the most commonly used form of pain relief in Sweden for the past twenty years, although it is less effective if not used from early labour onwards. Jenny found it helpful in her second labour in hospital in Portsmouth, until she wanted to have a bath: there was no one available to reapply the electrodes when she got back. Supporters said they particularly liked being able to control the intensity of the current.

Acupuncture and hypnosis will only work with those women who have used either method successfully throughout pregnancy. Some women find that massage and breathing can help them control the level of pain they experience, and there are several herbal remedies for use before and during labour. Raspberry-leaf tea helps tone the uterus and reduces the risk of haemorrhage during labour, poppy-head and lime-blossom tea are both pain relievers and Bach Flower Rescue Remedy might help in transition. Homoeopathic remedies vary for different sorts of labour, and since they are specific both to you and to the sort of labour you find yourself experiencing, it's advisable to contact a homoeopath to discuss options.

## Pre-Labour Fears

Other women – Jane, Lynne and Debbie – worry less about the pain than about something going wrong at this very last stage: not so much that their baby will suddenly die just before delivery, but more that some medical mistake will lead to brain damage at birth. As one remarked, 'you've been looking after this baby perfectly, wonderfully, for 9 months, now someone else might spoil it all.'

The number of avoidable disasters that happen in industrialised countries at birth is extremely low, but of course it is a natural fear. The fear is really borne of the idea that the situation will spiral out of control, the forerunner to worries about being able to care for your child adequately once it has been born.

Lynne, who had been terribly worried about Michelle's safety throughout the pregnancy, found the last few weeks extremely difficult to cope with and was very weepy. 'I was like a tap almost permanently on.'

She also had split abdominal muscles at 38 weeks, which felt like exposed nerves. Combined, all this fuelled her growing panic and fear that labour would be disastrous and that Michelle would not be born safely. Siân too felt a growing sense of unease in both countdowns to labour.

The closer I got to the birth the more I worried about something going wrong, because you suddenly realise that this baby is going to be with you soon, so you actually think about it as an entity more towards the end. And that's when your fears grow. They increased even to the point that with Alexander I went into hospital too early in labour because I hadn't felt him move for a while.

Several women had dreams about giving birth to children that they couldn't love. Lisa dreamed about already having robust five-month-old twins and somehow giving birth to a newborn baby who looked scrawny and helpless. She couldn't love it as much as her healthy babies and, in her dream, she gave it away to her mother and sister to look after.

Dreams – imagining the worst – are *not* omens or portents. For some, they are more a way in which your subconscious mind explores, preparing your conscious mind for what is the most dramatic and instant shift that anyone can experience.

For many women the fear of something going wrong at delivery was focused around physical and emotional fear at the thought of having a caesarean. Although most women said they would choose the operation if their baby's life was in danger, few want the operation unless it is absolutely necessary and many women talk of having an emotional need to go through the process of actually giving birth via vaginal delivery. For a few, there's also an instinctive sense that something as momentous as the arrival of one's child should be accompanied by an extreme physical experience.

Sue went into false labour at 37 weeks in her third pregnancy, with Lottie. The doctor started talking about an emergency caesarean if her contractions started again and the head still wouldn't engage. Lynne was fearful of going through labour then having to have a caesarean under general anaesthetic right at the end. Pam, who knew that her fibroid made a caesarean likely in any case, kept her hopes of a vaginal delivery alive until she was actually in the operating theatre.

> I didn't feel that I'd prepared myself. I didn't feel that it would be a slow transition because I think that's what labour does.

## The History of the Caesarean

Birth by caesarean is an ancient method, mentioned in religious and literary works from the Talmud to Shakespeare's *Macbeth*. There are even illuminated medieval manuscripts depicting wise women (*sages femmes*) and surgeons performing caesarean operations. According to legend, it was the method by which Julius Caesar himself was born, hence the name (although since Caesar's mother survived in an era long before medical technique was capable of preserving the lives of both mother and baby, the true derivation is more likely to be from the Latin, *caesura*, a cut). In Ancient Rome the law required that every pregnant woman dying in late pregnancy should be given a caesarean; and in 1608 the Senate of Venice made it a criminal offence for any physician not to perform the operation on a pregnant woman thought to be dead.

The first recorded successful European caesarean was performed in 1500 by a Swiss pig-gelder, Jacob Nufer, on his wife. (This is not as terrifying as it sounds, since in many cultures butchers were the first surgeons.) Not only did the baby survive, but Frau Nufer went on to give birth vaginally to four more children. Rumours of successful caesarean operations surfaced over the next three centuries, but even if the baby did survive the overwhelming majority of mothers died either from massive haemorrhaging or because of blood poisoning.

The first modern version was performed by Max Sänger, a German doctor, in 1882. The work of Pasteur and Lister had explained the causes of infection, antiseptic techniques were more widely available and anaesthetic was increasingly being used. Sänger sutured the uterine wall as well as the abdominal wall with silk threads, and used aseptic methods. Operating predominantly on women with deformed pelvises, he reported an 80 per cent success rate.

Even so, until the development of antibiotics between the two world wars, it was an operation with a high maternal mortality rate. Today the twin dangers of any surgical operation are still the risk of infection and post-operative haemorrhage.

The operation itself takes about 45 minutes, although the baby is delivered in the first 5 or 10 minutes or so, and it can be performed under epidural or general anaesthetic. The obstetrician first makes a small, usually horizontal, cut along what books still insist on calling the bikini line. She or he then cuts through the lower part of the uterus where there are no main blood vessels. If the membranes are still intact, they will be broken and the amniotic fluid sucked away. The surgeon then puts her or his hands into the uterus and gently rotates the baby's head until it appears in the incision. The baby is then eased out, often using forceps. If there is excessive bleeding a drug to help stem the flow might be administered at this point, before the delivery of the placenta and the sewing up.

In the developed world it is now a relatively safe operation, if a painful one from which to recover: research in America suggests that while 72 per cent of women who give birth vaginally regain their normal energy by six weeks after the birth, only 34 per cent of caesarean mothers feel back on form by the same stage.[12]

Maternal deaths are thankfully rare in the UK, but the fact remains that women who have a caesarean are really five times more likely to die than women who give birth vaginally.[13] An elective (planned) caesarean is safer than an emergency operation, but the risk to the mother is still between two and four times greater than in a vaginal delivery.

## Medical Reasons for the Operation

Caesarean sections have saved the lives of countless women and their babies. These days there is a growing fashion for requesting an elective caesarean à la Victoria Beckham, but the medical consensus is that there should still always be a valid medical reason for having one: pre-eclampsia; placenta praevia; the woman's pelvis simply being too small to allow the baby through; the woman herself being disabled so that vaginal delivery is impossible; the baby lying awkwardly; fetal distress either before the onset of labour or because labour is not progressing effectively enough. From the 1950s onwards there has been a steady increase in the number of caesareans performed, peaking in 2004–5 at 23 per cent.[14]

Doctors' fear of being sued for negligence if something goes wrong is one possible reason given for the rise. In a random sample of 400 obstetricians in Britain, 47 per cent of them admitted that fear of litigation over a difficult vaginal birth was their primary reason for performing a caesarean.[15]

Leading American obstetrician Dr Jonathan Scher takes a less cynical view of his colleagues' motivations.

In obstetric science the 1970s was the decade of the fetus. We turned our concern from the fate of the mother and

directed our energies and resources into improving the
condition and health of the fetus. The rise in indications
for caesarean section has resulted largely from that shift
in emphasis.[16]

Others were harsher, feeling that the regularity with which
the operation was performed was symptomatic of the mysti-
fication and medicalisation of birth, with increasing dominion
being exercised over women's bodies by the male medical
establishment. In 1986 the obstetrician Wendy Savage was
suspended from her consultant's post at a London teaching
hospital. She performed fewer caesareans than her colleagues,
and the implication was that she was endangering life. Her
defence was that she based her decision on the individual
woman (and of course there are those who are delighted not
to have to labour). The resulting inquiry found her record of
maternal health and infant survival at least as good as that
of her colleagues, and she was cleared. Hundreds of women
who had been delivered by Dr Savage staged a protest outside
the hearing.

Statistics show that women over 35 are more likely to have
caesareans, often because they are automatically seen as 'high-
risk'. Some doctors are reluctant to let women go into labour
if they have had a previous caesarean section because of the
very small risk of the scar rupturing. However, the tide does
finally seem to be turning. Leading obstetricians are agreed
that the caesarean rate in some maternity units is too high
and, in 2004, NICE published guidelines to help ensure that
women only have caesareans when they really need them.

## Vaginal Birth After Caesarean (VBAC)

During the first part of the twentieth century the phrase 'Once
a caesarean, always a caesarean' was in common usage among

doctors. Towards the end of the century, though, midwives and obstetricians started to question the need for women who had had one caesarean to automatically have another for subsequent babies. In 1992, a study carried out by St Mary's Hospital Medical School in London revealed that 71 per cent of women who had their first child by caesarean successfully gave birth vaginally second time round. Later studies suggest that as many as 80 per cent of women who attempt a vaginal birth after having a caesarean succeed.

While these figures are encouraging, obstetricians are loath to recommend VBAC out of hand because of the small risk of scar rupture it carries – somewhere in the region of 0.5 to 3.3 per cent. Having said that, research also suggests that VBAC is, in general, just as safe for mother and baby as having a repeat elective caesarean. At the end of the day it is up to each individual woman to decide which option is best for her.

## Multiple Pregnancies

Some doctors automatically expect women with multiple pregnancies to have caesareans, regardless of the nature of the pregnancy or the health of the babies themselves. Sharon's 34-week twins were delivered by caesarean section after a badly mismanaged labour. To avoid being railroaded, Nicki had sought out a female consultant who she thought would be more sympathetic to her desire to have a vaginal delivery for her twins unless it was medically unwise. But from 16 weeks onwards the consultant made comments like, 'have you ever seen a mentally handicapped person?' or 'do you want to be doubly incontinent?' Nicki resented the constant implication that she was deliberately and irresponsibly intending to endanger the twins' lives. Later she discovered that the consultant had written a book advocating elective (planned) caesareans for all multiple pregnancies. As Lee commented, in different circumstances:

> They think you're going to go and put your baby's life at risk on the day when you've gone through nine months of tender loving care, as if you're going to jeopardise your baby.

## Physical Changes

But worries about what could happen do not necessarily spoil what can be a happy and restful time. Many women look forward to labour. There's no doubt that one of the cleverest things about the design of pregnancy is that after nine months' carrying you can cope with the idea of pain, if only so that you will be able to reclaim your body and life once more: at the beginning the whole idea seems pointlessly barbaric.

Once Felix had moved down into my pelvis and his head had engaged I was less breathless. Although I felt as if I had an orange wedged between the tops of my thighs, physically I was much more comfortable. It was also the beginning of autumn. I have never been able to shake off that beginning of a new school year excitement, and this added to my sense of expectation.

Several women talked about feeling extremely excited, sexual even, in the last couple of weeks, as if they were poised on the edge of a new adventure. Lee felt positive, continuing to prepare physically right up until the day of Hannah's birth, as did Sasha, who was practising squatting and massaging her perineum with oil to help it stretch during labour. Nicki felt excited, being interviewed and taking on two new free-lance jobs in the weeks before Anna was born. Lisa found that she was very weepy – 'enjoyable tears' – which she found cleansing rather than upsetting: 'I was rather looking forward to labour, actually. I saw it as climbing a mountain, running a marathon, a great physical test.'

## Guilt About Your Older Children

At this stage it is common for women having second children to have nightmares about something awful happening to their existing child, a sort of subconscious way of worrying about not having enough love to go round. Sue worried greatly about how Nick would feel when Hannah was born, as well as that she wouldn't have enough love for the new baby. 'Then my grandmother told me not to worry and that children brought their own love with them. It helped a lot.'

Sarah was a little preoccupied by the idea of what things would be like when Abigail was born: 'I was more concerned and apprehensive about how she would fit in with Kirsty.'

Sasha had the difficult situation of Lou's older children starting to make demands on his time at about the time that Freddy was due. They were 16 and 14, and the younger of the two obviously felt threatened by the idea that Lou would love a new baby better than them.

> After all I'd been in her life since she was four; I was just Sasha, I wasn't going to do anything to shake things up. Then suddenly a baby was about to arrive.

In my dreams Martha was kidnapped, killed or taken away from me. By 39 weeks I was terrified, not only that I wouldn't be able to love another child as much as her, but also that our relationship would never be the same again.

> 6 OCTOBER 1992: feel prickly behind the eyes all the time. My emotions are running riot, and merely looking at Martha – straightening her glasses, organising imaginary

picnics, trying to get her pyjamas, 'on myself' – just makes
me overflow. Today she whispered to me to stop crying,
in her serious little way, and told me that everything was
all right. Will she still love me – us – like this when the
baby comes?

Once we had borrowed a baby bath and the Moses basket,
Martha became keener on talking about being a big sister,
how she was going to carry 'her baby' and help us bath it.
She liked to sit for hours in the basket on the floor, keeping
it warm, and loved to drag out photographs of herself sleeping
in the same cot when tiny. She too had waited long enough
and wanted Felix to arrive.

## When D-Day Comes ... and Goes

What happens when the sun rises and sets on your due date
without you experiencing so much as a twinge? Joanne was
excited on the actual day, especially since Rowan's head had
been deeply engaged since week 38, but nothing happened.
Every day that followed was increasingly depressing. Pam
had set her heart less on things starting on time, but each
successive day seemed to have 25 hours, then 26, then 27 ...
'The due date came and went, and it wasn't until the first
week of being overdue that I started to worry.'

Sasha found the two weeks she was overdue unbearable,
'partly because I'd been expecting him for 4 weeks before his
due date anyway'.

Women with their second or subsequent children tended
to assume that the pattern would be repeated and indeed it
is not common for a woman who has had a straightforward
delivery to be more than two weeks earlier or later for her
next children.

Fran's son Matthew was born at 40 weeks, then her

daughter Rowan at 42. This was a little depressing following the scare of premature labour at 30 weeks. Siân gave birth to her first baby two weeks late. For her own peace of mind she had to assume – rightly – that Katherine would follow suit:

> I had to think that, otherwise it would have been awful again. The last two weeks when you go over are awful. You wake up thinking well, it really could happen any time now, then it just stretches on. Another week goes by, then you have to go into the hospital for those last few weeks and then they start talking about being induced. And that was a real low last time. You just think, Christ Almighty, this is my body, why won't it do something, because you don't understand why it won't start.

For some the waiting is simply depressing, especially when it is extremely hot; others get worried that something might be wrong and others are terrified by the thought of being induced. How long doctors are prepared to wait for a woman to start labour naturally varies from county to county and country to country. The worry is of postmaturity, that the placenta will have run its course and will increasingly be unable to nourish the baby adequately. The baby will be checked and if its heartbeat is steady and its feet, arms and elbows still thumping away, then seven days' latitude is fine. After that many hospitals insist on monitoring women every day and after two weeks may begin to suggest starting labour artificially.

## A Helping Hand

The most common medical method of inducing labour is prostaglandin pessaries, which are made up of various hormones that have an effect on the pregnant uterus. They look like waxy bullets and one is usually inserted at night with the hope that contractions will start naturally within the next few hours. Having had Joe at 37 weeks, Tessa was determined that Matilda would not be late. She arranged with her consultant that if she didn't go into labour herself on 6 February, her due date, then she would be induced two days later. The weekend passed with nothing more than a few Braxton Hicks contractions, so at 8 a.m. on the following Monday Tessa arrived at the hospital and was given a pessary. By four o'clock nothing much had happened, and they were discussing administering a drip. Then her waters broke and labour started in earnest.

> Everyone kept saying how much quicker it was second time round. Everyone I knew had four, five, six hour labours, having gone through twelve or fourteen hours before. But Matilda's labour followed almost exactly the same pattern as Joe's. She was born just before 10 that night.

### Sweeping the Membranes

Sweeping the membranes is a technique that has long been used informally by midwives to help get labour going. It involves placing one or two fingers just inside the opening of the cervix and gently 'sweeping' the membranes with the fingertips to separate it slightly from the cervix. This releases hormones called prostaglandins, which send signals to your brain to start labour.

Some women find membrane sweeping painful, but it is so effective that it is now offered routinely to all women who are still waiting to go into labour at 41 weeks of pregnancy. Those who choose to have it done have a higher chance of going into labour over the next couple of days and are less likely to need more medical methods of induction.

## The Caul

It is possible, though rare, for a baby to be born still inside the amniotic sac. In folklore this has always been considered extremely lucky, and in powdered form it was a potent ingredient used in witches' spells. The sac, or caul, was considered a powerful talisman, particularly against drowning, and was also said to confer the gift of the gab: sailors and lawyers paid high prices for them. David Copperfield's caul was sold for 15 guineas, and James I of England and Winston Churchill were both born in their cauls.

Felix's head was born in the sac, then as his shoulders came out the pressure burst the bag. His head was unmoulded, he was caked in thick vernix and he was very calm.

## Syntocinon

Synthetic oxytocin, syntocinon, administered by intravenous drip is the last resort when contractions fail to start. Oxytocin is the natural hormone from the pituitary gland in the brain. When the artificial substance is used contractions are often said to be stronger and longer with shorter periods of relaxation between them. You have to have a needle in your arm or hand, which will not be removed until after labour and, because of the rapid crescendo of contractions, it is likely that painkilling drugs will be needed. The incidence of epidurals and forceps or ventouse with syntocinon-induced labour is very high.

## Do-It-Yourself Induction

There are of course many natural ways to induce oneself. Sometimes they work, sometimes they don't. In seventeenth-century France petals were dropped into water to symbolise the opening body; in Russia in the nineteenth century knots were untied; in Pakistan bottles are opened and in Malaysia long hair is let loose. Some physical methods are more successful than others; weight lifting, exercise, retching, sneezing. The two best-known homespun remedies are curry and sex. The idea of purging, thus stimulating sympathetic contractions, is an old one. Castor oil was a firm favourite in Britain for many years but is generally frowned on by midwives as a method of induction these days.

Sex should be more fun. Semen contains prostaglandins similar to those used in Prostin pessaries, so have sex as often as possible, lying for at least half an hour afterwards on your back with a pillow or two under your bottom. Nipple stimulation can also help induce labour, since it releases oxytocin from the pituitary gland into the bloodstream. You may need to massage your breasts for up to an hour three times a day. Acupuncture always works, even if the cervix is not ripe, and homoeopaths might recommend Caulophyllum 200 taken as a single dose. Herbs for inducing labour include golden seal, pennyroyal, feverfew and sassafras: they should not be taken earlier during pregnancy.

## The Baby

Many women who are overdue try all sorts of methods to get things started, but still end up with a hospital appointment to be induced. The baby's pretty fed up by now as well. The layer of fat that has been building up under the skin is plump enough for it to be able to regulate its body temperature after birth. It is now a tight fit inside the uterus and, although at 38 weeks there is more amniotic fluid around the baby than at any other time, the volume decreases in the days before the baby is born. This reduces the cushioning both you and your baby feel and can result in a rapid weight loss of as much as 3lb. Your baby could weigh 6lb or it could weigh 11lb, and it is difficult to tell from examining the uterus exactly what size baby is going to come out! It is probably curled up into a ball, so rather than feeling rolling movements there will more likely be the odd thump here, the odd thump there, as it tries to settle itself down. Some babies are thought to quieten just before delivery; others never stop jigging around, even in labour.

An increase of Braxton Hicks contractions might make some women feel that labour is imminent: a couple of women, such as Jane and Siân who had not really been aware of them throughout the pregnancy, thought that they were going into labour proper. Other warning signs are having diarrhoea attacks and sudden energy spurts. Both Sue and Lisa rushed around without feeling tired the day before their children were born.

History records many ways of predicting the onset of labour, the most bizarre perhaps being the old custom of couvade, from the French meaning to hatch. Any aches and pains suffered by the husband were thought to aid the woman's delivery, and in Europe in the Middle Ages people thought that birth pangs could be transferred to the husband by the symbolic transfer of clothing or by the midwife's spells. In remote parts of southern India today men still wear their wives' saris during labour. Of course most women would rather wait for their bodies to tell them that the time has come than listen to their partners cataloguing the aches and pains they are starting to experience . . .

As with everything in pregnancy it is no more usual for a woman to have a sixth sense that labour is about to start than it is to be completely taken by surprise. It's easy to be wise in retrospect, but for many it is only when reliving the countdown hours afterwards that there seem to have been distinctive tell-tale signs. Some even allow their nervous minds to deliberately misinterpret the physical signals, as Sarah found with Kirsty's labour:

> Quite by coincidence I had a girlfriend round that evening, supposed to keep me company. She had all my books out and was saying 'you're definitely in labour', and I was saying 'I can't be, I can't be'. And she just went through ticking things off.

But don't worry. In the end nature always finds a way of telling you.

# Birth

> I thought you were my victory
> though you cut me like a knife
> when I brought you out of my body
> into your life.
>
> Anne Stephenson, from 'The Victory'[1]

The precise time, date and location of birth is believed by astrologers to have a significant bearing on a child's future. In earlier centuries it was customary for wealthy European families to have an astrologer in attendance so that an accurate prediction could be given immediately. For those with fewer financial resources a less sophisticated method of divination relied on rhymes that we still know today, such as 'Monday's child is fair of face . . .' Even a child's physical appearance at birth was significant, and there were many sayings reflecting contemporary folklore:

A dimple on the chin brings a fortune in; A dimple on the cheek leaves a fortune to seek.

Children born at the same time as a striking clock were thought to possess supernatural powers. Those born at midnight were believed capable of seeing ghosts or hearing the supernatural Wild Hunt and Chime Children. Those born as the clock was chiming the magical hours of three, six, nine and twelve were thought to be able to talk to fairies without being harmed, to be immune to ill-will and blessed with a knowledge of herbal lore and healing crafts. A more widely known superstition is that to be the seventh child of a seventh child is extremely lucky, although with falling family sizes in Europe and America the odds on being thus blessed are getting smaller and smaller.

Literature from all cultures and from all periods is scattered with fascinating references to good and bad omens attending birth. The book *Mamatoto* gathers together a beautiful and fascinating selection of birth rituals and superstitions from all over the modern world.[2]

There are now suggestions that babies born in particular months may be protected from some common childhood allergies, according to research published by doctors in Munich in 1993. September babies are less likely to develop a skin allergy to grass pollen – February, May and June babies more likely; October's children are at less risk of developing asthma, whereas those born in August are more likely; and babies with birthdays in November are less prone to hay fever, those born in May more.

Women give birth in many different positions, the most inefficient of which is lying flat on their backs. Until the eighteenth century, when Louis XIV insisted that his mistresses gave birth lying down so that he could see what was happening, the most common position was the supported squat. In Victorian England, propriety insisted that women in labour were covered by a modesty sheet. Tied around the woman's waist and at the doctor's neck, it ensured that no flesh whatsoever was glimpsed.

## The Three Stages of Labour

As labour begins, few women are thinking about anything other than their bodies and the task in hand. Leaving the supernatural and paranormal to one side, it's probably wise to concentrate a little on the physiological facts.

Labour is divided into three stages. The first stage can last anything from a few hours to several days. This is the time taken by the gradual opening of the cervix to a fully dilated 10cm, followed by a brief period of transition. The second stage is the pushing and delivery of the baby itself, which can last anything between a few minutes and a few hours. The third stage is the expulsion of the placenta. This stage is accompanied by contractions which can be more painful than those experienced earlier. The delivery of the placenta can be precipitated by an injection of syntometrine, a synthetic hormone, immediately after birth. Traditional methods of expelling the placenta include sneezing or, in Jamaica, blowing into a bottle.

First labours last an average of 12 hours or so; second and third labours are on average quicker and easier; complications may attend fourth or subsequent labours. But, as you would expect, these are just rough averages. It is important to go into your labour in a positive frame of mind without assuming that everything will happen as the textbooks suggest.

Most pregnancy handbooks run clearly through the distinctive physical characteristics of each stage, but less emphasis is placed on the emotions that might accompany them. We all give birth for the first time only once, and it is perhaps the most fundamental and astonishing of all experiences.

In the following pages I have laid out a selection of birth stories from the women I interviewed, a mixture of first and subsequent births. Here, labour is timed from the onset of contractions, although medically, full labour is deemed to have begun once the woman is 3cm dilated. The shortest one lasted two and a half hours, the longest twenty-two. There is a mixture of positive and negative memories which doesn't necessarily correspond to what you might wish for or dread. It is reassuring that length of labour, type of pain relief or place of birth do not seem to be the determining factors in whether or not a woman looks back on a particular labour as good or bad. What is crucial is how the woman feels about the experience.

Some of the women had a great sense of achievement, others were disappointed; some found their expectations met, others felt let down; some felt controlled, intimidated by the doctors and midwives, others felt supported and in control. Some women felt that they couldn't have got through it without their partners; others were disappointed when their partners failed to stand up to the wishes of the medical staff. As one woman said when her partner didn't back her up in a disagreement with the midwife, 'on two occasions during labour, very serious ones, he made me voiceless. It was easier for him not to act, to support but not act.'

Some women say that the birth itself was an anticlimax; others feel that it was the greatest moment of their lives. For me, giving birth is the greatest part of pregnancy. Overall, there were 22 hospital births (including 3 caesareans and one water birth) and 6 home births (including 3 water births). No one had their baby in the car or in an ambulance . . .

In these stories different things stand out as important for different women. For some with older children it is the comparison with previous experiences, for others the shock of the new. It is also true that it can be difficult to distinguish between the facts of what happens during a labour and what the woman (and her partner) feels has taken place. If a woman's memory of labour is, on the whole, good, then it is likely that four examinations during the course of a 12-hour labour will not seem unreasonable and the woman will say that she was left to get on with things at her own pace. For a woman who has experienced an upsetting labour during which she felt in conflict with midwives and doctors, four internal examinations will seem more like 44. The women interviewed have focused on the details that mattered most to them and that seemed most relevant when putting voice to their experiences.

## Eve
### Baby Annie, 37 weeks, hospital, 5lb 15oz

Eve had not felt she bonded with the baby throughout the pregnancy, almost pretending that it wasn't happening to her, but was still delighted when her waters broke just three days after she had started her maternity leave. She wanted to get on with it, not sit around wondering.

> I immediately thought of another woman in my NCT class who had woken in a bed soaked in pee which she mistook for amniotic fluid. I looked at the clock. 7.30 a.m. Slowly I got up to go downstairs to the loo. Water dribbled down my leg. I stopped. It started again. As I walked back upstairs it still dribbled.

Both she and Stephen felt like naughty children playing truant from school as they drove through Brighton to the hospital. There a doctor told her that if contractions didn't start within 24 hours they would induce her for fear of infection, despite the fact that the baby was not actually due for another three weeks. Eve was determined not to be induced, so she spent the day charging around.

> Active birth started here. Stuffed with sanitary towels I raced around Waitrose for red grape juice and honey to sustain me during labour. By teatime I had a dull ache in the pit of my stomach. As all the books promised, it felt just like a period pain.

The contractions rapidly became stronger, and by the evening she and Stephen packed themselves into the car armed with a beanbag, suitcase, tape machine and all the other bits and pieces she'd organised to get them through labour. The journey to the hospital was dreadful, with Eve thrown off balance by the extent of the pain she was experiencing.

> Every bump in the road was like a bludgeon. I felt like climbing out of the rear window. I was losing control and I tried to concentrate on breathing. But I was frantic when we arrived at the hospital, gasping, struggling to escape the pain, breathing too fast. It was 9 p.m.

Finally arriving on the labour ward, Eve was 8cm dilated already, feeling thirsty and irritated with everyone – especially Stephen – for not magically knowing that she was thirsty. She also felt extremely sick, particularly when the words gas and air were mentioned, but when she retched nothing came out.

Everything seemed to be happening a long way away. The urge to push was incredible, but someone advised her to wait because she still had a small lip where her cervix had not completely opened.

By 11.30 p.m., a glucose drip having been administered, they discussed using forceps and put Eve's feet in stirrups. Exhausted by then, all she wanted was for it to be over:

Another contraction, another heave. They all started cheering me on again. How many people had crowded round my battered, wet, naked body? Did I care? No. I was to have an episiotomy, one of my worst fears. Did I feel it? I felt my body sliced into sharp consciousness and splitting in two as Annie's head, then her shoulders emerged. I heard two screams, mine and my baby's, together. Then a silent slither. Suddenly she was on my chest, wrapped in my arms.

At this point, 12.30 a.m., Eve went into a dream, only having eyes for Annie (who she still thought was a boy until a midwife pointed out that if that was the case then there was a bit missing . . .). The placenta was delivered – without the help of syntometrine – and after the preliminary checks the three of them were left alone for an hour. The Registrar returned with her white-coated cheerleaders to do the stitching and, at about four in the morning on 11 October 1989, they were finally wheeled to the ward.

A night nurse offered to put Annie in the nursery so that I could get some sleep. What a strange thing to say. I hope I was polite as I refused her offer. Annie and I had the ward to ourselves. Stephen tucked us up in bed together, her in the crook of my arm keeping me as warm as I was keeping her, and kissed us goodnight, finding it hard to leave. He went, poor man, laden with the beanbag and tape recorder, the food and the drinks, which we hadn't had time to touch.

**Tessa**
**Baby Joe, 38 weeks, hospital, 7lb;**
**Baby Matilda, 40 weeks, hospital, 6lb 10oz**

With Joe, Tessa had hoped to be early – not least because it was a boiling hot summer – but had prepared herself to be late on the advice of her gynaecologist. On 2 August 1989 she and Mark went to bed and made love. She was woken by a 'pop' a few hours later. She roused Mark, rang the hospital who said that they should come in, then stood up. She was astounded at the amount of amniotic fluid cascading from her body: 'The bed was flooded, the lift was flooded, the car was flooded, the hospital was flooded, the examining table . . .'

They arrived at the hospital at about six in the morning, with Tessa desperate to go to the loo. It was only then that she realised that the stomach pains weren't contractions but a mixture of constipation and nerves. At about 9 a.m. bad period pains set in and by ten they were really bad. She remembers being surprised that the pains were excruciating so quickly. No position – kneeling, crouching, walking – seemed to help. At 11 a.m. true contractions started. 'They were all over the bump, like it was being pulled from above and pulled down.'

An internal examination revealed that she was only 1cm dilated, and by two o'clock in the afternoon she'd had enough. (Mark's hand had also suffered not inconsiderably as she squeezed it blue through each agonising surge.)

Tessa had always intended to have an epidural, so had indicated as much on her birth plan. By three o'clock an anaesthetist had set the drip, fetal scalp monitor and everything in place. 'I felt the relief quickly, literally within two minutes.'

For the next eight hours Tessa felt calm, dreamlike. They

watched television. She was topped up from time to time, talked, dozed. Then at eleven that evening the consultant examined her and, telling her that she was ready to push, did a quick episiotomy. After a couple of tries Joe shot out. The atmosphere was completely friendly and unworried, where Tessa had expected it to be more heightened, dramatic: 'I thought I would cry, but I only cried when I saw him – I didn't cry when he came out.'

The medical team wiped Joe and sucked out his nose and mouth then helped Tessa deliver the placenta before passing her the baby.

I was amazed. I remember thinking almost immediately 'he looks just like Mark and I'll love Mark more because I have a son who looks like him, and I'll love my son so much because he looks like my husband.'

She couldn't move her legs for about an hour and a half, they were just too heavy. But she didn't mind any of this, she just felt like a queen. At 12.30 a.m. her mother arrived, carrying a bunch of lilies (just in case it was a girl, since Lily was the name they'd chosen) and some wonderful Marks & Spencer's biscuits.

Mark and Tessa snuggled up together and slept. She feels that the labour and birth couldn't really have gone better.

**Me**
**Baby Martha, 36 weeks, hospital, 6lb 10oz;**
**Baby Felix, 40 weeks, home (water birth), 8lb 1oz**

I was so convinced that Felix would be early, like Martha, that psychologically I felt overdue from about 37 weeks onwards. And since I'd been so convincing telling everyone that Felix would never go to term, people stopped ringing at the end of September. Perhaps they thought something had gone wrong. My parents – who were on holiday in Turkey – admitted that they became more and more worried as the days went by and they still hadn't received the expected phone call.

Then ten days before Felix was born, Martha went from having a bad cough and cold to threatened pneumonia in the space of a few hours. Sitting in our doctor's surgery late on Friday afternoon – being told that if Martha's breathing became any more distressed she would have to be taken into hospital – Greg and I both had overwhelming visions of him sitting in Lewisham hospital with our sick daughter and me giving birth in our sitting-room with the midwives. It was a long 36 hours. What was most strange was that Felix, who had been in the same position since I was 20 weeks pregnant, suddenly moved. He went from a straightforward head down into a posterior position that would have made labour more prolonged and difficult. It was as if he was saying: 'It's OK. I can wait. You get your crisis over first.'

Martha was properly ill for nearly two weeks and I too became ill enough for Greg's mother Rosie to have to come to look after us all. But once it was all over, when we'd all recuperated just enough for me to start feeling bored with waiting again, Felix rotated back to his familiar position.

Because I felt overdue, I'd become obsessive about trying to identify the onset of labour, asking everyone I knew how theirs had started and trying to fit my physical and mental state into their patterns. The irony was that when it did start I failed to accept it.

I was expecting a show, or to have an attack of diarrhoea, or for my waters to break or for my Braxton Hicks contractions to get stronger and regular. Stupidly, I felt I knew exactly how my labour was going to be: my waters would break a couple of hours before kick-off; labour itself would last about seven or eight hours, starting around ten in the evening; Martha would wake up the following morning to be presented with her baby sister, Florence, along with her breakfast toast; and there would be just-tolerable abdominal pain. Things couldn't have been more different.

At about six in the morning on 8 October 1992, two days before my due date, I woke with nagging backache, exactly the same sort of backache that accompanied my periods every month. But it was strong enough to make it hard to go back to sleep, so I had a coffee and a hot bath, then went back to bed. When Greg and Martha surfaced I commented that I did feel as if something might be happening, but since it was obviously pre-pre-labour, Greg might as well pedal off on his bike for a normal day at college. He thought he'd take the day off, just in case.

I half-noticed that the pain came and went, but it was no more than slightly irritating. We dropped Martha at school then decided to do a long-overdue major food shop. As we walked around Sainsbury's I did accept that this backache was getting slightly stronger, about three bursts in an hour, but I still felt that it was my body cranking up for something that might happen later on that night or the following day. Encouraged by Greg I agreed to ring up Becky at eleven o'clock, one of my independent midwives, to warn her that she might be getting no sleep that night. I then worked, made a few phone calls and wondered whether this really was how labour started.

Becky rang to check progress at lunchtime. I still felt that this could be pre-labour pains or it could simply be late-pregnancy twinges (I'd suffered so many of those, after all). Within half an hour, though, I was experiencing strong backache contractions that had me dropping to the floor on all fours every three minutes. Greg paged Becky to get her to come immediately. I still feel exhilarated remembering that moment, when you realise that this is it.

It was at this point that I fleetingly wondered why I wasn't in hospital having a wonderful epidural like I'd had with Martha. Too late now. Greg was in the living-room erecting the birthing pool. It was the same shade of blue and had the same smell as a child's paddling pool. I couldn't decide whether this was comforting or somehow a little disquieting. What's more, the pool was due back the following day, since I'd booked it in line with my expectation of an earlier delivery.

The dry run we'd conducted a couple of weeks before had shown us it took only ten minutes to set the pool up empty, but there remained the not inconsiderable task of filling it with warm water. Now fully convinced I was in established labour I clutched the side, desperately asking how much longer it would take.

Actually I got in before the thing was full and the water was wonderful. In the photographs I look surprisingly relaxed, not least because between contractions I could sit back, warm and supported. As the contractions got stronger I put both hands on the floor of the pool and whirled round and round: Becky joked afterwards that at one point she was worried she wouldn't be able to catch the baby as I spun past her. Although the pain was still extreme and I did feel that my back was being broken in half, I'm convinced that I was eased by the support of the water, which helped me to move more freely and with more suppleness than I ever could have done on dry land. I keened, wailed, shouted, noises came from the back of my throat. Becky, and her colleagues Cathy and Lucyann, kept a record in my notes.

16.00: Kate doesn't like these contractions – 'no, no, no . . .' 'Down, down.' The baby has hiccups! 'The sun's come out,' says Kate.

At one point the hose adding hot water came loose, scalding my leg: it was strangely comforting to feel a familiar pain. There were a couple of suffocating contractions, then as I sat back on my heels saying weakly that I was feeling 'a little upset actually' – bland words completely inadequate to my emotions – Becky uttered the immortal word, 'transition'.

Because I had expected the first-stage contractions to go on for hours and hours, because I'd expected them to get closer and closer together until they gave me no respite from the end of one wrench to the beginning of the next, this filled me with a tremendous confidence. It was only 4.30 p.m. and yet I was going to begin pushing. With my forehead leaning on the rim of the pool, straight-armed on all fours like a baboon, I pushed for half an hour. It felt like I was shitting a cricket ball.

17.18: Very gently Kate blows out the baby's head, covered all over with the membranes. Difficult to see what's what for a moment. Then waters break, and the baby's face can be seen inside – beautiful.

One more push and the body slithered out like a bony octopus, accompanied by fierce, tearing pain. I rocked back on my haunches and, as Becky passed him up through my legs, sat back on the floor of the pool. As his head came out of the water he opened his eyes and lay there, gently starting to breathe and looking up as if he recognised me. A boy called Florence . . .

One of the most satisfying things about being delivered

by women you know is that you can all post-mortem the birth – what went right, what went wrong – in the days that follow. I learnt from Becky that she had a split-second of horror as Felix's head was being born because it felt all squidgy, not hard at all. I don't know – and actually don't care – if medical science would agree, but I am convinced that being born in his amniotic sac in warm water contributed to making Felix such a tranquil and contented baby.

Neither Greg nor I wept, as we had at Martha's birth. Then neither of us had ever really believed it possible that I would give birth to a live, healthy baby. This time it felt normal. Everything was as it should be. No fuss.

It was at this point that things started to go wrong. I looked down at the water – crystal clear throughout labour – to see that it now resembled feeding time at the shark house. I got out, feeling wonderful, fed Felix, then heard myself saying from a long way off that I was going to faint. The placenta took over an hour to deliver and the pains were worse than the contractions during the labour itself. I was so dizzy that finally I had to be held up under the arms by Greg with Becky pulling gently on the cord to dislodge it. For the next four hours I lay on the ground, sipping extremely sweet tea through a bendy straw.

No one was telling Greg that I was OK. I could hear debates between Becky, Lucyann and Cathy as to how much blood I had actually lost. They all kept asking me stupid questions – where was the tea? What time did I think labour started? – which I later understood was the easiest way of checking that I wasn't drifting off into unconsciousness. But at the time I was irritated. *I* knew I couldn't really be that ill if I was capable of feeling ratty, but no one believed me when I said I was fine.

Greg went to collect Martha and his mother Rosie from

their impromptu tea party at about 8.30 p.m. Lucyann held Felix as Martha ran to me lying on the sofa. She took my hand and asked me if the baby had come out yet and was she a big sister now? On being told that it had and that she was, she then solemnly got straight to the point and asked if the baby had brought her a present. After half an hour's excitement with the new Duplo farm animals, she asked to hold Felix. It was then I cried, watching her stroke his hands and kiss his head. Everyone else drank the wine and ate the chocolate that we'd snatched from shelves that morning at Sainsbury's. I was unable to lift up my head to join in.

At about eleven o'clock it took me 20 minutes to get upstairs. Supported by Greg I dragged my feet all of five yards to the sitting-room door, then had to lie down on the floor; then up the three steps into the hall; then to the bottom of the stairs; and so on until I was in bed. Felix slept all night, Martha slept all night, Greg slept on and off. I relived the day and bled . . .

## Sue
**Baby Nicholas, 40 weeks, hospital, 7lb 1oz;**
**Baby Hannah, 40 weeks, hospital, 7lb 9oz;**
**Baby Lottie, 38 weeks, home, 6lb 2oz**

The birth of Sue's second child, Hannah, was so quick – a mere three hours – and so painless, that she elected to have her third baby at home. After a false alarm at 37 weeks, Lottie was born after another three-hour labour, which the midwife nearly missed. These two labours were emotionally very different from her first experience, when she was only 22. Then, her strongest emotion had been fear, because of not knowing what to expect.

On 13 September 1983 Sue had a show, but since her midwife had told her that it was no indication of labour starting immediately, she went to bed normally feeling very tired and with a dull backache, at about 11 p.m. Her husband Max said that she did a lot of sleep-talking and moaning during the night, but she made it through relatively undisturbed until the morning.

> Then I was woken up at 6 a.m. with a contraction that was so violent it literally threw me out of bed. The contractions really started then, coming every seven minutes and quite regularly. I called the hospital and was told I probably had hours to go, but to come in as soon as I felt I really wanted to or as soon as my waters broke, whichever happened first.

It was a weekday, and since they lived a good 20-minute drive from the hospital, they decided to go straight in to avoid the London rush-hour traffic. At this stage Sue was calm, but scared. They arrived at 7.15 and bundled into a delivery room as all the first-stage labour rooms were occupied (all those tipsy Christmas accidents from nine months before . . .).

> The midwife examined me straight away and her exact words (which I will never forget) were, 'goodness me, you're 8cm dilated already. I go off duty at 8, let's see if you can have it by then!'

That only gave her 45 minutes and, despite everyone being so supportive, Sue was terrified by now. The midwife broke her waters and gave Max the gas and air to administer. He was so frightened that he stuck the mask over his own face and got smashed, so Sue had no pain relief because by the time he offered it to her the baby was already out.

One comment of his I do remember – and we both still laugh about it – was when he asked 'does it hurt?' just as I'd stopped yelling after a particularly bad contraction. I replied, 'of course it fucking hurts. Do you think I'd be making this much noise if it didn't?'

She had been adamant about not wanting an episiotomy, not least because she felt that they were performed a bit too often and more for the benefit of the midwife than the mother. But Nick's heartbeat was dropping dramatically after each contraction. As soon as they'd performed the episiotomy his head was born. It was 8.20 a.m. on 14 September and the original midwife had just gone off duty.

I was too busy yelling to care much, though on reflection it would have been nice to have had the same one the whole way through. However, they were all lovely – really supportive, really calm and reassuring and very unconventional. I could have had the baby standing on my head if I'd wanted to, but in fact I was on the bed with my knees up and my back supported by pillows and Max, because that was how I was most comfortable. I had all three kids in this position. I couldn't bear squatting during labour – it was too painful.

**Lee**
**Baby Hannah, 40 weeks, hospital**
**(breech birth), 6lb 12oz**

Lee had met considerable opposition from the gynaecologist at her local hospital in Nottingham about the idea of a water birth, but she had pressed ahead and most of the staff there were in fact excited: it was the first time for them as well as for Lee and Simon. She had strong Braxton Hicks contractions from 38 weeks so Simon had gone into the hospital to set up the tank, and the microbiologist had checked the water. Then the Braxton Hicks calmed down, the due date passed, and it was agreed that she would go in for a scan on 20 April 1990: they knew the baby was breech, and both major hospitals in Nottingham – City and Queen's – have an automatic policy that all first-time breech babies over 8lb are delivered by caesarean section.

They duly presented themselves at the hospital, but when Lee was examined internally the obstetrician told her that she was already 5cm dilated. 'What he said was, "Well, you're half-way to delivering your baby. We'd better get you across to the labour suite."'

Her waters hadn't broken, she'd had no show, and the only indication that labour might begin soon was that she'd had that odd, sort of floaty detached feeling a few days earlier. They kept offering her an epidural – she had to turn it down seven or eight times.

> I thought it ludicrous to be given pain relief when it wasn't needed, and this really would not have been my labour had I agreed.

She greatly resented the pressure she was being put under, especially the indication that because her baby was breech she was automatically endangering it since she was bound to need a caesarean in the long run: 'They must think you're completely irresponsible.'

When Debbie, her community midwife, arrived and broke her waters, the contractions started straight away. Simon put on the Mozart and filled the tank. The pains were low down, like bad period pains, and the warm water helped as Lee went into a trance, reassured by the sound of Simon's and Debbie's voices in the background. After about two hours Debbie asked her to get out so she could see how she was doing. Another internal revealed that she was now nearly 9cm dilated, but the agony of having to get out of the pool and the pain of the examination made Lee scream for any drug that was available. Quickly wheelchaired across to the labour suite, she was helped into a supported squat on the bed. Two contractions, and Hannah's bottom began to show, while Lee gulped the gas and air.

Because it was all happening so quickly the midwife decided to put Lee's legs in stirrups in order to do an episiotomy. One of the dangers associated with a breech delivery is that because the vagina hasn't been opened by the biggest part of the baby – its head – the body will be born and the head will remain stuck in the birth canal. The baby might even try to breathe when its chest comes out but its mouth and nose are still trapped inside. The obstetrician later told Lee that it was the fastest breech he'd ever delivered and Lee mentioned this in a piece she wrote on water birth for her local NCT group:

> I am aware of Simon's encouragement, but my full attention is with Debbie. Our eye contact is stronger than ever before. I see Hannah's legs and back being held up between my legs. I pant frantically, and Hannah's head is delivered without forceps. I feel slightly detached from the whole situation. Simon is beside me, crying, and I welcome Hannah onto my tummy. I can hear clapping and congratulations. I see smiles all around me, eyes wide and bright. I suppose I'd better smile too, it seems to be the right thing to do. I look at Hannah, she's the most beautiful thing in the world, then I tell Simon how much I love him.

**Fran**
**Baby Matthew, 40 weeks, hospital, 7lb 13oz;**
**Baby Rowan, 42 weeks, hospital, 8lb 8oz**

With both children Fran had severe contractions from about
seven months onwards, and with Matthew she had actually
been taken into hospital at 29 weeks in premature labour. For
the next eleven weeks she had regular strong contractions,
which of course made trying to spot the onset of labour even
more difficult than it is for most women first time round:
'With Matthew there were also a couple of false alarms at the
end, when I thought my waters had broken when actually
I'd wet myself!'

On 7 May 1989 she went to bed feeling a little uncomfortable, having had a show. By one o'clock in the morning the
contractions were painful, and by 5 a.m. she was convinced
that these were different from the sorts of contractions she'd
been suffering for the previous 10 weeks. She and Jim drove
to the park and walked around in the early May sunshine,
Fran leaning against trees and rotating her hips as the
contractions came. When they got to the hospital it was
depressing to discover that after nine hours she was only
2cm dilated. She tried gas and air, but after another half an
hour of pain she asked for an epidural, despite having previously decided against one. 'But it didn't work across the
top, so I had to have more gas and air to help me through
the contractions.'

Time passed, with reading, sleeping, playing cards. There
was even a power cut in the hospital, so the generators
kept turning on and off as if they were all in a disco. At
ten that night she was examined again and told to start
pushing. Unfortunately the epidural had just been topped
up . . .

They said 'push', but I mean it's easier moving a chair
across the room without touching it because you've got
no concept of where to push. So they said 'find your
bottom', but I had no bottom because I had no waist,
no legs, no feet. So then they said 'visualise your bottom',
which I did . . .

The midwives were very supportive, saying that there was no
hurry and that she should take things at her own pace. But
Matthew's heartbeat was starting to dip, so they started bran-
dishing huge forceps, gave her an episiotomy and said that
unless she could get him out immediately they'd have to do
a caesarean. Fran then pushed so hard that Matthew shot out
and was nearly dropped by the midwife. He was bruised, but
otherwise fine, and both she and Jim were choked with tears
that he was finally here. It was all exactly as she'd imagined.

With Rowan, Fran was demoralised. Because of the contractions from 30 weeks she'd been expecting her to arrive early,
but by 42 weeks still nothing had happened. It was also
extremely hot and Fran was uncomfortable and enormous.
Contractions started at ten in the evening of 25 August 1991,
and this time when she got to the hospital she was greeted
with the encouraging news that she was already 6cm dilated.
She felt very positive, giggly from the gas and air, and
continued to dilate quickly. Again the pain suddenly became
intense and, because it was too late for an epidural, she was
given a shot of pethidine.

It was peculiar, because one minute you're dealing with
the contractions and whatever, leaning on the back of
the bed, and the next minute you're asleep. The weirdest
thing was when the midwife said to me 'tell me when
you want to push', and I answered 'what's push . . . ?'

After only four hours Rowan was delivered, no stitches, no tears. But emotionally it just wasn't the same as the first time; it was all rather mundane and everyday.

> I didn't feel that great urge to pick her up, I was quite happy to put her down. With Matthew I wouldn't give him to anybody.

**Caroline**
**Baby Emma, 42 weeks, hospital, 7lb 12oz;**
**Baby Anthony, 40 weeks, hospital, 7lb 7oz;**
**Baby Richard, 40 weeks, home, 9lb;**
**Baby Jessica, 42 weeks, home, 7lb 15oz**

Having had four goes at it Caroline is able to say with confidence that giving birth is never the same experience twice and that it does get easier! She was only 19 when she had her first child, Emma, and despite her strong fear of hospitals and the sort of equipment housed there, it didn't occur to her to do anything other than go to the local hospital in Sussex where all her friends had gone.

> I hate hospitals and they scare me to death, but I wouldn't personally have a home delivery for a first baby because you don't know what it's going to be like. Also, I didn't know how I'd cope, and the pain was a lot worse than I'd thought it possibly could ever be.

Emma was not born until 42 weeks. Beforehand the doctors began talking about induction and this scared Caroline. But again she didn't feel she had any right to say that she would rather let things happen naturally.

Though it was her first go Caroline hadn't wanted an

epidural or any injections whatsoever, but during her seven-hour labour her blood pressure and pulse rate both went up so she was told that she would have to have either a pethidine injection or an epidural. The labour pains were very low down on the left-hand side, like a knife, and were more severe than anything she experienced during her other three deliveries.

It took three attempts before the anaesthetist administering the epidural succeeded in getting the needle into Caroline's spine and, although technically it did then work in that the pain was numbed, she really didn't feel that it was worth all the palaver of getting it in there. She hated the drip in her hand, the catheter, the strap with the monitor; everything felt unnatural and intrusive. 'I just didn't dare move a single muscle, even afterwards: I thought the needles were still there.'

A small patch at the top of her right thigh was unaffected. To combat this, the anaesthetist left instructions that she should be sitting when they topped up the epidural so that the drug would filter down and work everywhere. In fact Caroline was pleased to have this unaffected area, because it meant that she could feel when to push. But despite having negative feelings about the progress of the labour, the moment when Emma was born at 12.58 a.m. on 6 October 1984 was as astounding as she'd heard it could be: 'I felt awe and over-whelming pride that I'd actually managed to do it.' Her first question was 'is it all there?'

Despite her feelings about the hospital, Caroline didn't feel confident enough to ask for a home delivery second time round. She also thought it was 'old-fashioned' and that 'nobody had babies at home any more'.

She didn't believe she was in labour: it just didn't feel painful enough. This time she had general aching all over her abdomen rather than in just one place, and felt she could have done it all again straight away! Anthony weighed in at

7lb 7oz after a barely noticeable two-and-a-half-hour labour, another October baby. The pair of them left the hospital six hours later.

It was the ease and speed of Anthony's birth which decided her to summon up the courage to try for a home birth third time round. She was nervous about asking her GP because there had been a piece in the local paper, the *Chichester Observer*, about her GP refusing to do a home delivery. But the surgery offered her an alternative doctor who would be happy to look after her, and she was given a rota of midwives.

Caroline was a little upset by the idea that any one of a number of midwives might be attending her birth, since one of the reasons for opting for a home birth was to be delivered by someone she knew. But she was sure she didn't want a third hospital birth: she'd felt observed and judged all the time she was in the hospital and felt that she was unlikely to be treated like a mother of two but as a novice unused to newborn babies.

> I didn't feel that I had control over Emma, that she was mine, until I left the hospital. I felt as if everything I was doing they'd be watching to see if I was doing it wrong.

Richard's labour started in the morning, while Emma was at school and her husband had taken Anthony shopping. She'd half-hoped that he'd hang on another day, until 15 September, so that he'd share a birthday with her mother. 'I had these pictures of having to phone Sainsbury's and Malcolm getting called up over the tannoy and things.'

She phoned the midwife – luckily her favourite was on duty – then, predictably, her contractions stopped as soon as help was at hand.

This time Caroline had pain in her back, with her uterus being hard only at the bottom during contractions. She tried gas and air, having loved it with Anthony, but this time it made her feel sick. Richard, a hefty 9lb, was born at 4.55 p.m. Caroline works as a childminder in her own home and all she could think about just after delivery was that the father of the child she looked after was downstairs. Silently she prayed that he wouldn't want to come upstairs to see the new arrival. This time she lost a lot of blood and – for several days afterwards too – for the first time felt exhausted and faint.

Jessica was also due to be born at home, but by 42 weeks the hospital was insisting that Caroline go in to be induced. Often the threat of induction starts a woman's labour off and sure enough at three o'clock in the morning of 22 September 1991 – with the hospital expecting her to present herself to them five hours later – Caroline's body obligingly went into action.

Caroline dismissed the strong heartburn, feeling she wouldn't be allowed to escape going to hospital that easily. She sat downstairs in her kitchen sipping milk and inwardly bemoaning the fact that there were no Rennies left. She started to have contractions about 20 minutes apart, but they were no stronger than Braxton Hicks contractions so she went back to bed after having a catalytic bath: 'I had a bath, a really hot one, since I thought "it worked with Richard, so I might as well try it again."'

At 6 a.m. Caroline was woken by a massive contraction, followed by another five minutes later. This was it, just in time. She rang the midwives, then called her mother and sister, who arrived at 6.45 just after the two midwives and her husband's sister, who'd come to look after the older children. Richard, just two, was still asleep but six-year-old Emma and four-year-old Anthony were awake and very, very excited.

The midwives did an internal examination on arrival – 6cm dilated already – and artificially ruptured the membranes. Caroline wandered around drinking coffee and smoking. She stayed downstairs for as long as possible, knowing that the time would go very slowly for Emma and Anthony, but finally the contractions became too painful and she didn't want the children to be distressed.

Upstairs she knelt on the floor, leaning on her bed, with her back being rubbed and her husband setting up the video camera. As the pain got stronger her fingers started to clutch the bedspread during each contraction, then she started to curl her toes as well. After an hour or so she half-heard one of the midwives saying that the noises she was making sounded rather transitional and that they should try to get her on to the bed after the next contraction.

Caroline heaved herself on to the mattress by herself and propped herself half-sitting, half-lying against the headboard. The next contraction brought Jessica's head (which looked alarmingly blue to the watchers) and as her body was born the speed made Caroline's eyes ping open with shock. She heard one of the midwives say that the cord was round the neck and because she could see how blue the baby looked she thought that it was dead. But Jessica breathed after a few seconds and within ten minutes the whole family was up in the room admiring the new baby and having tea and toast.

Looking back, Caroline found this labour as painful as Emma's had been. She kept thinking, 'I'll have something for the pain after the next contraction', but somehow it was all so quick that she never really got the chance. Yet 'during labour I would almost rather go with the pain than have to talk to someone.'

## Joanne
### Baby Rowan, 41 weeks, home, 8lb 15oz

Joanne felt that pregnancy and birth were natural occurrences and so had no hesitation in electing to have her baby at home with independent midwives. She wasn't expecting to be early, having been told that most first pregnancies are about 41 weeks, but she and Georgina were a little disappointed when the due date came and went with nothing happening. On 23 November 1989 Joanne's waters burst – about a teacupful in her estimation – and she discussed with Georgina and the midwives what they would do if she didn't go into labour within the next few days. She then had strong Braxton Hicks contractions, which she mistook for early labour, so she rang Georgina's sister, Linda, who came from Bath to London to help.

Friday passed and, after a day trip to Whitstable to cheer her up, Joanne asked for an internal examination. She was told that her membranes were still intact. The midwives agreed to return the following evening, Sunday 26 November.

> I was so pissed off on Saturday evening that I went on a bit of a spring clean – achieved very little, but Georgina's sister took this as a sign that I was going into labour soon. I ate the hottest curry and a whole pineapple. Then I just sat watching late-night TV. Nothing happened until 4.30 when I had a very uncomfortable contraction. Five minutes later another, and then five minutes later another.

Joanne woke Georgina and Linda and was surprised to discover that all the things she'd imagined would comfort her in labour – warm baths, massage – irritated her: she just wanted to be left alone to get on with it. Linda was timing the contractions and, panicking slightly since they were now only three minutes apart, asked Joanne if she wanted to have the midwives.

> I said no. I had this idea that a normal first labour took about 12 hours and even though I had no idea how long I'd been in labour, I knew it wasn't 12 hours.

Linda rang them at five o'clock all the same. They agreed to be there at eight, but Linda had to ring back at 6.15 to say that Joanne thought she could feel the baby's head. When they did arrive at 6.30 they commented in her labour notes that she was in 'very fast, well-established labour, looking and sounding like transition'.

Although it was all generally as Joanne had expected, the pain was much worse. She experienced three or four contractions during transition, the memory of which made her vow months later that she would never go through labour again.

> At about 7 I asked for gas and air, but my midwife said that it would be best to wait because the contractions were coming so frequently that she could tell I would soon be in second stage. I was really pissed off and thought she was being unfair. At 7.30 I moved onto the birthing stool, Georgina supporting me from behind. Linda was on the left side, squeezing my hand during contractions and giving me a sponge soaked with water. The other midwife applied hot flannels and almond oil to my vulva. At 7.35 the head appeared (expulsive contractions). At 7.45 the head was clearly visible. I felt cross and dizzy, but not too painful. Encouraged to breathe slowly. At 8.05 the head came out followed immediately by the body – plopped onto the floor.

Joanne didn't feel amazing elation when Rowan was born, more a sense of relief that it was over. She looked down to see Rowan lying there with no overwhelming need to touch him or even to ask if he was all right or whether it was a she or a he. Georgina picked him up and cried out 'it's a girl!' Joanne then had a look herself, and disabused her. All this seemed to take hours, but from the labour notes she saw afterwards that it happened in the space of a minute.

Suddenly the midwife started 'punching Joanne in the stomach' with no explanation whatsoever. Joanne was bleeding quite heavily and, as her uterus was relaxed rather than hard, she later learnt they were worried about the placenta not delivering efficiently. After a syntometrine injection the placenta and membrances came out. Again it felt like hours had passed, but this all happened just a few minutes after Rowan's birth. The only damage was a small tear at the base of the lower labia, but no suturing was necessary. From start to finish labour had taken just over three and a half hours.

## Sasha
### Baby Freddy, 42 weeks, hospital (emergency caesarean), 6lb 7oz

Despite the persistent vomiting, Sasha behaved as if she wasn't really pregnant at all for the whole nine months. But despite hating most of it, she had strong and positive ideas of what the labour would be like. She also knew that the sort of labour she had was important to her. Things don't always go as planned. 'It's like some sort of terrible sort of parable, my story . . .'

Sasha had been convinced that Freddy would be early, so by the time his due date at Christmas had come and gone and

New Year was approaching she was thoroughly miserable. She was kept up all night by contractions on 31 December, although she didn't really feel that it was the real thing because it was a stabbing pain coming from the cervix and driving up through her body. She'd practised four levels of breathing and to get through this she was using level 2. Then the contractions stopped in the morning.

> I'd only seen pain as something I could deal with, with the right attitude, so I was surprised at the extent to which these felt real.

On New Year's Day 1990 the contractions started up again and Sasha and Lou decided to go to the hospital, not because Sasha felt in established labour but because she was worried that her waters had leaked and were slightly stained, a tea-like tinge. This discoloration can be caused by the baby excreting meconium – the thick, dark-green paste that precedes the yellow excretion normally associated with babies' nappies – while still inside the womb. Sasha was tested for meconium, everything was OK and, since she was only 1cm dilated, they sent her home. On 2 January Sasha and Lou got up and went for a long walk. By 11 a.m. Sasha was needing to lean on the sofa to get through the contractions.

> But I was in a world of my own, like I was on a trip or something. I felt wonderful, I felt totally confident, completely in control. I felt I was doing it right.

At lunchtime they went to the hospital and, since there was no room, she was left squatting in the corridor for a while, waiting for a delivery room to be free.

The breathing was like a drug. The contractions were so overwhelming that I couldn't take up any of these positions I'd rehearsed, but it just felt wonderful, rhythmic. I was in a sort of sea-world.

Sasha had said on her birth plan that she wanted as little interference as possible, but when they examined her and found that she was only 2cm dilated they announced that because of her age – 38 – they were going to put an electrode on the baby's head. Sasha tried to argue, but because Lou didn't back her up she felt voiceless and helpless. Trying to ignore the discordant voices, she again concentrated on her breathing. By eight that evening she was 8cm dilated and was taken into a delivery room. Birth seemed imminent. The midwife then announced: 'I examined you half an hour ago and you were nearly fully dilated, so you must be ready by now. Push.'

Sasha insisted that she didn't feel ready, that she knew she hadn't experienced transition, that the baby felt in an awkward position. But like many otherwise assertive and confident women, when the medical staff tell you to do something it is hard to resist, even if your body is giving you conflicting signals. The temptation – particularly for partners – is to think that because the doctors and midwives have witnessed it all many times before they must automatically be right. It never occurred to Sasha to ask for another medical opinion, she just kept saying, 'I know the baby's not even in the birth canal, I know he's not.'

After three hours of pushing, the Registrar, who had come in to examine Sasha, confirmed that she was not fully dilated, that she had given herself an anterior lip by pushing too early, and that the baby was in a posterior position anyway. Sasha's instincts had been right, yet the midwife said nothing. They put her on an oxytocin drip to try to blast out the baby, but by midnight Sasha was totally demoralised and no longer confident that she could give birth at all.

> My body was like I was having an electric shock, completely out of control. My arms and legs were jerking violently, it was like a fit.

Freddy was now showing signs of distress, so the decision was taken to do an emergency caesarean although they would try to get him out with forceps first. But there wasn't enough time for an epidural to take effect, so Sasha would have to be put under. She was terrified, but most of all just wanted to be put out of her misery.

> The funniest thing of all was that I was wearing nail varnish,* so in the middle of all this drama there were about ten people including Lou taking the varnish off my fingers and toes while I was signing a form.

When Sasha came round in the operating theatre, with icy feet and a dry throat, Lou wasn't even there. Someone told her that she had a son. Soon she was wheeled into a dark, sleeping ward where babies were crying, and Lou appeared with a photograph of their son in the special care unit. Freddy had grade-three meconium aspiration, his lungs and stomach clogged up, he was being fed through the nose and had been placed on an antibiotic drip. He stayed there for ten days and Sasha had to go home without him.

---

* One of the indicators of how well a patient is coping with a general anaesthetic is the colour they are under their nails. No woman I have spoken to was advised against wearing nail varnish in labour just in case a general anaesthetic had to be administered.

**Siân**
**Baby Alexander, 42 weeks, hospital, 7lb 15oz;**
**Baby Katherine, 42 weeks, hospital, 9lb**

Both Siân's labours were extremely quick. Katherine, her second baby, was almost born in the car . . .

Alexander's labour started with a show, then the following evening the contractions set in about 11 p.m. Siân was utterly fed up with the waiting, but was also slightly worried because she hadn't felt the baby move that day, so at three in the morning she and Peter went to the hospital. She was only 3cm dilated, so she was sent home. She managed to sleep through the contractions on and off until 9.30 the next morning. At half-past ten they were back at the hospital feeling sure that this was it.

> It was like being on a big dipper really, there was no turning back. You knew you were going to go through an experience whether you liked it or not. I didn't feel excitement so much as trepidation.

On examination the midwife told her that she was already almost fully dilated, and pretty soon she was in transition.

> There was the overwhelming urge to push, it was just unbelievable, and someone had told me you had to be careful not to push before you're fully dilated. You just cannot imagine beforehand the power of the feeling that you want to push, you want to bear down, but I was trying not to which is why I think my voice went squeaky. I was saying 'can I push, can I push?' and the midwife said, 'if your body's telling you to push, then push'.

She felt overwhelmed with relief to be pushing, although it was a hard couple of hours. She had no pain relief since there never seemed to be an appropriate moment to ask for anything.

> I thought, 'thank God, I must be somewhere near the end now', but there was this odd feeling that the baby went back up again. I remember thinking what a bloody cheek, how unfair; it's two steps forward, one step back; who designed this . . .

Siân hadn't expected the stinging, burning sensation when the head hits the perineum to be quite so strong, and when Alexander came out at about one o'clock her first feeling was not one of overwhelming affection:

> I had the injection to get rid of the placenta, then having coped with that I couldn't really cope with the baby as well. I couldn't really cope with the emotion of feeling I had to bond with this thing. Basically I just let the nurse and Peter do things with it while I just sat there thinking 'Thank God it's over.'

Alexander slept in the nursery the first night. The nurses were horrified when Siân asked if he could sleep in the nursery the second night, too. But she was so tired that she didn't even hear him crying in the cot next to her bed and a night nurse had to wake her up.

> She said, 'your baby's been screaming for the past twenty minutes and you obviously haven't heard it at all.' And the combination of those two things made me feel like a pretty bad mother.

The bonding – a much overused word – really began on the third day, the day before she left the hospital to go home.

## Pam
### Baby Jackson, 43 weeks, hospital (elective caesarean), 8lb 3oz

Pam had accepted that because of the fibroid in her womb it was likely that she would have to have a caesarean, but staff at the hospital were extremely supportive in agreeing that they would see if she went into labour naturally.

The first week after her due date came and went; during the second week she had a show; on the Wednesday of the third week her consultant said that although the baby's heartbeat was fine and Pam's blood pressure OK, they didn't feel they could let her go on beyond the Saturday, 18 April 1992. Pam was seeing her acupuncturist the next day and, since needling often seems to get labour going, the hospital agreed not to set the date for the operation until 8 a.m. on the Saturday morning. Sure enough, as soon as the acupuncturist put the needle in at the uterus point, Pam's waters burst, soaking the chair.

Everyone was delighted, but the rest of Thursday passed, Friday morning, Friday afternoon, Friday evening . . . Pam finally had to accept that the operation was going to happen. Her depression gave way to the fear of being cut open.

The hospital team was supportive and sensitive, knowing the importance Pam had attached to going into labour without artificial help, how much she had hoped to give birth vaginally. Gérard was calm, excited even, trying to buoy up her spirits. As they were preparing her for theatre, they offered her a choice of anaesthetic.

I said 'don't even consider a general anaesthetic. I can't give birth to my baby, I can't have labour, I can't do this, I can't do that, I can't do the other, so at least I'm damn well going to be awake when it comes out.'

Pam sat motionless as the epidural needle went in, expressionless. Then, as she lay on the operating table with the shadowless lamp above her and everyone milling around in their gowns, stroking her head, trying to reassure her, the emotion that she'd kept suppressed throughout the whole pregnancy erupted:

All of a sudden I gave this involuntary gasp, and the tears just came – and then I knew that I was really frightened.

Pam couldn't think about anyone but herself – not the doctors, not Gérard, not the baby. She felt nothing as they cut, no tugging, no stroking. She was blind too, her bump obscuring her view. But she saw the doctor's hands go in and both gynaecologists heave away. Then they held Jackson up, who gazed straight into her eyes. Everything was silent, as if suspended.

I don't know, because I haven't had it, but I would imagine that that's what the pain of the contractions is: it gets you into another frame of mind.

Jackson cried and they put him on Pam. Gérard cut the cord and there was a flurry of activity. Pam felt numbed, in shock, completely overwhelmed, and in staggering pain. It was then that they told her that there was a second fibroid, which the scan hadn't picked up. Months later this discovery helped Pam to come to terms with not having given birth vaginally.

* * *

The baby's head was actually lodged on the second fibroid. He would never have engaged, he would never have come down, I would never have gone into labour. That was why he was three weeks late.

# Now We are Three . . . Or More

## The First Few Days

Then waking at 6 in the evening from out of a stupor to see in my mothers [*sic*] arms a little piece of humanity all dressed in white which they told me was my little son! The sensation with which I touched my lips and my fingertips to his soft flesh only comes once to a mother. It must be the pure animal sensation: nothing spiritual could be so real – so poignant.

Kate Chopin, *1894 Diary*[1]

*Mamatoto*[2] describes how different peoples – from Africa and India to Siberia and Thailand – welcome newborn babies into their communities. Rituals to celebrate birth vary enormously from country to country and from age to age. In places where there is high infant mortality, celebrations rarely begin until the baby has negotiated the perilous first few weeks. And historical literature is littered with the rites that should attend the newborn babies, most importantly that a child must be baptised if its soul is not to be consigned to hell or limbo.

Many cultures today celebrate with special foods and drinks; others have songs to welcome a new baby and to celebrate motherhood. Traditionally mothers in many societies are seen as unclean and are isolated for the first few weeks. Romany gypsy lore dictates that the bed the baby is born on must be burnt, that the new mother has separate living quarters for a month, that she should not cook or touch anyone's food and that no men can eat with her or enter her quarters. Even the father cannot touch the child until after its christening. Male fear of the female power of reproduction is evident in many customs surrounding birth.

In Aboriginal culture, the placenta is buried near the birth site and a humpy (rough dwelling) built to house the mother and baby for a month until the bleeding stops. Only women visit during this time. Then a fire is made with a type of eucalyptus tree and the mother sits over the smoke, to heal and purify her. Most tribes believe that the husband will become ill if his wife doesn't do this.

But many of these rituals, both past and present, presuppose that every labour and birth will be similar and that every woman will feel the same emotions: in fact, that individual women will easily make the transition into motherhood, regardless of their own desires and reactions. In modern industrialised societies for the most part there is less of a sense of a child being born into a community anyway.

## Bonding

Many books and medical people seem to expect every woman to feel immediate overwhelming love and affection, a sense of selflessness as all other emotions fade into insignificance beside the mother/baby bond. And of course some women are lucky enough to be gripped by this sort of passion. Many fathers also fall helplessly in love with their child, directly after the birth, although most are more concerned with how their partner feels.

But many women talk about how guilty they felt when bonding didn't happen for the first few days, weeks, months and sometimes even years. Loving and caring lovingly for a baby are not at all the same thing as falling *in* love with your baby.

As Suzanne Moore, mentioning the provocative book *Mother – Infant Bonding: A Scientific Fiction*, written by the American psychologist Diane Eyer, wrote:

> Of course love at first sight does happen, but not always. It's an individual as well as a social process, not one, surely, that can be served by this all-purpose theory whereby mother and child are mystically glued together.[3]

Although ultimately it is the general health of the mother and the baby that matter, becoming a parent requires huge mental adjustment. For both partners. Not only does the sort of labour and birth experienced make a difference to one's initial, instinctive reaction to this tiny, dependent thing, but the reality of holding your flesh-and-blood baby in your arms for the first time is rarely exactly as imagined. Several women worried about the fact that there seemed to be no place for their husbands' feelings:

> It was OK for me to feel odd, but he was supposed to suddenly behave like a Dad, just like that. He was as shocked as I was.

At the moment of Martha's birth I was euphoric, engulfed by love for both her and Greg. Within a few hours this had been replaced by a sort of tender detachment. At four in the morning I looked over at this swaddled tiny thing lying in the cot next to me and found it hard to believe that it was the same baby who had been kicking me so robustly for the past few months.

Throughout that first night I kept putting my hand on my abdomen, expecting to feel movement, and grieving for my companion of the past eight months. I had thought I'd have eyes for nothing, for no one, but Martha. In fact my own emotions (not to mention physical ailments – a numb leg, excruciating stitches, afterpains, tiredness, heavy lochia*) were more real to me than she was. I felt weepy on day three as my colostrum gave way to my milk, bringing with it engorgement, a sort of flu-like sensitivity and unbelievably sore nipples. Funnily enough, this was also the day I fell in love with my baby: the intimate internal bond had gone, to be replaced by something more public and permanent.

With Felix it was all so normal in comparison. Physically I felt fantastic, considering I'd just given birth: I was a little anaemic, perhaps, but my vagina looked and felt fine. I had no drug-induced side-effects and, although the afterpains were much, much more painful than I'd remembered, my uterus had all but disappeared back into my pelvis within ten days. I'd read that afterpains could continue for two or three days after the birth, and that they got worse with each pregnancy. The irony was that having had no drugs during

---

* Lochia, the discharge of blood and uterine lining (decidua) from the uterus, remains red for the first three to six days because it contains blood from the big veins in the uterus that have been supplying the placenta. After about a week it will become paler, partly due to the presence of the white blood cells that have rushed to the uterus to protect it from infection. It may continue for up to six weeks, and increase after physical exertion or breastfeeding.

labour I needed strong, prescription drugs to cope with these contractions. But, despite this, I was able to fall in love with Felix immediately because I wasn't judging my feelings against somebody else's ideal. Second time round you don't worry about what you're supposed to experience, you just get on with dealing with your expanded family. On both occasions, however, the first mug of tea with three sugars was indescribably wonderful . . .

The women I interviewed had varied memories of their first few days. Not surprisingly, those whose labours and births had been easier than expected and for whom breast-feeding caused no problems felt confident and happy sooner than those who had problems to contend with. And, as with pregnancy itself, the gulf between expectation and reality was very undermining for some.

Sasha, whose labour and birth had been so mismanaged by the hospital staff, felt no connection with her baby when she saw him wired up in the special care unit for the first time. She had hoped to breastfeed, but Freddy was kept in for ten days. To try to ensure that she would have a milk supply when he finally came home, Sasha used a breast pump to express milk every three hours and spent her days charging back and forth to the hospital. Sadly, her milk supply never stabilised. Now with an adored healthy three-year-old son, Sasha is able to say that she didn't really bond with Freddy for the first year. And because she felt guilty, she is aware that she over-compensated by being worried by every sniff, every bout of crying.

> I was anaesthetised for a year. I used to go into his room when he was at the childminder's or something, and look at his things, and think I ought to feel a welling here, in his room. Where is it?

## Babies in Special Care

It is not uncommon for women whose babies are on the danger list not to bond at once. Perhaps it is a form of self-protection, a way of coping with the shock. Perhaps it is simply that not being able to suckle or touch one's hour-old child means that it is impossible to believe that one has crossed the divide and become a mother at all.

Sharon, whose twins were born at 34 weeks by emergency caesarean, had to argue with the hospital staff to be allowed to go to the special care unit. No one explained exactly why they were in there – Charlotte was 4lb 12oz, Katie 4lb 15oz – and, like many women who have to cope with the worry and disappointment of not having their newborn babies with them, she felt that there was an appalling lack of support and information from hospital staff. When at last they met, Sharon was in great pain, in a wheelchair, with two drips attached; the twins were both wired up to ventilators and Katie, although the bigger of the two, had all sorts of electrodes on her chest to help her kidneys and liver to function properly.

> When I first saw them I felt a bit let down. I felt, 'well, these are my babies', but they could have been anybody's. I expected to feel this wonderful rush of love and emotion, and it didn't happen.

Three days later she suddenly burst into tears, and everything fell into place. All she wanted was to be allowed to be alone with her daughters: she wanted to forget about her crumbling marriage, the fact that, despite expressing, her milk simply wasn't coming, and get on with coping with the shock of becoming a mother so much earlier than she'd expected.

Nicki insisted on being allowed to give birth to her twins vaginally, unless specific medical reasons made it unwise.

Max's birth was straightforward, but then her contractions stopped, and she knew

> that it was all down to me; that I had a couple of minutes to get this baby out or he'd have cerebral palsy. I'd taught a lot of brain-damaged children and I knew that they were damaged in the way that I was damaging my child at that time.

John's heartbeat had gone, and Nicki remembers feeling guilty that if only she'd been less interested in the quality of her experience and agreed to an elective caesarean none of this would be happening. It also flashed through her mind that if something happened to the second baby then she wouldn't want Max, because she'd expected two babies, two babies it would have to be, or nothing.

When the doctor arrived he said that he'd have to perform an episiotomy and use forceps, despite the fact that there was no time to give Nicki any sort of pain relief. John was pulled out blue, still and not breathing. Nicki thought he was dead. He was oxygenated, and the medical team worked for 45 minutes to resuscitate him. He didn't cry, but he did start breathing. But there was no relief, as the doctor said that the next ten days of his life would be crucial. 'Though they never explained what was wrong and why 10 days. I just couldn't get any answers.'

Given this background it is not surprising that Nicki had trouble bonding with John to start with. She was in a private room with Max, who was being fed breast milk through a tube because he was so small. But John was in special care and Nicki, whilst feeling guilty, also 'somehow felt cross with him too, for putting me through it'.

He made a wonderful recovery, and they were all discharged together after two weeks. Nicki's guilt then focused on the fact that she'd never sat up all night with John in special care and she feels now that their real intimacy only came three years later when he nearly died from an asthma attack at the age of three.

On the other hand Rachel, who also had an emergency caesarean at 34 weeks, did bond immediately with Rose who was in special care and mentally all right. Like Sasha and Sharon, Rachel had to battle with the hospital to be allowed to see her baby. They told her she'd have to wait a certain number of hours before they'd take her to the special baby unit, not least because she'd lost three pints of blood.

> It was as if time was passing without me in it. I just lay on this bed, not stoned any more, desperate to see the baby. And I couldn't believe I'd had one, and I couldn't believe she was all right. And I was in the delivery suite so I could hear other people in labour, so it was all a bit like torture.

She was counting the minutes when an unlucky nurse brought in a bunch of flowers. Hurling them to the floor, she screamed 'take these fucking flowers away and show me my fucking baby!'

So, 23 hours after the operation, in a wheelchair, on a drip and in agony, Rachel was taken to the special care unit. The minute she saw Rose she was swept away with love for her, but the fear that Rose might have sustained brain damage and the lack of information and counselling made the next few weeks incredibly difficult. Her husband Jeremy's optimism, which had so annoyed her during the pregnancy, was a lifeline now. Determined to breastfeed, Rachel expressed milk which was given to Rose hourly through a drip. A syringe was then put into Rose's stomach to draw up and assess how much she'd taken. For the first few days she lost weight and every ounce became crucial. Then astoundingly Rose rallied and was allowed to come home after only two weeks.

Rachel had gone home after only ten days, unable to cope with being in the hospital any more.

> I was put in a ward with other women who had their babies with them, which I knew at the time – although part of me cut off from it – is the cruellest thing you can do to someone.

## Baby Blues

Most women experience some sort of baby blues – known variously as childbirth blues, puerperal blues, postnatal blues, maternal blues, three/four/five-day blues – which may or may not affect how they feel about their child. Estimates vary that between 50 and 80 per cent of new mothers are affected to some degree, and in one study in which 50 per cent of women were found to have been affected, 66 per cent of these had symptoms within four days of birth and 26 per cent on the third day. Eating the placenta is a traditional, if unsettling, remedy for warding off the blues.

Often the feelings of depression, being unable to cope, bursting into tears because the hospital canteen has given you peas rather than carrots, coincide with the often painful business of milk arriving. The colostrum that nourishes the baby for anything from its first few hours to its first few days gives way to breast milk proper. Most women are amazed at the size of their breasts, and very few are lucky enough not to feel as if their nipples have been scraped with a potato peeler. But sometimes the depression is simply the understandable response to the extraordinary high that has accompanied the birth, the visitors, the flowers and the cards of the first few days.

As the world rushes in, the awareness of the new responsibility of being a parent can be just a bit too much. While it is right that friends and family come to pay homage to you and your baby, too many visitors are demanding, want to be entertained, and exert pressure on the new parents. The best visitors are those who arrive bringing a meal with them to be heated up later, admire you and the baby for ten minutes, then leave.

Tiredness also contributes to feeling ground down, but sometimes asking someone else to carry part of the load is counter-productive. Although it can be extremely useful on a practical level to have a friend or relation come to help out for the first couple of weeks, this can arrest the development of the new family unit. It can set a precedent whereby the mother and helper – often the mother's mother – become the established babycare experts whilst the partner remains shut out on the sidelines, a bumbling amateur. Once this pattern is set it is hard for the couple to take equal responsibility in future.

Many women admit that worries about the division of labour between them and their partner start as early as three or four days after the birth, contributing to the fear of being unable to cope. Statistics suggest that women's fears are not unfounded, in that the majority of men who had taken equal responsibility for the household during pregnancy fail to carry this over into parenthood itself.[4] Parenthood should irrevocably alter the lives of both parents, but if there is a third person fielding phone calls, making meals, pacifying the crying baby, then some partners will be tempted to behave as if nothing has changed.

In the short term the partner's continuing freedom may seem a good thing: he or she can continue to work as usual, come home and relax in the evening, continue to get enough sleep. But the danger is that in these circumstances some men simply do not adjust to being a father at all during the first crucial weeks. Patterns of who does what are set from the moment of birth. Neither men nor women are born with innate nappy-changing skills, but if the new mother – or her helper – always does it then pretty soon she will be the expert . . .

There are many, many conscious and subconscious emotions exacerbated by physical and practical considerations that might collude to bring on baby blues. In a few cases, however, these feelings are not simply a transient, self-limiting emotional upset but indicate the beginning of postnatal depression.

## Postnatal Depression

The existence of postnatal (postpartum) depression was recognised by early physicians such as Hippocrates who, almost comically, attributed it to suppressed uterine discharge. The eleventh-century gynaecologist Trotula, in trying to explain why some women were affected and others were not, suggested that the cause was an excessively moist womb. American psychiatrists virtually abandoned the concept of postpartum mental illness in the twentieth century and it simply disappeared from the A–Z of diseases. As psychiatrist and postpartum expert James A. Hamilton, professor at Stanford University, comments:

> The vast majority of physicians trained in psychiatry between 1950 and 1990 were taught that the adjectives postpartum and puerperal were archaic when applied to mental illness.[5]

Postnatal depression is a much overused and inaccurately used phrase, but perhaps is most helpfully defined by

Katharina Dalton in her accessible *Depression After Childbirth.*[6] She calls it:

> the first psychiatric illness requiring medical treatment, occurring in a mother within six months of delivery.

Postnatal depression is recognised in British law under the Infanticide Act of 1939, which states that a mother cannot be found guilty of the murder of her own child within 12 months of delivery as the 'balance of her mind is so disturbed by reason of her not having fully recovered from the effects of giving birth'.

I suspect many women feel uncomfortable that enshrined in law is the idea that a woman's physical state renders her mentally unbalanced. Yet few people understand how devastating postnatal depression can be until they – or someone they know – suffers from it.

## Theories of Causes

Postnatal depression – or postnatal unhappiness as some prefer to term it – is estimated to affect 10 per cent of mothers, and can require hospital treatment. Broadly speaking there are two schools of thought as to what causes it. Some doctors, such as Dr Brice Pitt of Imperial College, London, think that the syndrome is organically determined, perhaps due to the precipitous fall in the progesterone and oestrogen levels after delivery. A woman's hormone levels are affected within hours of conception and the levels of progesterone and oestrogen (and the luteinising hormone LH), instead of falling as at the beginning of a period, continue to rise. But at birth, the levels that have been building up over the nine-month period drop back within hours.

Other medical practitioners feel that the triggering cause

is psychological, exacerbated but not caused by the vast physical changes. After all every woman's hormonal level changes dramatically postpartum but only a small proportion of women suffer from postnatal depression.

When it comes to potential causes or, at least, influencing factors, the Royal College of Psychiatrists suggests women are more likely to experience postnatal depression if they have had depression before; if they do not have a supportive partner; if their baby is premature or sick; if they lost their mother as a child or if they have recently experienced a lot of stress in a short amount of time.

## Treating Postnatal Depression

Many women are reluctant to seek help when the depression doesn't lift, particularly when the symptoms are relatively mild. They and others around them may dismiss the symptoms as a failure to cope rather than a problem that can be treated. Two women interviewed who suffered from depression that needed treatment described themselves as zombies for the first few months after the birth.

In serious cases of postnatal depression the physical symptoms may include loss of appetite, heart palpitations, sleeplessness and extreme tiredness. Emotional symptoms may include an inability to enjoy anything (including your baby), irritability, guilt, anxiety and the feeling that you cannot cope. About one mother in 1000 is estimated to suffer from the condition of postpartum psychosis: she may suffer paranoia, nightmare hallucinations and think about harming herself or her baby. Friends and family often think that if only they could say the right thing, everything would return to normal. The woman's symptoms are put down to the tiredness that affects all new parents. It takes courage on everyone's part to acknowledge that outside medical help is needed.

Debbie feels that she suffered from mild postnatal depression after the birth of her eldest son, although at the time she simply felt guilty that she wasn't coping. She had an extremely unpleasant 30-hour labour, 18 hours of which were spent in the hospital under instructions not to move until there was a free delivery room. Her waters were broken after two excruciating attempts, and she was subjected to eight internal examinations.

> I did manage to push him out finally, but as soon as he was born I was just sick again. And then they put me up in stirrups to sew me up, and I was sick again.

Jack needed help to cry, and although Debbie thought he was wonderful she was too tired even to breastfeed. Bad baby blues came on the third day, and once home she felt isolated, inexperienced and inadequate.

> He just used to cry the whole time. And I thought 'Is there ever going to be a moment when he doesn't cry?' I thought I'd be able to cope better than I did, and I found for about 18 months I just couldn't cope with Jack at all really.

Despite her strong love for her son, it took a lot of courage on Debbie's part to decide to have another child. She chose to go to a smaller local hospital rather than return to the big teaching hospital.

> With David, although it was painful, it wasn't the same experience at all. I suckled him immediately, he cried immediately. It's healed the wounds, somehow.

Pam, whose elective caesarean at 43 weeks was due to a fibroid growth in her womb, found the first four months of

Jackson's life extremely difficult. She doesn't categorise her feelings as postnatal depression, but was still aware of huge anger and resentment vying for space with the love and absorption she felt for her baby.

> It took me quite a while to be honest with myself, to admit to and name the feeling. I didn't feel resentment towards the baby, but towards the state of motherhood and my part in it. The fact that the whole procedure of giving birth and the end result is a shock to the system is an understatement . . .

Some women manage to find their own way out of the mists of postnatal depression with the support of family and friends. For others the answer is counselling while some find medication helpful. For all women affected by postnatal depression, recognising and accepting that they need help is the first step to recovery.

### Breastfeeding

Initial problems with breastfeeding (including mastitis* of both breasts within three weeks of leaving the hospital) obviously highlighted Pam's worries about how to cope. Siân too had problems with breastfeeding Alexander, to the degree that she decided to bottle-feed her second baby, Katherine, rather than put herself through the same emotional mill. Lee suffered dreadful mastitis, as did Lisa, and it is difficult not to feel miserable if you are in pain! 'It felt like a cheese grater being drawn across my nipples. I felt like a bit of a failure.'

---

* Mastitis is an acute, agonising infection of the milk ducts and breast tissue which may result in a pus-filled lump (abcess) in the breast.

All the evidence – both scientific and commonsensical – says that breast is best. Breastfed babies have fewer respiratory infections, ear infections, allergies and tummy upsets, and are less prone to diabetes, obesity and heart disease in later life. Research initially seemed to suggest that breastfeeding boosted babies' IQs as well, but a large study published in November 2006 showed that breastfed babies are indeed brighter, but only because their mothers' tend to be more intelligent and their babies inherit this intelligence.[7] But for all that, it is not something that suits everyone. It is an issue where physiological capabilities should not be seen as synonymous with emotional ones.

Breastfeeding was first officially encouraged in Britain in the 1920s, partly as a way to combat newborn ill-health at a time when 1 in 6 babies did not survive beyond their first birthday. In 1975, only 51 per cent of mothers breastfed at some point. By 2000, the number of new mothers breastfeeding was up to 69 per cent and in 2005 it was 76 per cent. But only 42 per cent of mothers are still breastfeeding after six weeks.[8]

An ability to breastfeed is not evidence of being a good mother any more than bottles of formula are indications of a bad or inadequate mother. Good mothering is about loving your child, touching, caring, providing for it to the best of your ability. Some women have difficulty breastfeeding: they may be ill, or receive no support and encouragement. Others find it easy, fulfilling, and enjoy the intimacy.

MARCH 1990: I'm moved by the warmth of Martha nuzzling up to me to feed in the nights. I light a candle, so she knows it's not time to get up, and half doze as she sucks. It's a peaceful, intimate time. I didn't expect to find it so fulfilling.

But breastfeeding in itself will not determine a woman's emotional relationship with her baby. There is too much guilt in mothering anyway without women torturing themselves that because they breastfed their daughter for three weeks less than their son they will be shoring up huge therapist's bills when she reaches her teens.

## I Don't Know What to Do . . .

The most important thing for any new parent is to acknowledge that few women and even fewer men are immediately confident with their brand-new baby and that most new parents worry about being inadequate. 'How can we tell the difference between hungry cries, tired cries, wet cries and constipated cries?' 'What will we do if it chokes?' 'Is it too hot, or too cold?' 'Why won't it stop crying?' These are all standard questions in the new parents' lexicon. And although many women, like Caroline and Jane, found the hospital staff intrusive and dictatorial, others remember feeling safe in the hospital being shown how to bath and change their babies. When tiny Annie wouldn't feed, Eve rang the night bell to ask the nurse what her baby wanted.

> I was terrified of changing her nappy because I thought I'd break her legs and she hated being unwrapped.

I thought that Martha had some horrible disease at two days old when run-of-the-mill feeding blisters appeared on her upper lip. I was astounded that they were going to let Greg and me take this baby home unsupervised. As Tessa put it, 'my God, they're letting us out. What do we know? We don't know anything . . .'

But leaving specific practical or physical problems aside, most women are lucky enough to fall in love with their babies which helps make them confident. With her third child, Lottie, Sue felt on top of the world:

> Once I had made up my mind to have her I felt pretty guilty about even thinking of abortion. And when she was born I was even more horrified because she was so tiny and helpless. My immediate thoughts when she was delivered were delight and excitement. I wanted to run up and down the street screaming 'I've had a beautiful girl!' I enjoyed her early months so much. It was like having a first child without the worry of being inexperienced.

Lynne's daughter Michelle was contented and quiet and fed easily. Looking at her over the first few days, Lynne cried with happiness and disbelief that everything was all right. She sat in her flat, as workmen traipsed in and out fixing the ceiling that had caved in, completely in love with her 'brand new' daughter.

Despite the trauma of John's birth, Nicki and her husband Mike felt confident with the twins and Anna at once, it all felt natural. Joanne also found everything straightforward with Rowan, and she was up and about by day nine. Caroline felt clever and happy on all four occasions, and described looking down at a tiny baby in her arms as one of the most fulfilling feelings in the world. All the worries about being able to love a baby disappeared the minute Jenny held James.

Eve, who'd felt little connection with her baby during the pregnancy, was also bowled over by the immediate passion she felt for Annie. She wouldn't leave the house for the first few weeks, since everything felt a little intimidating and frightening, but nestled happily with Annie in bed.

One morning poor Stephen took her downstairs, and I screamed from the top of the stairs 'bring that baby back to me straight away'. I felt terribly that she was mine, and everything was right.

## Older Sisters and Brothers

The reaction of older children can also make the first few days an incredibly happy and contented time for everyone. Sarah had not enjoyed her second pregnancy, and had recurrent worries about being able to love a second child as much as she loved her two-year-old daughter. She gave birth to Abigail at home.

> Before Mike brought Kirsty into our room I had made sure that the baby was in her own bed. I asked her where the baby was, which would normally have brought her straight to my tummy, but not this time. She started looking round the room and eventually went to the Moses basket. At first she couldn't see anyone underneath the blankets, but soon spotted her new baby sister, went 'ooh' and stood smiling and pointing at her. We all got back into bed together and had a good family cuddle.

Fran's 27-month-old son Matthew had been interested in the idea of a potential sister or brother throughout the pregnancy, and Fran was extremely eager to see how he would react to the real thing.

> He was very inquisitive. He looked at her for a couple of minutes then went and played with his cars on the floor. But when I actually came out of hospital he wanted to hold Rowan, was fine doing that and was very good.

He used to come and lie down next to the baby when
I was feeding, which was lovely.

Martha's reactions to Felix – loving and accepting without
being excessively interested – made everything easy. He
behaved like a baby in a book, so made it easy for her too.
He ate a lot in one go, rather than snacking every couple of
hours, slept happily at night and generally he didn't complain
when plonked down on floors, sofas or beds when phones
rang or washing machines flooded.

## PKU Test

The first time Felix cried properly was when Becky did his
PKU test, also known as the Guthrie test, which involves
pricking a heel and then squeezing four large drops of blood
on to a card for analysis. In Britain it is routinely carried out
on babies between 8 and 14 days old to check the amount of
the amino acid phenylalanine in the blood: a concentration of
above 20 milligrammes per millilitre indicates that phenylketonuria may be present. This is an inherited disorder in
which phenylketonuria accumulates in the blood and tissues,
usually leading to severe brain damage unless treated. It is
extremely rare, and can be completely cured by treatment.

## Vitamin K

In some hospitals vitamin K is given to newborn babies, especially premature babies, since they lack the intestinal bacteria
that produce the vitamin which is essential for the formation
in the liver of substances that promote blood clotting.
However, in 1992 there were suggestions that there might be
links between the administering of the drug and child cancers,
although a report in the *British Medical Journal* in August 1992

claimed that the risk was linked to vitamin K injections not oral treatment. Some units now offer the choice of a single large dose of vitamin K adminstered by injection, or a lower oral dose which will need following up. You can also choose not to have vitamin K for your baby if you wish.

Recent research has suggested that colostrum is rich in vitamin K, which should offer a certain level of natural protection. Most formula milks also have a higher added vitamin K content. Ask your midwife or GP for advice if you are worried, especially if you are booked at a hospital that has an automatic policy.

### The Fun Starts Here

The most valuable advice any new parent can be given is to take each day as it comes. You might feel wonderful for the first two weeks, then dreadful for the next three; you might feel unable to cope with a daughter who never sleeps, but tomorrow she might drop off for the whole night and you'll find yourself instead creeping up to the cot to poke her, fearful that she's somehow died; you might feel that you can run the world for six months and succeed!

The transition from non-parent to parent is easy for some, difficult for others, but we can each only do our best. It doesn't matter if the woman down the road is back at work within ten days; it doesn't matter that friends think you're mad for feeding on demand rather than every four hours; it doesn't matter if you don't get dressed until lunchtime – if at all. Give yourself and your partner a chance to revel in parenthood by following your own instincts. Seek help if you need it, listen to advice if you want it. But otherwise, it's your baby, your life. Stick to your own way of doing things. Most of all, let yourself enjoy your baby.

During the day Cassie would sleep when she wanted and get up when she wanted. She always went into the nursery and gazed at her son, sinking down beside his cot, just staring at him. Sometimes she would lift his covers and run her fingers over his skin, letting him feel her touch, sometimes she would sketch him. She was aware that Nanny felt that her passion for her child was quite improper. Her displeasure made Cassie laugh.

*Mothers & Other Loves*, Wendy Oberman[9]

# Biographical Details

The interviews were carried out between June and September 1992, based on a questionnaire divided by theme: the Decision to Conceive; Physical Changes; Charting Your Pregnancy; Relationship with your Growing Baby; Fears; Work and Money; Relationship with your Partner; Labour and Birth; and the First Few Days.

Some names have been changed for reasons of confidentiality. Ages and details below were accurate at time of first publication in October 1993.

**Caroline** is 28. She is a full-time mother, and works mornings at a local playgroup. She met Malcolm (32), who works on a turkey farm, when she was 14 and they have been married for ten years. They live in Bognor Regis, and have four children – Emma (9), Anthony (7), Richard (4) and Jessica (2).

**Debbie** is 32 and a primary school teacher. Her husband Patrick (31) is also a teacher, and they have been together for twelve years. They live in Northern Ireland with their two sons – Jack (5) and David (18 months).

**Debra** is 35 and a full-time parent. She and Hugo (28), a set constructor, have been together for nine years, and married two years ago. They live on a houseboat in Surrey and have one son, Edward (1).

**Eve** is 34 and works three days a week as an editor in a book publishing company. She has been with Stephen (44), a lecturer, for eleven years, married for four. They live in Brighton with their daughter, Annie (4), and are expecting a second baby in November.

**Fran** is 31 and a junior school teacher. She has been with Jim (32), a postman, for five years and they married 18 months ago. They live in London and have two children – Matthew (4) and Rowan (2).

**Jane** is 34 and works four days a week as an office administrator. She has been married to Matt (44), a journalist, for three years and they have one daughter, Sophie (3). They live in London.

**Jenny** is 31 and works part-time in a legal publishing company. She has been married to Bruce (31), a management consultant, for four years. They live near Portsmouth and have two children – James (3) and Douglas (10 months).

**Joanne** is 33 and a music teacher from Australia. She has been with Georgina (37), a solicitor, for eleven years and they have one son, Rowan (3). They live in London.

**Lee** is 31. She had been with Simon for nine years before marrying in 1988, and they are both full-time parents. They have one daughter, Hannah (3), and live in Nottingham.

**Lisa** is 33 and a lawyer. She and Rob (41), an architect, have been together for three years and they have one son, Harry (14 months). They live in London.

**Lynne** is 33 and a part-time health visitor. She has been with John (35), who is self-employed, for fourteen years, and married 10 years ago. They have one daughter, Michelle (4). They live in Reading.

**Nicki** is 34 and has a job-share working as a manager in a college catering for children with special needs. She and Mike, a carpenter, have been together for nine years and they live in London with their three children – Max and John (6) and Anna (4).

**Pam** is 43 and a freelance video stylist. She got divorced after a 14-year marriage, and has been with Gérard (38), a French actor, in London for the past four years. They have one child, Jackson, (18 months).

**Rachel** is 32 and works in the City. She met Jeremy (32), a librarian, ten years ago and they married three years later. They have one daughter, Rose (3), and are expecting a child in October. They live in London.

**Sarah** is 33 and has been married to Mike, a company director, for four years. She is a full-time mother and training to be a part-time antenatal teacher for the National Childbirth Trust. They have two children, Kirsty (3) and Abigail (16 months) and live in London.

**Sasha** is 42 and an artist. She has been with Lou (47), also an artist, for fourteen years and they married in 1989. They have one son, Freddy (3) and Lou has two teenage children from a previous relationship. They live in Oxford.

**Sharon** is 33 and works in local government. She has 8-year-old twins – Charlotte and Katie – and is divorced, having left her husband a few weeks after the girls were born. She lives in Kent.

**Siân** is 32 and a television producer. She and Peter (31), a writer, have been married for seven years and live in London. They have two children – Alexander (3) and Katherine (1).

**Sue** is 33 and a freelance journalist. She has been married to Max (37), a company director, for ten years, and they live in London with their three children – Nick (10), Hannah (8) and Lottie (3).

**Tessa** is 32 and a script executive. She has been married to Mark (35), who works for a charity, for five years and they live in London with their two children – Joe (4) and Matilda (8 months).

# Notes

## Introduction

1 Adrienne Rich, *Of Woman Born: Motherhood as Experience and Institution* (Virago, London, 1977)
2 *Guardian*, 2 September 1992

## Chapter 1 If and When . . .

1 Office for National Statistics, *Population Trends*, Autumn 2004
2 Office for National Statistics, *Family and work*, 2004
3 Phyllis Ziman-Tobin, *Whether or Not to be a Mother* (Fawcett-Columbine, New York, 1994)
4 Social Trends 2006
5 *Guardian*, 16 February 1993
6 Wolfson Institute of Preventive Medicine, 2006
7 Bruno Bettelheim, *A Good Enough Parent* (Thames & Hudson, London, 1987)
8 Dr Zena Stein, *Journal of Epidemiology*, 1985
9 *Guardian*, 6 November 1995
10 Ibid.
11 Katherine Gieve (ed.), *Balancing Acts* (Virago, London, 1991)

12 United Nations, *World Fertility Report 2003*

13 Social Trends, 2006


## Chapter 2 Is it Positive?

1 Katherine Gallagher, from 'Firstborn' in *Passengers to the City* (Hale & Ironmonger, Sydney, 1985)

2 J. W. Hutton, *Caste in India* (Cambridge University Press, Cambridge, 1946)

3 Oliver Wendell-Holmes, 'Currents & Counter-Currents in Medical Science', in a collection of the same title (London, 1860)

4 *Guardian*, August 1989

5 NICE, *Fertility assessment and treatment for people with fertility problems*, February 2004

6 *Human Reproduction*, December 2005

7 BBC News Online, October 2005

8 *Daily Express*, 29 April 1992


## Chapter 3 I Feel Sick

1 Lynne Reid Banks, *The L-Shaped Room* (Penguin, London, 1962)

2 *RCOG, The management of tubal pregnancy*, May 2004

3 *American Journal of Obstetrics and Gynecology*, March 1998

4 *Mother & Baby*, January 1992

5 Department of Health, 2006

6 ONS, 2004

7 Department of Health, op. cit.

8 Department of Health, op. cit.

9 Angela Neustatter with Gina Newson, *Mixed Feelings: The Experience of Abortion* (Pluto Press, London, 1986)


## Chapter 4 I Didn't Expect to Feel Like This

1 Meena Alexander, from 'Young Snail' in *The Virago Book of Love Poetry* (Virago, London, 1990)

2 Social Trends, 2006
3 *British Medical Association Complete Family Health Encyclopedia* (Dorling Kindersley, London, 1990)
4 Tommy's, 2006
5 BMA, *Smoking and reproductive life*, 2004
6 Action on Smoking and Health (ASH), *Smoking and reproduction*, 2006
7 Ibid.
8 BMA, op. cit.
9 'Healthy Pregnancy', *Independent* supplement, 3 September 1996

## Chapter 5 A Safe Pair of Hands

1 Jessica Mitford, *The American Way of Birth* (Gollancz, London, 1994)
2 ONS, Birth Statistics, 2006
3 Report of Expert Maternity Group, *Changing Childbirth* (1993)
4 Ibid.
5 'Healthy Pregnancy', op. cit.
6 Sheila Kitzinger quoted in *The American Way of Birth*
7 ONS, *Mortality statistics*, 2003
8 Albany Midwifery Practice, 2006
9 *British Medical Journal*, March 1992
10 Social Trends, 2006
11 Ibid.

## Chapter 6 Tests, Tests, Tests

1 Audre Lorde, from 'Now That I Am Forever With Child' in *Chosen Poems Old and New* (W. W. Norton, New York, 1982)
2 aidsmap.com, accessed October 2006
3 Health Education Authority, 'Life Will Never Be the Same Again', July 1992
4 ONS, 2006

5  Contact the Multiple Birth Foundation for further details about DVDs, books and leaflets

6  www.wolfson.qmul.ac.uk, accessed October 2006

7  www.wolfson.qmul.ac.uk, accessed October 2006

8  H. V. Firth et al., 'Analysis of Limb Reduction Defects in Babies Exposed to CVS', *Lancet*, 1994

9  G. E. Robinson et al., 'Psychological reactions to pregnancy loss after prenatal diagnostic testing: preliminary results', *Journal of Psychosomatic Obstetrics & Gynaecology*, 1991


## Chapter 7 Girl or Boy?

1  UN Statistics, 1980–90

2  'The Intendedness and Wantedness of the First Child' in *The First Child and Family Formation* (Carolina Population Center, Chapel Hill, 1978)

3  D. W. Winnicott, *The Child and the Family: First Relationships* (Tavistock, London, 1957)

4  ONS, 2006

5  DEMOS Report, Spring 1996

6  Cabinet Office, 2003


## Chapter 8 Anyone for Sex and Love?

1  Jeremy MacClancy, *Consuming Culture* (Chapmans, London, 1992)

2  Results for the National Perinatal Epidemiology Unit, Radcliffe Infirmary, Oxford, June 1993

3  Dr Thomas Verny and Dr John Kelly, *The Secret Life of the Unborn Child* (Time Warner, London, 2004)

4  C. P. and P. A. Cowan, *When Partners Become Parents* (Basic Books, New York, 1992)

5  Equal Opportunities Commission, *Dads and their Babies: a household analysis*, June 2006

6  C. F. Clulow, *To Have and to Hold: Marriage, the First Baby &*

*Preparing Couples for Parenthood* (Aberdeen University Press, Aberdeen, 1982)

7 British Social Attitudes Survey, 1996

8 Economic and Social Research Council, February 2006

9 *When Partners Become Parents*, op. cit.

10 Ibid.

11 The Body Shop, *Mamatoto* (Virago, London, 1991)

12 Paul Ferris, *Sex and the British: A Twentieth Century History* (Michael Joseph, London, 1993)

13 National Survey of Sexual Attitudes and Lifestyles, 1993

14 Sheila Kitzinger, *A Woman's Experience of Sex* (Dorling Kindersley London) 1983

15 Juliet Rix, *Is There Sex After Childbirth?* (Thorsons, London, 1995)

## Chapter 9 Who Am I?

1 Lesley Saunders, from 'Voices' in *One Foot on the Mountain: An Anthology of British Feminist Poetry 1969–79* (Onlywomen Press, London, 1980)

2 *Mamatoto*, op. cit.

3 Eva Zajicek, from 'The Experience of Being Pregnant' in *Pregnancy: A Psychological and Social Study* (Academic Press, London, 1981)

4 Naomi Lowinsky, *Stories from the Motherline: Reclaiming the Mother-Daughter Bond, Finding Our Feminine Souls*, (J. P. Tarcher, Los Angeles, 1992)

5 *Vanity Fair*, July 1991

6 *Whether or Not to be a Mother*, op. cit.

## Chapter 10 Visualise Your Bottom

1 Patricia Beer, from 'Jane Austen at the Window' in *Selected Poems* (Hutchinson, London, 1980)

2 'Life Will Never Be the Same Again', op. cit.

3 Janet Balaskas, *New Active Birth* (Unwin, London, 1989)

4 *The National Childbirth Trust Book of Pregnancy, Birth & Parenthood* (Oxford University Press, Oxford, 1992; revised 1996)

5 Dr Miriam Stoppard, *The Pregnancy & Birth Handbook* (Dorling Kindersley, London, 2005)

6 Margaret Llewelyn Davies, *Maternity: Letters from Working Women Collected by the Women's Cooperative Guild, 1915* (Virago, London, 1978)

7 A. Saari-Kemppainen et al., 'Ultrasound screening and perinatal mortality: controlled trial of systematic one-stage screening in pregnancy', *Lancet*, 1990

8 Elizabeth Noble, *Having Twins* (Houghton Mifflin, Boston, 1991)

## Chapter 11 Build Up, Count Down

1 David Widgery, *Some Lives! A GP's East End* (Sinclair-Stevenson, London, 1993)

2 H. Whent, 'Smoking and Pregnancy – A Guide for Purchasers and Providers', Health Education Authority, 1994

3 Dr Foster Good Birth Guide, 2005

4 F. Alerdice et al., 'Labour and Birth in Water in England and Wales', *British Medical Journal*, 1995

5 *Evening Standard*, 29 April 1996

6 RCOG / Royal College of Midwives, Joint statement No. 1, Immersion in Water During Labour and Birth, April 2006

7 F. Burns and K. Greenish, 'Pooling Information', *Nursing Times*, 1993

8 E. Burke and A. Kilfoyle, 'A Cooperative Study of Waterbirth', *Midwives Chronicle*, January 1995

9 C. J. Howell et al., 'Randomised study of long-term outcome after epidural versus non-epidural analgesia during labour', *British Medical Journal*, 2002

10 J. H. Maccaulay et al., 'Epidural analgesia in labour and fetal hyperthermia', *Obstetrics and Gynaecology*, 1992

11 ONS, NHS Maternity Statistics, England: 2004–05
12 C. Francombe et al., *Caesarian Birth in Britain* (NCT and Middlesex University Press, London, 1994)
13 G. Lewsi et al., *Why Mothers Die*, RCOG Press, 2001
14 ONS, NHS Maternity Statistics, England, 2004–05
15 Dr Jonathan Scher and Carol Dix, *Pregnancy, Everything You Need to Know*, Penguin, London, 1985
16 Ibid.

## Chapter 12 Birth

1 Anne Stephenson, from 'The Victory' in *The Bloodaxe Book of Contemporary Women Poets: Eleven British Writers* (Bloodaxe, Newcastle-upon-Tyne, 1985)
2 *Mamatoto*, op. cit.

## Chapter 13 Now We are Three . . . Or More

1 Kate Chopin's 1894 Diary, in the notebook 'Impressions', reprinted in *Kate Chopin's Private Papers* (Indiana University Press, Bloomington, 1992)
2 *Mamatoto*, op. cit.
3 *Guardian*, 29 January 1993
4 *When Partners Become Parents*, op. cit.
5 *Guardian*, 31 January 1992
6 Dr Katharina Dalton, *Depression After Childbirth: How to Recognize and Treat Postnatal Illness* (Oxford University Press, Oxford, 1980; revised 1989)
7 G. Der et al., 'Effect of breastfeeding on intelligence in children: prospective study, sibling pairs analysis and meta-analysis', *British Medical Journal*, November 2006
8 National Childbirth Trust, 2006
9 Wendy Oberman, *Mothers & Other Loves* (Heinemann, London, 1989)

# Addresses & Contacts

**Abortion Rights**
18 Ashwin Street
LONDON E8 3DL
0207 923 9792
www.abortionrights.org.uk

**Action for Sick Children**
36 Jacksons Edge Road
Disley
STOCKPORT SK12 2JL
0800 0744519
www.actionforsickchildren.org
*Campaigns to make sure that sick children get the best possible treatment*

**Action on Pre-Eclampsia**
84–88 Pinner Road
Harrow
MIDDLESEX HA1 4HZ
0208 863 3271
www.apec.org.uk
*Information and support for women with pre-eclampsia*

**Action on Smoking & Health (ASH)**
102 Clifton Street
LONDON EC2A 4HW
0207 739 5902
www.ash.org.uk
*Campaigns against smoking, passive smoking and other related issues; provides information; publishes leaflets*

**Action against Medical Accidents (AvMA)**
44 High Street
Croyden
SURREY CR0 1RB
0208 667 9065
www.avma.org.uk
*Advice for parents wishing to take legal action*

**Active Birth Centre**
25 Bickerton Road
LONDON N19 5JT
0207 281 6760
www.activebirthcentre.com
*Classes, groups and practical information for parents interested in active birth; birthing pool hire; list of teachers*

**Alcoholics Anonymous (AA)**
PO Box 1
Stonebow House
Stonebow
YORK YO1 7NJ
0845 769 7555
www.alcoholics-anonymous.co.uk
*A national network of self-help groups for those battling with excessive drinking; find your local group in the phone directory*

**Antenatal Results and Choices (ARC)**
73 Charlotte Street

LONDON W1T 4PN
0207 631 0285
www.arc-uk.org
*Support and information throughout the antenatal testing process*

**Association of Breastfeeding Mothers**
PO Box 207
Bridgwater
SOMERSET TA6 7YT
0870 401 7711
www.abm.me.uk
*Telephone advice and support groups for mothers who breastfeed – or wish to*

**Association for Improvements in Maternity Services (AIMS)**
5 St Ann's Court
Grove Rd
Surbiton
SURREY KT6 4BE
0870 765 1453

Scotland: 40 Leamington Terrace
EDINBURGH EH10 4JL
0870 765 1449
www.aims.org.uk
*Support and information about parents' rights and available choices; advice about complaints procedures; publishes a quarterly journal on current issues in maternity care*

**Association for Post-Natal Illness**
145 Dawes Road
LONDON SW6 7EB
0207 386 0868
www.apni.org
*Self-help groups offering one-to-one support to mothers*

**Association of Radical Midwives (ARM)**
16 Wytham Street
OXFORD OX1 4SU
01243 671673
www.radmid.demon.co.uk

**Association for Spina Bifida and Hydrocephalus (ASBAH)**
ASBAH House
42 Park Road
Peterborough
CAMBRIDGESHIRE PE1 2UQ
01733 555988
www.asbah.org
*Information and support for parents and families*

**Asthma UK**
70 Wilson Street
LONDON EC2A 2DB
08457 010203
www.asthma.co.uk
*Advice on all aspects of asthma*

**Baby Life Support Systems (BLISS)**
2nd & 3rd Floors
9 Holyrood Street
LONDON SE1 2EL
0207 378 1122
www.bliss.org.uk
*Practical and emotional support for parents whose babies need special care*

**Babyloss**
PO Box 1168
SOUTHAMPTON SO15 8XZ
www.babyloss.com
*Support for anyone affected by the death of a baby during pregnancy, at birth, or shortly afterwards*

**BirthWorks**
58 Malpas Road
LONDON SE4 1BS
0208 244 9785
www.birthworks.co.uk
*Information on and hire of portable birthing pools*

**British Acupuncture Council**
63 Jeddo Road
LONDON WI2 9HQ
0208 735 0400
www.acupunture.org.uk

**Diabetes UK**
Macleod House
10 Parkway
LONDON NW1 7AA
0207 424 1000
www.diabetes.org.uk

**Epilepsy Action**
New Anstey House
Gate Way Drive
Yeadon
LEEDS LS19 7XY
0808 800 5050
www.epilepsy.org.uk

**British Homoeopathic Association**
Hahnemann House
29 Park Street West
LUTON LU1 3BE
0870 444 3950
www.trusthomeopathy.org

**British Pregnancy Advisory Service (BPAS)**
4th floor
Amec House
Timothy's Bridge Road
STRATFORD-UPON-AVON CV37 9BF
0870 365 5050
www.bpas.org
*Offers pregnancy testing, counselling, abortion, vasectomy, sterilisation; see phone directory for local services*

**Brook**
421 Highgate Studios
53–79 Highgate Road
LONDON NW5 1TL
0800 0185 023
www.brook.org.uk
*Advice on contraception, pregnancy and abortion for young people*

**Caesarian Support Network**
55 Cooil Drive
Douglas
ISLE OF MAN
IM2 2HF
01624 661269
*Emotional support and advice for women who have had – or may need – a caesarean section*

**Child Support Agency**
Helpline 08457 133 133
www.csa.gov.uk

**Employers for Childcare**
87 Main Street
MOIRA BT67 0LH
0800 028 3008
*Advice on childcare for employers and parents*

**Cleft Lip and Palate Association (CLAPA)**
First floor
Green Man Tower
332B Goswell Road
LONDON EC1V 7LQ
0207 833 4883
www.clapa.com
*Support and information for parents and families*

**The Compassionate Friends**
53 North Street
BRISTOL BS3 1EN
0845 123 2304
www.tcf.org.uk
*Support for parents whose children have died*

**Confederation of Healing Organisations**
27 Montefiore Court
LONDON N16 5TY
0208 800 3569
www.confederation-of-healing-organisations.org
*Will provide a list of all alternative medicines and therapies*

**CRY-SIS**
BM CRY-SIS
LONDON WC1N 3XX
08451 228 669
www.cry-sis.org.uk
*For parents whose babies cry excessively or have difficulty sleeping*

**Disability Information Trust**
Mary Marlborough Lodges
Nuffield Orthopaedic Centre
Headington
OXFORD OX3 7LD
01865 227592

**Disabled Parents Network**
81 Melton Road
West Bridgford
NOTTINGHAM NG2 8EN
08702 410 450
www.disabledparentsnetwork.org.uk

**Down's Syndrome Association**
Langdon Down Centre
29 Langdon Park
TEDDINGTON TW11 9PS
0845 230 0372
www.downs-syndrome.org.uk

**Eating for Pregnancy Helpline**
0845 130 3646

**Equal Opportunities Commission (EOC)**
Arndale House
Arndale Centre
MANCHESTER M4 3EQ
0845 601 5901
www.eoc.org.uk
*Support and legal advice on all aspects of employment rights; pursues cases of discrimination*

**Family Planning Association**
50 Featherstone Street
LONDON EC1Y 8QU
0845 310 1334
www.fpa.org.uk
*Information on all aspects of family planning and contraception*

**Foresight**
178 Hawthorn Road
West Bognor

WEST SUSSEX PO21 2UY
01243 868001
www.foresight-preconception.org.uk
*Information and advice on pre-conceptual care*

**Foundation for the Study of Infant Deaths (FSID)**
Artillery House
11–19 Artillery Row
LONDON SW1P 1RT
0207 233 2090
www.sids.org.uk
*Research into causes of neonatal death; support and advice*

**General Medical Council**
44 Regent's Place
350 Euston Road
LONDON NW1 3JN
0845 357 8001
www.gmc-uk.org
*Investigates complaints about professional misconduct of doctors and consultants*

**Gingerbread**
307 Borough High Street
LONDON SE1 1JH
0800 018 4318
www.gingerbread.org.uk
*Self-help association for one-parent families; see phone directory for local groups*

**Harris Birthright Centre for Fetal Medicine**
Kings College Hospital
Denmark Hill
LONDON SE5 9RS
0203 299 9009
*Carries out neo-natal research*

**Independent Midwives Association**
89 Green Lane
Farncombe
SURREY GU7 3TB
0870 850 7539
www.independentmidwives.org.uk
*For advice and lists of local independent midwifery services*

**Institute for Complementary Medicine**
PO Box 194
LONDON SE16 7QZ
0207 237 5165
www.i-c-m.org.uk

**In-Touch Trust**
10 Norman Road
Sale
CHESHIRE M33 3DF
0161 905 2440
*Telephone advice for families affected by genetic disorders*

**Kith & Kids**
The Irish Centre
Pretoria Road
LONDON NI7 8DX
0208 885 3035
www.kithandkids.org.uk
*Advice and support for parents of disabled children*

**La Leche League**
PO Box 29
West Bridgford
NOTTINGHAM NG2 7NP
0845 456 1855
www.laleche.org.uk
*Support and counselling for breastfeeding problems; advice on local groups*

**Marie Stopes**
153–157 Cleveland Street
LONDON W1T 6QW
0845 300 8090
www.mariestopes.org.uk
*Advice on contraception, pregnancy and abortion*

**Meet-a-Mum Association (MAMA)**
7 Southcourt Road
Linslade
LEIGHTON BUZZARD LU7 2QF
0845 120 3746
www.mama.co.uk
*Self-help group for new mothers; will put women in touch with local women and/or local support groups*

**Midwives Information and Resource Service (MIDIRS)**
9 Elmdale Road
Clifton
BRISTOL BS8 1SL
0800 581 009
www.midirs.org
*Information service primarily for midwives; non-members may buy copies of research papers*

**Miscarriage Association**
c/o Clayton Hospital
Northgate
Wakefield
WEST YORKSHIRE WF1 3JS
01924 200799
www.miscarriageassociation.org.uk

**Multiple Births Foundation**
Queen Charlotte's & Chelsea Hospital
Du Cane Road

LONDON WI2 0HS
0208 383 3519
www.multiplebirths.org.uk

**Narcotics Anonymous**
202 City Road
LONDON EC1V 2PH
0845 373 3366
www.ukna.org
*Self-help organisation for those battling with drug addiction; advice on local groups*

**National AIDS Trust**
New City Cloisters
196 Old Street
LONDON EC1V 9FR
0207 814 6767
www.nat.org.uk

**National Association for Maternal and Child Welfare**
40 Osnaburgh Street
LONDON NW1 3ND
0207 383 4541

**National Association of Nappy Services**
0121 693 4949
*Information on local nappy service; delivery and collection*

**National Association of Parents of Sleepless Children**
PO Box 33
Prestwood
Gt Missenden
BUCKS NH16 0HZ
*Answers individual postal enquiries; publishes leaflets*

**National Childbirth Trust (NCT)**
Alexandra House
Oldham Terrace
LONDON W3 6NH
0870 444 8708 (breastfeeding)
0870 444 8709 (pregnancy and birth)
www.nct.org.uk
*Information support on all aspects for parents-to-be; runs ante- and postnatal groups nationwide; breastfeeding support; publishes books and leaflets giving advice on all aspects of pregnancy and birth*

**National Childminding Association**
Royal Court
81 Tweedy Road
Bromley
KENT BR1 1TG
0845 880 0044
www.ncma.org.uk
*Information on finding a registered childminder*

**National Council for One-Parent Families**
255 Kentish Town Road
LONDON NW5 2LX
0800 018 5026
www.oneparentfamilies.org.uk
*Information on benefits, rights during pregnancy, taxation and social security*

**NHS Direct**
0845 4647
www.nhsdirect.nhs.uk
*Advice on all health problems*

**Parliamentary and Health Service**
Ombudsman
Millbank Tower

Millbank
LONDON SW1P 4QP
0845 015 4033
www.ombudsman.org.uk
*For complaints against the NHS*

**Patients' Association**
PO Box 935
Harrow
MIDDLESEX HA1 3XJ
0845 608 4455
www.patients-association.org.uk
*Advice and information; campaigns on behalf of NHS patients*

**Positively Women**
347–9 City Road
LONDON EC1V 1LR
0207 713 0222
www.positivelywomen.org.uk
*Advice and support for women who are HIV+/have AIDS*

**Pre-Eclampsia Toxaemia Society (PETS)**
Rhianfa
CARMEL LL54 7RL
01286 882685
www.pre-eclampsia-society.org.uk
*Support and information for women with pre-eclampsia; send s.a.e.
with enquiry*

**Quit**
Ground floor
211 Old Street
LONDON EC1V 9NR
0800 00 2200
www.quit.org.uk
*Advice on stopping smoking; details of local support services; recorded
message outside office hours*

**Relate**
Herbert Gray College
Little Church Street
RUGBY CV21 3AP
0845 456 1310
www.relate.org.uk
*Confidential counselling for relationship problems; look in phone book for local groups*

**Royal College of General Practioners**
14 Princes Gate
LONDON SW7 1PU
0845 456 4041
www.rcgp.org.uk

**Royal College of Midwives**
15 Mansfield Street
LONDON W1G 9NH
0207 312 3535
www.rcm.org.uk

**Royal College of Obstetricians and Gynaecologists**
27 Sussex Place
LONDON NW1 4RG
0207 772 6200
www.rcog.org.uk

**MENCAP**
123 Golden Lane
LONDON EC1Y 0RT
0207 454 0454
www.mencap.org.uk

**Samaritans**
Emergency 24-hour line: 08457 90 90 90

*See phone book for local addresses and numbers*
www.samaritans.org.uk

**Scope**
Head Office
12 Park Crescent
LONDON W1
0171 636 5020; free helpline 0800 626216
www.scope.org.uk
*Advice and information about cerebral palsy*

**Sickle Cell Society**
54 Station Road
LONDON NW10 4UA
0208 961 7795
www.sicklecellsociety.org
*Support and information for parents of children with sickle cell*

**Single Parent Action Network (SPAN)**
Millpond
Baptist Street
BRISTOL BS5 0YW
0117 951 4231
www.spanuk.org.uk

**Society of Homeopaths**
11 Brookfield
Moulton Park
NORTHAMPTON
NN3 6WL
0845 450 6611
www.homeopathy-soh.org

**Society of Teachers of the Alexander Technique**
1st floor
Linton House
39–51 Highgate Road

LONDON NW5 1RS
0845 230 7828
www.stat.org.uk
*Can provide information about local teachers/groups*

**Splashdown Water Birth Services**
17 Wellington Terrace
Harrow-on-the-Hill
MIDDLESEX HA1 3EP
08456 123405
www.waterbirth.co.uk
*Supplies birthing pools nationwide*

**Stillbirth & Neonatal Death Society (SANDS)**
28 Portland Place
LONDON W1B 1LY
0207 436 5881
www.uk-sands.org
*Information and a nationwide network of support groups for bereaved parents and families*

**Terrence Higgins Trust**
314–320 Gray's Inn Road
LONDON WC1X 8DP
0845 12 21 200
www.tht.org.uk
*Information on HIV/AIDS*

**Twins and Multiple Birth Association (TAMBA)**
2 The Willows
Gardner Road
GUILDFORD GU1 4PG
0800 138 0509
www.tamba.org.uk
*Self-help organisation for parents of twins and more; advice on local support groups*

**Vaginal Birth After Caesarian (VBAC)**
01256 704871
www.caesarean.org.uk
*Information and support for women wishing to avoid a repeat caesarean delivery*

**Wellbeing of Women**
27 Sussex Place
Regent's Park
LONDON NW1 4SP
0207 772 6400
www.wellbeingofwomen.org.uk
*Charity research arm of the Royal College of Obstetricians and Gynaecologists; looks into health of women and babies*

**Women's Therapy Centre**
10 Manor Gardens
LONDON N7 6JS
0207 263 7860
www.womenstherapycentre.co.uk
*All forms of therapy, counselling and advice for women*

**Working Families**
1–3 Berry Street
LONDON EC1V 0AA
0207 253 7243
www.workingfamilies.org.uk
*Advice and information on parents' rights in the workplace*

# Further Reading

## Fertility & Conception

*Beating the Biological Clock* – Pamela Armstrong

*The Abortion Pill* – Etienne-Emile Baulieu

*Older Mothers: Conception, Pregnancy & Birth After 35* – Julia Berryman, Karen Thorpe & Kate Windridge

*Preparation for Pregnancy* – Suzanne Gail Bradley with Nicholas Bennett

*Our Stolen Future: How Man-Made Chemicals are Threatening our Fertility, Intelligence & Survival* – Theo Colborn, Dianne Dumanoski & John Peterson Myers

*Sooner or Later? The Timing of Parenthood in Adult Lives* – P. Daniels & K. Weingarten

*The Manual of Natural Family Planning* – Dr A. M. Flynn & Melissa Brooks

*Endometriosis* – Suzy Hayman

*Conceiving Your Baby: The Essential Guide for Couples Considering Assisted Conception* – Sally Keeble

*The Fertility & Contraception Book* – Julia Mosse & Josephine Heaton

*Infertility* – Roger Neuberg

*Preparing for Motherhood* – Ray & Dorothea Ridgway

*In-Vitro Fertilization* – Geoffrey Sher, Virginia Marriage Davis & Jean Stoess

*Safer Childbirth?* – Marjorie Tew

*Getting Pregnant: The Complete Guide to Fertility & Infertility* – Professor Robert Winston

*Making Babies* – Professor Robert Winston

## Abortion & Miscarriage

*Abortion: Between Freedom & Necessity* – Janet Hadley

*Coping with a Termination* – Dr David Haslam

*Hidden Loss: Miscarriage & Ectopic Pregnancy* – Valerie Hey, Catherine Itzin, Lesley Saunders & Mary Anne Speakman

*Unplanned Pregnancy: Abortion, Adoption, Motherhood* – Debby Klein & Tara Kaufmann

*Miscarriage: The Facts* – Gillian C. L. Lachelin

*Coping with Miscarriage* – Mimi Luebbermann

*Mixed Feelings: The Experience of Abortion* – Angela Neustatter

*Miscarriage* – Ann Oakley, Ann McPherson & Helen Roberts

*Experiences of Abortion* – Denise Winn

## Pregnancy & Birth

*New Active Birth: A Concise Guide to Natural Childbirth* – Janet Balaskas

*The Encyclopedia of Pregnancy & Birth* – Janet Balaskas & Yehudi Gordon

*Water Birth: The Concise Guide to Using Water During Pregnancy, Birth & Infancy* – Janet Balaskas & Yehudi Gordon

*Mamatoto: A Celebration of Birth* – The Body Shop

*Pregnancy* – Gordon Bourne

*Twins, Triplets & More* – Elizabeth Bryan

*Where to be Born: The Debate & the Evidence* – Rona Campbell & Alison Macfarlane

*Your Natural Pregnancy: A Guide to Complementary Therapy* – Anne Charlish

*The Caesarian Experience* – Dr Sarah Clement

*Childbirth Without Fear* – Grantley Dick-Read

*So You're Going to be a Dad* – Peter Downey

*Healthy Mum, Healthy Baby* – Wendy Doyle

*What to Expect When You're Expecting* – Arlene Eisenberg

*Aromatherapy for Pregnancy & Childbirth* – Margaret Fawcett

*Healthy Eating for You & Your Baby* – Fiona Ford, Robert Fraser & Hilary Dimond

*Is My Baby All Right? A Guide for Expectant Parents* – Christine Godsun, Kypros Nicolaides & Vanessa Whitling

*The Mothercare Pregnancy Book Week by Week* – Nina Grunfeld

*The Great Ormond Street Book of Baby & Childcare* – Tessa Hilton with Marie Messenger

*The Experience of Childbirth* – Sheila Kitzinger

*Homebirth: And Other Alternatives to Hospital* – Sheila Kitzinger

*New Pregnancy and Childbirth* – Sheila Kitzinger

*A Woman's Experience of Sex* – Sheila Kitzinger

*Having a Baby* – Nancy Kohner

*Painless Childbirth* – Fernand Lamaze

*The Baby Bible*: Choosing the Best for You & Your Baby – Juliet Leigh

*Pregnancy & Birth the Alexander Way* – Ilona Machover & Angela & Jonathan Drake

*The National Childbirth Trust Book of Pregnancy, Birth & Parenthood: The Complete Guide to Having a Baby* – NCT

*Having Twins* – Elizabeth Noble

*Antenatal Education: A Dynamic Approach* – Mary Nolan

*Women's Bodies, Women's Wisdom* – Dr Christine Northrop

*Birth Tides: Turning Towards Home Birth* – Marie O'Connor

*Birth Reborn* – Michel Odent

*The Real Pregnancy Guide* – Vivienne Parry in association with *Practical Parenting*

*Your Body, Your Baby, Your Life* – Angela Phillips with Nicky Leap & Barbara Jacobs

*The New Our Bodies, Ourselves* – Angela Phillips and Jill Rakusen

*Drugs in Pregnancy & Childbirth* – Judy Priest

*Protecting Your Baby-to-Be* – Maggie Profet
*Natural Pregnancy* – Lee Rodwell
*Coping with Caesarians & Other Difficult Births* – Wendy Savage and Fran Reader
*Conception, Pregnancy & Birth* – Dr Miriam Stoppard
*Everywoman's Life Guide* – Dr Miriam Stoppard
*The Pregnancy & Birth Handbook* – Dr Miriam Stoppard
*Every Woman's Birth Rights* – Pat Thomas
*The Secret Life of the Unborn Child* – Thomas Verney with John Kelly
*Pre-Eclampsia: The Facts* – Isabel Walker & Chris Redman
*Alternative Maternity: A Comprehensive Guide to Natural Home Birth* – Nicky Wesson
*Therapies from Conception to Post-Natal Care* – Nicky Wesson

## Disability

*The Baby Challenge* – M. Jain Campion
*Past Due: A Story of Disability, Pregnancy & Birth* – Anne Finger
*Musn't Grumble: Writings by Disabled Women* – Lois Keith (ed.)
*Pride Against Prejudice: Transforming Attitudes to Disability* – Jenny Morris (ed.)
*Understanding Your Handicapped Child* – Valerie Sinason
*Babies with Down's Syndrome: A New Parents' Guide* – Karen Stray-Gundlersen (ed.)

## Breastfeeding

*Is Breast Best?* – Nicky Adamson
*The Experience of Breastfeeding* – Sheila Kitzinger
*The Politics of Breastfeeding* – Gabrielle Palmer
*Breastfeeding* – Mary Renfrew, Chloe Fisher & Suzanne Arms
*The National Childbirth Book of Breastfeeding* – M. Smale/NCT
*Breast is Best* – Drs Penny & Andrew Stanway

## Parenting Advice & Handbooks

*Twins in the Family* – E. Bryan
*Depression After Childbirth* – Dr Katharina Dalton with Wendy M. Holton
*You & Your Premature Baby* – Barbara Glover & Christine Hodson
*The Crying Baby* – Sheila Kitzinger
*The Year After Childbirth* – Sheila Kitzinger
*Babyhood* – Penelope Leach
*The Parents' A–Z* – Penelope Leach
*Cot Death* – J. Luben
*Coping with Cot Death* – Sarah Murphy
*Is There Sex After Childbirth?* – Juliet Rix
*Depression: The Way Out of Your Prison* – Dr Dorothy Rowe
*The New Baby Care Book* – Dr Miriam Stoppard
*The Working Mothers' Handbook* – Working Mothers' Association


## History, Sociology & Psychology

*A Good Enough Parent* – Bruno Bettelheim
*The Reproduction of Mothering* – Nancy Chodorow
*Partners Become Parents: Talks from the Tavistock Marital Studies Institute* – Christopher Clulow (ed.)
*When Partners Become Parents* – Carolyn P. & Philip A. Cowan
*Mothers* – Dr Ann Dally
*Balancing Acts: On Being a Mother* – Katherine Gieve (ed.)
*Mother Courage: Letters from Mothers at the End of the Twentieth Century* – Christine Gowdridge, Susan Williams & Margaret Wynn (ed.)
*Lesbian Motherhood in Europe* – Kate Griffin
*The Second Shift: Working Parents & the Revolution at Home* – Arlie Hochschild
*The Midwife's Tale: An Oral History from Handywoman to Professional Midwife* – Nicky Leap & Billy Hunter
*The American Way of Birth* – Jessica Mitford
*New Generations: 40 Years of Birth in Britain* – Joanna Moorhead/NCT

*From Here to Maternity* – Ann Oakley

*Women, Medicine & Health* – Ann Oakley

*Motherhood: What it Does to Your Mind* – Jane Price

*Of Woman Born: Motherhood as Experience & Institution* – Adrienne Rich

*A Mother's Eye: On Motherhood & Feminism* – Anne Roiphe

*The Tentative Pregnancy: Amniocentesis & the Sexual Politics of Motherhood* – Barbara Katz Rothman

*The Adoption Reader* – Susan Wadia-Ells (ed.)

*Babies & their Mothers* – D. W. Winnicott

# Index